HERBAL
PRESCRIPTIONS
for
BETTER HEALTH

HERBAL PRESCRIPTIONS
for
BETTER HEALTH

Your Everyday Guide to Prevention, Treatment, and Care

DONALD J. BROWN, N.D.

PRIMA PUBLISHING

Prima Publishing™ and its colophon are trademarks of Prima Communications, Inc.

ILLUSTRATIONS BY HELENE D. STEVENS

Library of Congress Cataloging-in-Publication Data

Brown, Don (Donald J.), 1956–.
  Herbal prescriptions for better health / Don Brown.
    p. cm.
  Includes index.
  ISBN 0-7615-0114-2 (hardcover) ISBN 0-7615-0323-4 (paperback)
  1. Herbs—Therapeutic use—Popular works. I. Title.
RM666.H33876   1995
615'.321—dc20

95-32966
CIP

96 97 98 99 00 AA 10 9 8 7 6 5 4 3 2 1
Printed in the United States of America

HOW TO ORDER

Single copies may be ordered from Prima Publishing, P.O. Box 1260BK, Rocklin, CA 95677; telephone (916) 632-4400. Quantity discounts are also available. On your letterhead, include information concerning the intended use of the books and the number of books you wish to purchase.

To
GABY, MILES, AND ARI
for their love,
encouragement,
and reminding me to eat.

It was suggested that I used unconventional methods and there is nothing a professional group mistrusts so nervously as it does anything that appears unconventional, and that has not been thoroughly written up in journals. It may be quackery. Worse still, it may be effective. And if it is both quackery and effective it is utterly hateful.

—ROBERTSON DAVIES, *The Cunning Man*

Contents

PART 3

QUESTIONS COMMONLY ASKED ABOUT HERBAL MEDICINES

PART 4

CATEGORIES OF HERBAL MEDICINES

PART 5

COMMONLY PRESCRIBED HERBAL MEDICINES

Contents

x

PART 6

HERBAL PRESCRIPTIONS FOR COMMON HEALTH CONDITIONS

Contents

Preface

My Herbal Odyssey

HERBS and I didn't get off to a good start during my early childhood. While playing outside our house in Buena Park, California, I managed to run a rather substantial sliver of wood under a thumbnail. My mother, after failing to get the intruder out with tweezers, called her mother, who was working as a nurse at the time. I was whisked to maternal grandmother's abode and promptly set up in the kitchen among some stainless steel utensils not commonly associated with eating and a ton of gauze.

Four hours later, after my screams had exhausted her, grandmother declared that amputation was the only rational option. Shielded by my equally hysterical mother, I was transported to my paternal grandmother, whose primary claim to fame was her pot roast. She calmly informed my mother that all my ill-fated thumbnail needed was a healthy application of herbal salve. The herbal salve, according to grandma, would draw the splinter out from under the nail. After telling me to shut up (which was anesthesia that could rival morphine), she proceeded to anoint my finger with salve and then wrap it with gauze. She then proclaimed that the pot roast was calling and that we should hit the road. Instructions were given for replacing the salve and wrap every day.

The salve didn't work and three days later my infected thumb felt as though a two-by-four was embedded under the nail. My mother sat me down on the couch with a root beer float and we shared a Kodak moment—watching *The Ozzie and Harriet Show*. Empowered by Ricky Nelson's song at the end of the show (which always had mom chirping like a bird), she grasped my thumb, subdued me with a forearm stranglehold, and removed the splinter.

It took a good ten years for me to develop a truce with herbs. My initial interest grew out of my study of American Indians and their healing systems. Two years later, I was given a copy of *Back to Eden* by Jethro Kloss. I began brewing exotic herbal teas and identifying local plants that had medicinal properties. An herbal student was born!

A number of divergent paths have contributed to my current interest in herbal medicine. Studies in Jungian psychology led to further exploration of the healing systems of different cultures. Work with emotionally disturbed children and adults led to critical thinking regarding drug therapy and the limitations of our health care system. My studies in naturopathic medicine took the tradition and mysticism of herbal medicine and paired it with modern scientific scrutiny. This was a wonderful discovery and helped decide the path I'm currently pursuing.

This book represents my development in herbal medicine to date. The primary focus is on safe and responsible use of herbal medicines. The secondary focus is on herbs that have a track record of modern clinical studies or a reliable history of clinical use to ensure their effectiveness in the treatment of human illness. Last, but not least, I hope the book inspires you to become a more critical consumer and student of herbal medicine.

Thanks for reading. I'm off to perfect grandma's herbal salve!

Acknowledgments

Helene Stevens, for the wonderful illustrations and for fostering my interest in herbs; Nick Gallo, for working his magic with the text; Michael Danko, for reminding me when it was soda time; Linda Moss, for trying out many of the herbs covered in the book; Joe Pizzorno, N.D. and Steve Austin, N.D., for providing a model of natural health care education that has successfully merged science and tradition; my students at Bastyr University for assisting my growth as a teacher and student of natural medicine; Karen Blanco, Leslie Yarborough, Natasha Kern, and Mike Corrigan for their roles in making the book happen.

part I

THE CHANGING FACE OF
HERBAL MEDICINE

HEALTH CARE CONSUMERS SPEAK OUT!

HALFWAY through the current decade, the prognosis for herbal medicine in the United States is excellent. Many thousands of health care consumers have made an informed decision to include herbs and alternative therapies in the treatment of their health problems and in their efforts to stay well. In fact, a recent study indicates that well over one-third of the adults in the United States are incorporating some form of alternative therapy (the study, completed at Harvard, uses the unfortunate term "unorthodox") in their health care plans.[1] Your actions have largely been responsible for new legislation that allows for clearer and more accurate information about the way herbs function in the body.

Herbal medicine is undergoing a renaissance in the United States. Access to clinical research on herbs, conducted primarily in Europe and Asia, has encouraged U.S. health care providers to consider prescribing herbal therapies for conditions that have largely baffled the medical community. Herbal therapies offer hope for conditions as varied as the common cold and Alzheimer's disease. As more research information becomes available, increasing numbers of health care professionals are recommending herbal treatment for their patients.

This dramatically improved access to quality information on herbs, while good, is not enough to achieve a full integration of herbal therapy into "mainstream" medicine. More is required:

SELF-EDUCATION Health care consumers—that's you and I—in the United States must educate themselves so as to make informed choices about herbal medicines. The World Health Organization has published guidelines for the education of the health care consumer about the medicinal use of herbs.[2] These guidelines constitute a model by which consumers can access clear information about issues of safety and effectiveness of herbal medicines.

EDUCATION OF HEALTH CARE PROVIDERS Health care professionals need education, too—particularly in the area of using herbs to treat illness.

NATUROPATHIC MEDICINE LEADS THE WAY

A huge stumbling block in the evolution of herbal medicine in this country is the shortage of health care professionals who are knowledgeable about prescribing herbs for health concerns. I'm pleased to say that this shortage appears to be lessening. Growing numbers of medical doctors, pharmacists, osteopaths, and chiropractors are choosing to incorporate herbal medicines into their practices.

A profession leading the way is naturopathic medicine. Naturopathic physicians are trained in four-year, postgraduate institutions that combine orthodox medical science (pathology, microbiology, and physical diagnosis) with clinical training in nutrition, herbal medicine, homeopathy, and hydrotherapy. There are currently four naturopathic medical colleges in North America:

- Bastyr University (Seattle, Washington)
- National College of Naturopathic Medicine (Portland, Oregon)
- Southwest College of Naturopathic Medicine and Health Sciences (Scottsdale, Arizona)
- The Canadian College of Naturopathic Medicine (Etobicoke, Ontario, Canada)

Naturopathic physicians are medical experts in the use of herbs to treat illness. Graduates of the above-mentioned schools take 150 to 175 classroom hours of herbal medicine. These classes cover pharmacology, clinical conditions, and toxicology. State licensing examinations for naturopathic physicians include a section on herbal medicine and herb toxicology. In states with active licensing laws, naturopathic physicians are allowed to diagnose illness and use herbal medicines as part of their treatment alternatives. States with naturopathic licensing laws include the following: Alaska, Arizona, Connecticut, Hawaii, Montana, New Hampshire, Oregon, and Washington. In addition to these states, Florida and Utah have older laws under which some naturopaths continue to practice.

Naturopathic medical schools and physicians are also leading the way in the integration of herbs back into our health care system. The colleges are now promoting clinical research in herbal medicine. Naturopathic physicians have become herbal emissaries and are working increasingly with orthodox medical professionals to promote the best use of herbal medicines. What's more, they have become a vital source of information for health care consumers wishing to use herbs and other alternative therapies to treat illness.

A LEGAL VICTORY FOR HERBAL SUPPLEMENTS

I would be remiss not to mention a landmark event that occurred at the end of 1994. The passage of the Dietary Supplement Health and Education Act of 1994 (DSHEA) marked a profound change in government policy toward the regulation of dietary supplements, which had previously been regulated as mere foods. The DSHEA establishes a clear legal definition of a dietary supplement. It includes provisions that allow for the flow of information to consumers about the way that supplements work in the body. It also mandates more uniform assessment of safety.[3]

Best of all, this law protects the right of consumers to choose dietary supplements as part of their health care plans. This is particularly critical for herbal supplements, which have long been viewed with suspicion by the Food and Drug Administration. The following summarizes congressional reasoning for the passage of the DSHEA:

- Improving the health of U.S. citizens is a top national priority.
- Dietary supplements have been shown to be useful in preventing chronic disease, and their appropriate use will help limit the incidence of chronic disease and long-term health care costs.
- Consumers should be empowered to make informed choices about preventive health care programs; these choices should be based on scientific studies relating to dietary supplements.
- Almost 50 percent of Americans use dietary supplements to improve their nutrition.
- Consumers are placing greater reliance on nontraditional health care providers, because of the high cost of traditional medical services.
- The federal government should not take any actions to impose unreasonable barriers limiting or slowing the flow of safe products and accurate information to consumers (but should take swift action against unsafe products).
- Dietary supplements are safe within a broad range of intake, and safety problems with dietary supplements are relatively rare.
- Legislative action is necessary to protect the consumer's right of access to safe dietary supplements to promote wellness.

For the herbal supplement user, the DSHEA allows two exciting developments:

STRUCTURE–FUNCTION CLAIMS   Herbal supplement manufacturers can now make what are known as "structure–function" claims. Most structure–function claims describe the way an herb or one of its constituents alters or helps maintain a bodily structure or function. The DSHEA now allows an herbal supplement label to contain this kind of information; that is, how the herbal supplement affects the body. However, manufacturers are still not permitted to make claims for an herbal supplement regarding treatment or prevention of a specific disease.

A good example is *Ginkgo biloba* (see Part 5); an extract made from the leaves of this tree has been shown to increase circulation to the central nervous system and to the extremities. The new law concerning structure–function claims now allows this information to appear on herbal preparation labels. Another example is garlic, which has been shown to lower serum cholesterol and triglycerides. It's now legal to provide this information on the label of herbal preparations of garlic.

It's critical to note that these structure–function claims must be based on sound scientific information and not on someone's impressions of the ancient Greek applications of the herb. Herbal supplements backed by solid research will feature these claims and become the standard for further development of products. This should also help weed out companies that sell products based more on marketing hype than real science.

THIRD-PARTY LITERATURE   The DSHEA's other aspect that is important to consumers is the "Third Party Literature" provision. This portion of the law allows herb companies and stores to provide publications on herbs, so long as they do not advertise a particular brand. This means that chapters from books, articles, and official abstracts from peer-reviewed scientific publications may be used in conjunction with the sale of herbal supplements. The provision is certainly a step forward in empowering herbal consumers through education.

part 2

European Phytotherapy: A Rational Model for the Future

We see the position which medicinal plants should hold in modern medicine: before the major chemotherapeutic agents, and indeed before surgery, in any case in their own position and in their own right. The sequence also establishes the degree of seriousness and danger of the different interventions, being a progression from the least invasive to the most invasive.

RUDOLF FRITZ WEISS, M.D.

WHAT'S A "PHYTO"?

WHEN searching for a model to spur the further development of herbal medicine in this country, one need go no further than the herbal system employed by European countries such as Germany and France. Certainly, the herbal products that have been developed in these countries meet the requirements for clinical effectiveness and safety stated in the Dietary Supplement Health and Education Act of 1994 (DSHEA; see Part 1). The system of herbal regulation in these countries (particularly Germany) offers the most rational approach to the integration of safe and effective herbal medicines into our health care system.

The term used to describe the modern clinical use of herbs in many European countries is *phytotherapy*. Phytotherapy is the science of using plant medicines to treat illness. Efforts in this field have successfully combined modern medical practice with herbal medicine. As a result, countries such as France, Germany, and Italy have adopted a regulatory climate that nurtures extensive research on herbs and encourages acceptance of their use in their health care systems.

PHYTOTHERAPY: HISTORICAL PERSPECTIVE

The French physician Henri Leclerc (1870–1955) is often credited with being the "father of phytotherapy." He published numerous papers on the use of herbal medicines in the clinical setting. His works are summed up in his textbook, *Précis de Phytothérapie*, which continues to be a primary reference in modern phytotherapy.

The real mover and shaker, however, was the German physician Rudolf Fritz Weiss (1898–1991). Dr. Weiss inspired the organization of a group of professionals dedicated to phytotherapy, and also published the highly influential textbook *Lehrbuch der Phytotherapie* (Textbook of Phytotherapy).

This has become the leading reference book on the use of herbs in medical practice. Now in its seventh edition in Europe, the sixth edition is available in the United States under the title *Herbal Medicine*. Dr. Weiss also founded the *Zeitschrift für Phytotherapie* (Journal of Phytotherapy), devoted to research on applications of herbal medicines in the health care setting.

INFLUENCE OF HERBAL MEDICINE ON EUROPEAN HEALTH CARE

Like pharmaceutical drugs in the United States, herbal medicines used in European phytotherapy undergo extensive laboratory testing and clinical trials prior to approval for use by humans. Known as *phytomedicines*, these herbal products have become an important part of the health care delivery system in many European countries.

Phytomedicines are used largely as supportive therapies for chronic illness or for the treatment of minor ailments that do not require drug therapy. Many phytomedicines are also used to prevent disease. Subsequently health care costs in areas such as geriatric medicine and gynecology have fallen.

The "mainstreaming" of phytotherapy into clinical practice in Germany and France has led to significant numbers of physicians and pharmacists recommending phytomedicines to their patients. More than 70 percent of general practitioners in Germany prescribe phytopharmaceuticals and many of these are covered by national health care insurance. This has led to a market for phytopharmaceuticals in Germany that is estimated at $3 billion annually. Total sales of herbal medicines in the European Union represent approximately one-half of the yearly sales of herbs worldwide.[1]

Table 2.1 lists the top-selling phytomedicine products in Europe. Table 2.2 lists the phytomedicines most commonly prescribed in Germany. Many of these products are now sold in the United States.

HOW HERBS ARE REGULATED IN EUROPE

We would be wise to look to Germany and France for a successful model of how to regulate herbal medicine. For example, herbal medicines in Germany are reviewed by a commission of professionals from a variety of

Table 2.1
LEADING EUROPEAN PHYTOMEDICINE PRODUCTS

Product	Manufacturer	Plant
Tebonin (EGb 761)	Schwabe	*Ginkgo biloba*
Ginsana	Pharmaton/Boehringer Ingelheim	Ginseng
Kwai	Lichtwer Pharmaceuticals	Garlic
Efamol	Scotia Pharm.	Evening primrose
Echinacin	Madaus AG	*Echinacea purpurea*

Source: *HerbalGram* 34: 64, 1995.

European Phytotherapy: A Rational Model for the Future

Table 2.2

PHYTOMEDICINES MOST FREQUENTLY PRESCRIBED IN GERMANY

Phytomedicine	Body system or conditions addressed
Ginkgo biloba extract	Circulation and central nervous system
Horse chestnut extract	Circulation through the veins
Hawthorn extract	Heart and circulation
(nettle root)	Urinary tract and prostate
St. John's wort extract	Antidepressant
Echinacea	Immune system stimulant
Valerian	Sedative

Source: *HerbalGram* 34:65, 1995.

health care disciplines. They are responsible for the creation of the Commission E monographs on plant medicines. Similar to official summaries used to regulate drugs in the United States, these herbal monographs describe the plant medicine, its health care applications, appropriate dosage, and safety information. To date, more than 300 monographs have been published by this group. These monographs represent the most comprehensive information available on the use of herbs in the modern health care setting. I will be referring to them frequently in Part 5.

PHYTOMEDICINES IN THE UNITED STATES

In Part 1, I suggested that the structure–function claims allowed by the new DSHEA legislation will best suit those herbs that have been well researched. As opposed to many of the herbal medicines previously sold in this country, phytomedicines are poised to fill that bill. It would not be surprising if this were to be the largest area of growth in herbal sales over the next five years.

Phytotherapy and phytomedicines are already making their mark on herbal medicine in this country. We are gaining greater access to European research on herbs. Phytotherapy textbooks are being incorporated into the training of naturopathic physicians and are also being used in a variety of clinical settings.

Of the utmost significance, however, is the growing influx of European phytomedicines backed by extensive research and an impressive track record of clinical studies and medical use. Examples include bilberry, hawthorn, *Ginkgo biloba*, milk thistle, *Vitex agnus-castus*, and valerian. One *Ginkgo biloba* extract has been the subject of more than 400 clinical reports and numerous textbooks! It is hoped that these herbal preparations will open the door to expanded medical use of herbs in the United States. They should also set new standards of excellence for herbal research and manufacturing.

THAT'S PHYTO, NOT FIDO!

About three years ago I was asked to be a guest on a San Diego talk show dedicated to natural health care. The first half-hour was spent covering current trends in herbal medicine. To impress the host and his listeners, I began extolling the wonders of phytotherapy and phytomedicines such as gingko, milk thistle, and echinacea.

The second half of the show was open to callers with questions. The first caller was a woman who, based on the volume of her voice, was probably a bit hard of hearing. She began by praising the show, the host, and the health benefits she had gained by listening over the year.

She then turned her attention to me. She politely complimented my knowledge of natural health care and particularly herbs. Her voice, however, took on a more serious tone as she added, "I do have some serious concerns about this new therapy using dogs!"

I explained that it was "phytotherapy," not "fidotherapy." She concluded her call with, "Never mind."

---

part 3

QUESTIONS COMMONLY ASKED ABOUT HERBAL MEDICINES

RIGHT now Americans are still learning about herbal medicines—particularly their use in health care. The following questions about herbs are commonly asked by consumers, retailers, and health care professionals. They run the gamut from safety issues to questions about quality and choosing the right herbal supplement.

I'm a medical professional, not an herb grower or manufacturer. As such, I urge you to call companies selling herbal supplements with your questions. Most of them have customer service departments to serve you.

And remember: the purpose of this book is to help you choose herbal medicines with a sound résumé of clinical research and "real-life" use for different conditions. These criteria should play a major role in your choice of herbal medicines.

Do herbs really work?

Eighty percent of the world's population can't all be wrong! That's the estimated number of people worldwide who use herbal medicines to stay well. In many countries herbs are used primarily as folk medicines, but developed countries such as Germany, France, China, and Japan have successfully incorporated herbal medicine into their health care systems. Why? Because they work!

These countries have created a model for the effective use of herbal medicine. Thanks to their efforts, we need no longer refer to herbal medicine as "folk medicine." Folklore gave us clues to the medical use of herbs, but the modern research conducted in these countries has provided us with scientific support for their use in modern medical systems.

If herbs are so effective, why don't doctors regularly recommend them in the United States?

The bottom line is that medical doctors in the United States don't receive any training in herbal medicine. As mentioned in Part 1, naturopathic medicine represents one way in which herbal medicines might be successfully integrated into a medical system. We also have a very strong role model in the health care systems of France and Germany, where doctors and pharmacists receive training in herbal medicine. Herbal medicines are a core part of their treatment options (see Part 2).

In the next decade, we're going to see huge growth in educational opportunities for health care professionals in herbal medicine. Paired with the introduction of herbal medicines with a strong history of research and clinical use, I expect herbs to be welcomed back into our health care system.

In the meantime, educate your doctor—share books like this and those listed in "Herbal Medicine Resources." Also, the references can provide doctors with answers to their questions.

Why aren't herbs labeled as to what they do and what conditions they treat?

Until the end of 1994, herbs were regulated like foods by the Food and Drug Administration. This regulation disallowed health claims of any kind, including which actions an herb has in the body or which condition it might be used to treat. The result: a consumer wanting to buy an herbal medicine often knew less about its actions than he or she did about a potato's.

As mentioned in Part 1, the passage of the Dietary Supplement and Health Education Act in late 1994 is starting to reverse this trend. Consumers will now begin seeing labels that explain how an herb influences different actions in the body. But the labels still can't tell you anything about treating specific conditions with an herb.

The law also offers you greater access to "third-party" literature, that is, unbiased reviews of research that shed light on which conditions respond best to herbal medicine.

Where do herbs fit in my health care program?

Herbal medicines are usually more gentle in their action than commonly prescribed drugs. They may take longer to act and often work to support or influence balance in a body system, instead of doing its job for it. This makes them ideal for prevention of illness.

For many individuals, they also offer means of recovery from illness. Again, the nudge is usually gentle and based on support rather than on overwhelming your body's own ability to get well.

Herbal medicines are also a wonderful way to address many chronic conditions that are not responding to drug therapy. Examples include eczema, rheumatoid arthritis, premenstrual syndrome, and benign enlargement of the prostate. Once improvement occurs, the herbal prescription generally is a safer alternative for continued treatment.

Remember, the best way to decide how herbs fit into your health care program is to find a health care professional trained in herbal medicine to act as your guide.

Can herbs be taken with prescription or over-the-counter drugs?

The answer is usually yes. Many herbal medicines will support body systems during drug therapy. A classic example is the use of echinacea during and after antibiotic therapy to keep the immune system functioning optimally.

Herbs can also reduce the side effects of some drugs. For example, milk thistle extract can help keep the liver functioning normally when a person is taking antidepressant or anticonvulsive drugs.

There are exceptions. I wouldn't recommend using St. John's wort while you're taking a prescription antidepressant. Also, it wouldn't make sense to take saw palmetto while taking a prescription drug for benign prostate enlargement. These are examples of herbal *alternatives* to drug therapy.

Herbs are typically not aggressive enough for use in the treatment of many acute or emergency situations. Notable are bacterial infections, which are best treated with antibiotics.

Can herbs act as substitutes for prescription or over-the-counter drugs?
Well, we've already mentioned St. John's wort and saw palmetto. Even these two herbal alternatives, however, are best thought of as treatments for milder forms of the conditions they address. Other examples include vitex for premenstrual syndrome and infertility, valerian for insomnia, kava for mild anxiety, and hawthorn for early-stage congestive heart failure.

Medical care in this country stands to improve dramatically if we could start phasing herbal prescriptions into the early treatment of many conditions before they become more serious. We could save precious health care dollars by slowing the progression of conditions that ultimately require expensive medical interventions.

When I begin taking an herb, how do I know what dosage to use and how long to take the product?
Part 5 of this book highlights herbs that have received the scrutiny of modern research. The best attempt has been made to determine the most effective doses. Use this information to select standardized herbal preparations that offer a clear dosing schedule.

However, such standardized products are currently in the minority. Other herbal preparations can be effective when taken at the proper dosage. Use the recommendations in Part 6 as a guide; also, compile a list of quality reference books on herbal medicine (see References).

Like most drugs, herbs affect people in different ways. When taking a product for the first time, you may want to start with a low dose and work up over time to the desired dose. It may take some experimentation before you determine how long to take a product. The guidance of a qualified health care professional or herbalist can help guide you.

Note: Seek professional help when deciding on the proper dosage for your child.

Should I take my herbal supplement at mealtimes or between meals?
We don't know for sure with every herbal medicine. Some herbs probably benefit from mealtime consumption because digestion and assimilation will be at their peak. Oil-based preparations derived from plants such as evening primrose and flax should always be taken with food.

There are always exceptions to the rule. If you're using bromelain to relieve inflammation, take it between meals. Taken during meals, it acts as a digestive enzyme and will offer little antiinflammatory activity.

I've heard that because herbs are from plants, they're basically safe.
Do I have to worry about any side effects?
Most of the herbs covered in this book have few side effects. These are usually mild and affect a small minority of people. Some people may be allergic to an herb or one of its constituents.

If you take an herbal product and have a bad reaction, contact your doctor first. Notify herb companies, also. This feedback provides them with important information about their products. Like the drug industry, herb companies should track side effects of their products.

The adage that herbs are safe just because they are from plants is a dangerous one. Herbal laxatives such as senna, aloe, and cascara should be used with the caution afforded any drug. When consumed in large amounts on a regular basis, licorice root products can cause high blood pressure and water retention. Comfrey root may cause damage to the liver when consumed in large amounts.

While the scare tactics employed by government agencies to make herbs look dangerous are usually overblown, use the same caution with herbs that you would with any medication. Most of the serious side effects I've been called about over the past five years have stemmed from overuse or misuse of an herbal medicine. Use herbs sensibly and you'll usually avoid trouble. If you're not sure, seek the help of qualified professionals.

Can a pregnant or lactating woman take herbal medicines?
As is true with many drugs, the answer is both yes and no. Herbs that have been clearly shown to be dangerous during pregnancy or lactation

should bear a warning on the label (I wish I could say this is always the case). Examples include stimulant laxatives such as cascara and aloe. Strong astringent herbs such as horse chestnut and witch hazel, as well as herbs with hormone-like substances (black cohosh and Asian ginseng), should be avoided.

Most commercial herbal products currently sold don't include information about pregnancy and lactation. If the label of an herbal preparation doesn't say anything, seek the opinion of a health care professional well versed in herbal medicine before taking an herbal supplement.

In Part 5 of this book, I address contraindications during pregnancy and lactation. The great legal two-step is to say "not contraindicated" instead of "safe." Herbs such as evening primrose oil, bilberry, echinacea, and ginkgo are among those that can be used during pregnancy or lactation. I've depended on the German Commission E monographs for this information. Another good resource is naturopathic physicians trained as midwives.

Can children take herbal medicines? Is the dosage the same?

My clinical experience, which is strongly oriented to pediatrics, says that children respond beautifully to herbal medicines! The big concerns are proper dosage and getting kids to take the often foul-tasting herbal medicine.

Dosage

Most pediatricians adjust drug prescriptions for children on the basis of weight. This can be done with some of the standardized herbal preparations we'll discuss in Part 5. However, with many traditional preparations this is difficult, because we often don't know what the optimal dosage is even for an adult. It's sometimes comforting to know that the pediatric dosage of some herbal medicines does not drop significantly; echinacea is a classic example.

Some herbalists use Young's formula, which bases estimated dosage on a child's age. I favor dosage based on weight. While Young's formula is easy to use, the room for error is large. What if your five-year-old weighs the same as most eight-year-olds?

I may sound like a broken record, but when in doubt, seek professional help!

Delivery

This is the hard part—an herbal medicine will benefit your child only if you can get it into them. Liquids are the best form of delivery for young children, but they often taste bad and are high in alcohol (a concern for infants less than one year of age). Try mixing these in juice. Glycerin-based, liquid preparations are a good-tasting alternative but are often weak in strength (see the following description of *tinctures*). Powdered herbs can be mixed in applesauce or sweet potatoes.

Be creative and patient. I'm not the best advisor, since my son thinks anything or anyone called "herb" should be avoided!

Are herbal medicines addictive?

The commercial herb industry is not allowed to sell herbal supplements that are addictive. Obviously, many addictive drugs come from the plant kingdom (e.g., opium, heroin, and cocaine) but fortunately they aren't sold in your friendly health food store or natural health section of your pharmacy.

One trend that makes me very uneasy is the growing use of herbs high in caffeine for weight loss and energy. Caffeine certainly rates as a mild addiction and has the down side of making people edgy. With time it also runs down your adrenal function (see the section on stress and fatigue under Endocrine System in Part 6). Products promising "escalation" or "acceleration" belong on espresso stands and not in health food stores.

Do herbs contain steroids or hormones?

This is a widely held misconception. Some herbs (e.g., black cohosh and ginseng) contain compounds that may act like hormones, albeit weakly. Others (e.g., wild yam) contain some of the chemical precursors of a hormone. However, they do not have the strength of actual hormones such as estrogen or progesterone.

Some herbs actually support glands that produce hormones and steroids. These products will often work on the endocrine system, which includes the thyroid, adrenal glands, and reproductive organs. Examples include vitex, eleuthero (Siberian ginseng), and licorice.

What form of herbal medicine is most effective?

This is another question without a clear-cut yes or no answer. Herbal medicines come in many forms. You can have garlic, ginger, or turmeric with your meals. You may choose to have some chamomile tea for your upset stomach. Goldenseal tincture will probably soothe your sore throat better than a capsule. A concentrated extract of ginkgo in tablet form, however, will be far more effective than a tincture in treating poor circulation.

Commercial herbal preparations are available in many different forms: bulk herbs, teas, tinctures, fluid extracts, powdered herbs in capsules and tablets, and solid extracts. Let's consider each of these.

Herbal Powders

Usually available in capsules or tablets, herbal powders typically have minimal processing and are reasonably priced.

Teas

Herbs are often prepared as medicinal teas. Practitioners of traditional Chinese medicine often use a form of medicinal tea called a *decoction*. A decoction is made by combining bulk herbs in water and boiling them together. The mixture is then strained and the liquid consumed. Decoctions make stronger, more concentrated medicinal teas.

Infusions

To make an infusion, pour boiling water over the herb and let it steep. Chamomile is commonly prepared in this manner. Tea bags are the most common form of infusion used in the United States.

Note: Many plants have active constituents that are not soluble in water. You're better off taking a liquid or solid extract in such cases.

Tinctures

Tinctures are an extremely popular form of herbal preparation in the United States. You make a tincture by letting an herb soak in a solvent (usually alcohol or water) for several hours, days, or even weeks, depending on the herb. Tinctures are most commonly made with alcohol.

Over the past few years, glycerin has been used to make "alcohol-free" tinctures. While far more tasty than grain alcohol, glycerin is not as good a carrier as alcohol and results in somewhat weaker preparations. If you're concerned about alcohol in tinctures, try placing the alcohol-based tincture in a tea, and take it that way. This will dilute and even evaporate some of the alcohol.

Tinctures are typically a 1:5 or 1:10 concentration. This means that one part of the herbal material is prepared with five to ten parts (by weight) of the liquid. A tincture is therefore usually considered a more diluted herbal preparation.

Fluid Extracts

Fluid extracts are more concentrated than tinctures. Like tinctures, they are often made with either water or alcohol, but sometimes other solvents may be used in an extraction. The final product is concentrated by distilling some of the solvent and thus increasing the herbal concentration. Fluid extracts are typically a 1:1 concentration.

Solid Extracts

A solid extract represents the most concentrated form of an herbal product. It results when *all* of the solvent is evaporated off, leaving a solid residue. These residues are usually available in powdered form. An exception would be oil-based preparations containing fatty acids, such as saw palmetto extracts. Solid extracts are typically 2:1 to 8:1 concentrations.

Standardized Extracts

Many of the herbal medicines discussed in this book have taken the extraction process one step further. *Standardization* means guaranteed levels of a certain constituent or group of constituents in the final product. This is usually expressed as a percentage of the total weight of the extract. Standardization allows for accurate dosing based on a measured amount of the proven, active constituents. For example, milk thistle extracts contain 70 to 80 percent silymarin. The recommended daily dose of silymarin is 420 milligrams. Thus 600 milligrams of the extract will provide the recommended dose. Other examples of standardized herbal medicines are bilberry, ginkgo, and kava.

There's a lot of overlap among the categories. Ask fifteen herbalists or doctors about which preparations they prefer, and you'll probably hear fifteen different opinions. Standardized liquid or solid extracts offer the most reliable dosing forms. Medical professionals looking for measured and often quicker results will usually opt for this form of herbal medicine. You may also want to start here if you're treating a specific health condition.

Tinctures and powdered herbs, while weaker in their effect, do offer a cost-effective alternative for treatment of minor ailments. They can also be employed as part of your daily supplement program.

If I choose to use a tincture or fluid extract, how can I compare dosage with a solid extract?

One gram of a 10:1 solid extract equals 10 milliliters of a 1:1 fluid extract and 100 milliliters of a 1:10 tincture. Remember that some standardized extracts can have very high concentrations. A 50:1 extract of ginkgo leaves would require 50 milliliters of a 1:1 fluid extract and 500 milliliters of a 1:10 tincture to be in the ballpark!

Please keep in mind that these are rough comparisons. A standardized extract has a carefully measured amount of active constituent(s) also. Just because you produce an equal amount of fluid extract or tincture doesn't mean you're guaranteed a proper amount of these active constituents.

Are single herbs or herbal combinations better?

Once again, the answer is an unequivocal, "It all depends." If you're taking herbs to help round out your optimal diet and supplement program, then herbal combinations are often an ideal way to go. There's less concern here with therapeutic dosages.

My scientific mind and impatient nature have biased me in favor of using single-herb preparations or small combinations for the treatment of health conditions. Most of the herbal medicines discussed in Part 5 are effective therapeutic agents on their own merits without being combined with other herbs. When we start combining herbal preparations, we lose some of our assurance about the way an individual herb will work in the body. The bottom line is, when you know it works a certain way by itself, use it by itself.

This doesn't mean that I oppose using herbal combinations. I find these valuable when a condition presents a combination of symptoms. I may choose to combine echinacea with goldenseal for a cold with a sore throat. A person with high cholesterol and intermittent claudication will benefit far more if he combines garlic and ginkgo.

A key concern about combinations is whether they deliver sufficient dosages of the recommended herbs. If you've got a product with every-thing but the kitchen sink in it, you're probably looking at a rather weak cumulative effect.

In addition to having sufficient amounts of the featured herbs, an herbal combination should have a rationale for the combination. Combining *Drosera* and thyme for a dry, spasmodic cough makes sense. So does gentian and yellow dock to help with digestion. But putting ginkgo in a formula with valerian and other herbs and claiming it's good for hyperactive kids is senseless.

Here again, a health care professional can be a useful guide. Also, finding a retail outlet with an educated staff will make your decision easier.

When I decide to buy an herbal medicine, how do I know which one is best?
The answers to the next few questions should help you decide what herb companies sell quality products and provide accurate and reliable infor-mation. This is a good starting point in deciding "best" products.

Products from companies that have formed liaisons with European, Asian, and Indian companies that produce high-quality and well-researched products should be at the top of your list. These companies are attempting to bring you the best available form of the herb. Liaisons of this sort also give you greater assurance that the herbal preparation matches the form used in research and clinical settings.

Use the advice of an expert in herbal medicine. This person could be a naturopathic doctor or an herbalist. The resources listed in References can help you find further research in the scientific literature.

Are there standards that companies in the herb industry must follow?

The herb industry has its own trade organization, known as the American Herbal Products Association (AHPA). Membership in the organization is voluntary. Companies that belong to the AHPA work together to set standards of quality for the growing, harvesting, storage, and manufacturing of herbal products.

Another trade organization of interest is the National Nutritional Foods Association. They have a "True Label" program that assures accuracy in label claims. Many herb companies participate in this program.

Which companies produce the best products?

Your first criterion should be quality control. A quality herb company buys the best raw materials and maintains the strictest quality assurance in its manufacturing methods. This includes testing raw materials for adulterants, heavy metals, pesticides, and bacteria. Assaying for levels of active constituents, when applicable, is also important. A quality herb company will continue to test for contaminants and bacteria during manufacturing. Lastly, its labels and packaging will accurately depict the contents of the product and its shelf life. This includes the content of the herb(s) in the product as well as any fillers and excipients. For example: if it's a liquid product, what is the concentration of alcohol or glycerin?

Next, look for companies that are committed to education. Companies that hire employees who are trained in herbal medicine are more likely to offer accurate information. Their labels will be based on research and clinical information instead of hype. These companies spend a great deal of money educating the people from whom you buy herbs in the retail store. This is an important link to you, the consumer. Educated retailers help ensure that you receive accurate and reliable information.

Last, some personal biases. I believe that a quality herb company commits a portion of its resources to research. We desperately need to do more clinical research on herbal medicine in the United States. Such research will influence, perhaps critically, how herbs will be integrated into the U.S. health care system.

A quality company committed to excellence in their products should also have a global perspective. This means support for commercial growing of native herbs in their countries of origin. This creates financial opportunities for many countries. Also, supporting programs that work to save natural habitats for plants is critical. Without a healthy environment, we can hardly expect a healthy future for herbal medicine.

What do the designations "organically grown" or "wild-crafted" mean?
An herbal product that bears the designation "organically grown" means that no pesticides, herbicides, chemical fertilizers, or irradiation were used to produce, grow, or preserve the plant. Most herb companies strive to buy organically grown herbs whenever possible.

"Wild-crafted" usually means that the herb is not grown in a controlled setting, such as a farm. Wild-crafted herbs are usually picked in the wild by an experienced herbalist. While this is often romantically perceived as being the best way to harvest herbs, it is fraught with potential problems. The first problem is the environmental impact. If every herb company depended on wild-crafting, our natural supply of wild plants would be so greatly diminished that many herbs would face possible extinction.

The second problem is consistency in wild-crafted herbs. Different growing conditions can significantly change the concentration of medically active constituents.

Large herb companies in the United States and Europe rely primarily on herbs that have been grown under controlled situations. This means less impact on our wild plants, as well as better quality control. Many U.S., European, and Asian herb companies have developed plant strains and optimal growing conditions that guarantee a higher plant yield and greater concentration of important medical constituents in the herbs.

Where can I obtain accurate and reliable information on herbal medicine?
See the list of resources listed in References. In addition, health food stores and other retail outlets can provide you with educational materials. Herb companies can even send you information, provided it doesn't make claims for treating illness.

Be a critical reader!

part 4

CATEGORIES OF
HERBAL MEDICINES

BEFORE diving into commonly prescribed herbal medicines in Part 5 and herbal prescriptions for common health conditions in Part 6, let's take a look at some general categories of herbal medicines to describe their actions in the body. Some of these actions will be familiar (astringents and laxatives) and some unfamiliar (carminatives and demulcents). Herbs in the adaptogen and antioxidant categories effect a broad spectrum of actions in the body.

These categories give you a framework for the way groups of herbal medicines act in the body. For example, if you're having trouble properly digesting food and suffer a lot of bloating after a meal, you may want to consider a digestive bitter such as yellow dock. If you're run down from stress and overwork, adaptogenic herbs such as eleuthero (Siberian ginseng) or astragalus are extremely useful. These categories are widely accepted and used by health care professionals who prescribe herbal medicines.

Remember that herbs like to defy labels. Some will end up in more than one category. For a more thorough review of herbal categories, I highly recommend Chapter 3 in David Hoffman's *The Herbal Handbook: A User's Guide to Medical Herbalism* (Healing Arts Press, Rochester, Vermont, 1988).

ADAPTOGENS

It's fitting to begin a discussion of herbal categories with a term that embodies herbal medicine's amazing diversity. An *adaptogen* is a substance that increases the body's resistance to stress and exerts a balancing effect on various systems of the body, including the immune, nervous, and cardiovascular systems.

Adaptogens can trace their descent from the herbal tonics commonly used in the traditional herbal healing systems of China and India. A prime example is Asian ginseng, which we'll cover in Part 5. Two Russian scientists, I. I. Brekhman and I. V. Dardymov, first applied the term adaptogen to Asian ginseng and later to its Russian relative eleuthero (Siberian ginseng).[1] Their expanded definition of an adaptogen includes the following three criteria:

- An adaptogen must show a nonspecific effect and raise the powers of resistance to toxins of a physical, chemical, or biological nature.
- An adaptogen effects a normalizing or balancing action independent of the type of pathological condition.
- An adaptogen must be harmless and must not influence normal body functions more than necessary.

The following herbal medicines qualify as adaptogens:

Asian ginseng	Schizandra
Eleuthero (Siberian ginseng)	Ashwagandha
Astragalus	Codonopsis ("Dangshen")

While most of these herbs have an illustrious career in traditional herbal medicine, they may be even more applicable in today's stress-filled world than they were hundreds of years of ago. Adaptogens enhance health by performing the following actions:

Stress reduction (adrenal support)
Enhancement of brain and central nervous system activity
Immunomodulation
Antioxidant activity

Liver protection and antitoxin activity
Improved blood sugar metabolism
Increase in stamina and endurance

The core of an adaptogen's diverse actions is its ability to help the body deal more effectively with stress.[2] The key here is support for the adrenal glands. The adrenals, which sit atop the kidneys, are responsible for helping us respond to stress. They also help us rebound from stress. When the adrenals become overwhelmed, we lose this edge and different systems in the body begin to break down.

If you're experiencing chronic stress, the number one condition you'll note is fatigue. You'll also experience problems with blood sugar metabolism, sluggish immune function, and even general aches and pains in the muscles and joints. Chronic fatigue syndrome is a classic example of exhausted adrenals.

Adaptogens serve to recharge exhausted adrenal glands. When this central task is discharged, they continue to support adrenal action and optimize our ability to deal with stress in its many forms.

I'll let the chapters on eleuthero and Asian ginseng in Part 5 serve as an introduction to some of the potential health care applications for adaptogenic herbal medicines. The actions of adaptogens also make them ideal for resisting illness. They should be an important consideration for any supplement regimen aimed at optimizing health.

ANTIOXIDANTS

A popular topic in health care today is the role that free radicals play in many diseases. Particular attention has been focused on age-related conditions such as atherosclerosis, Alzheimer's disease, and macular degeneration.

As opposed to small pictures of Huey Newton or Abbie Hoffman circulating in our bloodstream, free radicals are actually highly reactive groups of atoms that repeatedly undergo chemical reactions without change to themselves. We all produce them and have substances in the body known as *antioxidants* to keep them in check. When free radicals form in excess, naturally occurring antioxidant substances produced by the body (such as glutathione and superoxide dismutase) can be overwhelmed. Damage to cells in the body ensues.

Modern society produces a lot of contributors to free radical formation. These include pesticides, environmental pollution, and second-hand cigarette smoke. Free radicals also rise with overexposure to ultraviolet rays produced by the sun. Stress can raise the level of free radicals, as can chronic illnesses, such as human immunodeficiency virus (HIV) infection. Also, as we get older, our defense systems become less aggressive and free radicals have more opportunity to cause harm.[3]

Unless you've been living in seclusion on some deserted island (although the *New York Times* probably has delivery there), you know that antioxidant nutrients can help counter free radical production in the body. Vitamin C, vitamin E, selenium, and a variety of carotene-like substances provide this antioxidant support.[4]

Many herbal medicines also offer antioxidant support. The herbal constituents that shine in this area are the *bioflavonoids*. Occurring in a wide variety of edible plants (including herbs), bioflavonoids are one of nature's most potent antioxidants. In fact, the average bioflavonoid is probably several times more potent in this regard than vitamin E.[5,6]

Start adding bioflavonoids to your free radical defense program by way of your diet. Apples, green tea, onions, cherries, and blueberries are excellent sources of bioflavonoids. High consumption of bioflavonoids in the diet is associated with lowering the risk of cardiovascular disease.[7]

Many herbal medicines have complex bioflavonoid structures as medically active constituents. Examples in Part 5 include bilberry, hawthorn, ginkgo, and milk thistle. Owing to research on the way these particular bioflavonoids work in the body, we've also been able to establish a "tissue-specific" effect for many of them. Table 4.1 lists herbal medicines, their active bioflavonoids, and the body systems they support. All of these are discussed in greater detail in Part 5.

Bioflavonoids have become a priority of herbal medicine research. In the next decade these important plant constituents promise to lead the way in further unlocking the preventive and therapeutic potential for antioxidants.

Table 4.1
TISSUE-SPECIFIC BIOFLAVONOIDS

Herbal medicine	Bioflavonoids	Body system
Bilberry	Anthocyanosides	Eyes, circulatory system
Hawthorn	Oligomeric procyanidins	Heart, circulatory system
Ginkgo biloba	Ginkgo flavone glycosides	Brain, nervous system, cardiovascular system
Milk thistle	Silymarin	Liver and gallbladder

ASTRINGENTS

If you drink straight black tea, you'll notice a tightening sensation inside your mouth. This is because of substances known as *tannins* inside the black tea. In fact, milk is commonly added to tea to counteract the activity of tannins.

Tannins are the primary component of herbal medicines commonly labeled "astringents." Tannins actually get their name from their use in tanning hides (animal, not human!). When tissue comes in contact with tannins, proteins coagulate, causing a tightening effect. This creates a protective barrier and also helps add "tone" to the tissue.

Tannin-containing herbs are useful in the treatment of inflammation of the skin and mucous membrane (another name for the lining inside the respiratory and gastrointestinal tracts). Inflammation occurs in topical conditions such as eczema and leg ulcers. Internally, tannins add tone to the gastrointestinal tract, helping to stop diarrhea and soothing irritated tissue.

Tannin-containing astringent herbs are commonly applied in the treatment of poor circulation in the veins. Because they improve sluggish blood flow in the veins, astringents are particularly useful for the treatment of hemorrhoids and varicose veins. The constricting effect of tannins also provides relief for many sports injuries. They also reduce edema (fluid accumulation associated with inflammation) following surgery.

Table 4.2
HEALTH CARE APPLICATIONS FOR ASTRINGENTS

Herbal astringent	Application
Horse chestnut	Varicose veins, hemorrhoids, leg ulcers, postoperative swelling, and hematomas
Witch hazel	Eczema, hemorrhoids, and varicose veins
Tormentil	Diarrhea

Commonly used astringent herbs include witch hazel leaves, horse chestnut, oak bark, and English walnut leaves (see Table 4.2 for some of the health care applications of these herbs). *Note:* Internal use of astringents is contraindicated during pregnancy.

CARMINATIVES

Carminative herbs soothe and tone the digestive system. Typically high in volatile oils, these herbs are used in cases of gastrointestinal upset, irritation, and cramping. They help relieve excess gas and bloating.

Two classic examples of carminative herbs are peppermint and chamomile. As we will note in Part 5, chamomile is revered in Europe and is one of the most commonly prescribed herbs for digestive tract problems. Health care applications for these herbs include irritable bowel syndrome, indigestion, heartburn, and infant colic. Other carminative herbs include anise, caraway, and fennel. On the basis of our discussion in Part 5, ginger may also be considered a carminative.

The key to the gastrointestinal actions of carminatives is their volatile oil content. Since volatile oils are not water soluble, the typical teacup of peppermint or chamomile is medicinally weak. Unless you're brewing a highly concentrated tea of dried chamomile flowers or fresh peppermint leaves, you're better off using concentrated fluid extracts or alcohol-based tinctures. These will offer a more reliable source of medically active volatile oils.[8]

CHOLAGOGUES

An area that has long been the focus of natural medicine is healthy liver function. The liver, as we will note in the chapter on milk thistle in Part 5, is the primary organ of detoxification in the body. In addition, it works with the gallbladder to digest and assimilate fats. One key to proper fat digestion is *bile:* when bile production in the gallbladder and flow from the liver become impaired, many people experience a sense of fullness or bloating following the consumption of fats in the meal.

Herbs classified as *cholagogues* have two primary actions. The first is to stimulate the production of bile. The second is to stimulate the proper flow of bile. Some herbal texts refer to the second action as "choleretic." By improving bile production and flow, these herbs also reduce the risk of gallstone formation. They are also associated with improving fat digestion and promoting healthy liver function.[9]

Listed here are commonly prescribed cholagogues:

Dandelion root	Milk thistle
Turmeric	Artichoke
Goldenseal root	Chelidonium

Note again the overlap of categories. Many digestive bitters (see the section "Digestive Bitters") can also be classified as cholagogues.

DEMULCENTS

Demulcents are herbs that are high in *mucilage* (a slimy, soothing substance). These herbs are noted for their ability to soothe or protect irritated mucous membranes inside the body. When applied topically to the skin, a demulcent herb is commonly referred to as an *emollient*. These herbs have demulcent properties:

Marshmallow root	Slippery elm
Mullein flowers	Aloe leaves (only the mucilaginous part)
Plantain leaves	Fenugreek seeds

The slimy mucilage in these herbs produces remarkable effects on the body. A demulcent[10]

- Eases irritation in the bronchioles secondary to a cough
- Reduces irritation in the gastrointestinal tract secondary to diarrhea
- Relaxes and eases urinary tract irritation
- Soothes skin irritation and inflammation and speeds wound healing

Naturopaths prescribe demulcent herbs to ease the following conditions:

Sore throats
Dry, irritating coughs
Diarrhea
Irritable bowel syndrome
Inflammatory bowel conditions
Urinary tract irritation (e.g., following an infection)
Burns

Note that some herbal texts list comfrey and coltsfoot as commonly prescribed demulcents. These herbs contain a group of constituents known as pyrrolizidine alkaloids, which are potentially harmful to the liver.[11,12] Internal consumption of comfrey and coltsfoot is not recommended.

DIGESTIVE BITTERS

My 11-year-old son would argue that all herbs are bitter and taste like something intended to poison him. His perspective is clouded by the fact that his dear old dad used to try out different vile-tasting herbal tinctures on him during naturopathic training.

The bitter taste associated with many herbs (particularly the root or rhizome portion) is the basis for using them to stimulate digestion. When a bitter substance hits your tongue, taste buds tell the brain to signal the mouth to produce more saliva, and the stomach to release more acid to help break down food. Some research on bitters also suggests a stimulating effect on the pancreas and increased production of digestive enzymes. As mentioned previously (see "Cholagogues"), these herbal bitters also stimulate bile flow. The bottom line is that one feels hungrier and digests better after consuming an herbal bitter.

If your digestion is sluggish due to poor production of stomach acid, you'll find bitters particularly useful. If you notice a lot of bloating and gas after eating a meal high in protein, try taking an herbal bitter immediately before eating. Stomach acid production also has a tendency to decrease as we age. Herbal bitters are frequently prescribed for elderly persons who produce less stomach acid and experience sluggish digestion.

Commonly prescribed herbal digestive bitters include:

Gentian root and rhizome	Dandelion root
Yellow dock	Blessed thistle
Centaury	Barberry bark

IMMUNOMODULATORS

More attention is being paid to the effect that many herbs have on the immune system. Examples in Part 5 include echinacea, eleuthero (Siberian ginseng), and Asian ginseng.

Immunomodulation describes the ability of an herb, nutrient, or other substance to promote healthy immune function. Our immune systems are a complex interplay of cells that dictate the body's resistance to infections. These include macrophages, lymphocytes (B and T), and other factors known as cytokines (e.g., interleukin, interferon, and tumor necrosis factor). Lymphocytes, the body's primary defense against viral infections, have been a primary area of focus with regard to HIV infection.

A common denominator among immunomodulating herbs is the presence of complex sugar molecules known as *polysaccharides*. Polysaccharides improve the activity of lymphocytes and other cells of the immune system, thus strengthening the overall immune response.[12]

Perhaps the most well-known example of an immunomodulating herb is echinacea. As we will note in Part 5, echinacea simply increases all aspects of the immune response. This makes it valuable for strengthening a potentially healthy immune system to resist infections such as colds and flu. It can also speed the body's recovery from infections and reduce the recurrence of bacterial and yeast infections. Echinacea is the perfect short-term boost that many immune systems require from time to time.

However, a "get busy" immune stimulant like echinacea is not for everybody. If your immune system is already overactive, as is the case with autoimmune diseases, you should avoid echinacea. It's also not recommended for progressive diseases such as multiple sclerosis. Finally, the jury is still out on whether echinacea should be used by persons with HIV infection.

It's my opinion that these conditions are the domain of the adaptogenic herbs listed above. Adaptogens such as astragalus and eleuthero (Siberian ginseng) tend to enhance the immune system by way of a balancing approach, as opposed to the more nonspecific approach taken by echinacea. This means adaptogens can be used to treat conditions in which the immune system is either depressed or overactive. The following list of immune-related conditions may be treated with herbal adaptogens:

HIV infection
Chronic fatigue syndrome
Chronic hepatitis
Cancer patients recovering from radiation or chemotherapy
Systemic lupus erythematosus

Keep in mind that with most of these conditions, immune-enhancing actions represent only one aspect of a complete health care program.

Some mushrooms, including shiitake, reishi, and maitake, contain a high concentration of polysaccharides. These polysaccharides, like those of immunomodulating herbs, affect the immune system. Traditionally employed as tonics, these mushrooms have many of the same applications as the herbal adaptogens.

LAXATIVES

By the time you finish this book, you may be thinking laxative. From prunes to good ol' Ex-Lax, laxatives are among the most commonly sold over-the-counter remedies in both the United States and Europe. Herbal laxatives are sold most often.

Herbal laxatives are usually placed into two categories: stimulant or bulk-forming. Table 4.3 gives common examples of the two categories.

BULK-FORMING LAXATIVES

Bulk-forming laxatives, which are high in fiber as well as mucilage, expand when they come in contact with water (try leaving some psyllium seeds in a bowl of water for a couple of days). As they increase in volume in the bowel, they stimulate a reflex contraction of the walls of the bowel, followed by emptying. This class of laxatives exerts a milder effect than stimulant laxatives and are most suitable for long-term use.

Since they are high in fiber, bulk-forming laxatives also contribute to keeping cholesterol in check. Research also suggests that diabetics can benefit from the dietary fiber in guar gum, psyllium, and fenugreek. The dietary fiber helps lower blood sugar in people with non-insulin-dependent diabetes (also known as adult-onset or type II diabetes).[13]

STIMULANT LAXATIVES

Stimulant laxatives increase bowel movements, owing to the presence of active constituents known as *anthraquinones*. Anthraquinones increase the contraction of the muscles of the bowel wall primarily by acting as mild irritants. This is not dissimilar to a cough in response to a throat irritant.

Stimulant laxatives are wonderful short-term cures for constipation. However, long-term use is not recommended without medical supervision. Long-term overuse of stimulant laxatives can cause dehydration

Table 4.3
HERBAL LAXATIVES

Bulk-forming	Stimulant
Psyllium seed	Senna leaves
	Cascara bark
	Aloe (latex from the leaves)

and also create a dependence on laxatives for a normal bowel movement. Stimulant laxatives are normally not recommended for pregnant or lactating women (senna is the exception). These laxatives should be avoided if you have an inflammatory bowel disease such as ulcerative colitis or Crohn's disease.

The best researched and most widely used stimulant laxative is senna. One of the best products for treatment of chronic constipation in elderly people is a combination of senna (18 percent) and psyllium (82 percent). In a study of seventy-seven elderly patients in a nursing care home, the use of this combination was found to be far more effective and cost-efficient than a synthetic laxative (lactulose) in the treatment of chronic constipation.[14]

Cascara, another laxative, is milder in action than senna. Aloe is an extremely potent laxative and is usually employed only when senna or cascara are not effective.

part 5

COMMONLY PRESCRIBED
HERBAL MEDICINES

PICKING herbal medicines that meet my criteria for excellence was easy. Keeping the list to a manageable size, however, was not. It reminded me of the time someone asked me to name my favorite jazz albums of all time. Unfortunately, I only had five choices!

The herbal medicines presented here won primarily on the strength of clinical research, history of clinical use, safety, and a lot of personal bias. Most of them fill gaps not currently addressed by our medical system. As I look them over, I'm struck by how easily they would fit into the U.S. health care system. Wouldn't it be great to have gynecologists recommending vitex as a therapeutic starting point in the treatment of menstrual disorders? How about hawthorn extracts being recommended by cardiologists for early stages of congestive heart failure and angina?

The herb chapters that follow are formatted with a quick-reference introduction that summarizes the particulars on each herb, including common uses, notes on recommended use and proper dosage, and safety issues. The text that follows tells the story behind each herb, with a focus on how it might fit into your health care choices.

Also, please remember the following guidelines before deciding to use any of the following herbal medicines:

- Do not self-diagnose. Many of the herbal medicines are recommended for conditions that require proper medical diagnosis and close monitoring by your physician. Once this part of the picture is clear, discuss your desire to use herbal medicines with your doctor. A naturopathic physician or medical doctor, osteopath, or chiropractor trained in natural health care is an optimal choice.
- Don't discontinue any prescription medications without first discussing it with your doctor.
- Don't be afraid to share your herbal education with your doctor. Most physicians are concerned that you may be self-medicating with something that may potentially harm you. Share books like this one and those recommended in "Herbal Medicine Resources" with them. Once they become familiar with the fact that most of these herbs are approved for medical use in other countries and have extensive clinical research, they may choose to become students of herbal medicine also!
- Herbal recommendations, like drugs, don't stand alone in our approach to health. Try to integrate them into a comprehensive health care program that focuses on diet and lifestyle factors.

Bilberry

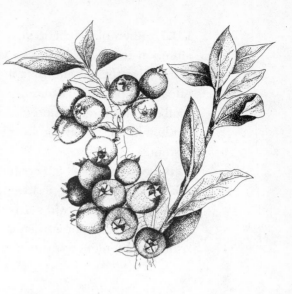

BOTANICAL NAME *Vaccinium myrtillus*
PART USED The ripe berries

COMMON USES
- Poor night vision and poor visual adaptation to bright lights
- Prevention and treatment of diabetic retinopathy
- Easy bruising
- Varicose veins and hemorrhoids during pregnancy

ACTIVE CONSTITUENTS Anthocyanosides (a bioflavonoid complex)

HOW IT WORKS Like other bioflavonoids, anthocyanosides are potent antioxidants. In addition, they assist with normal formation of collagen in connective tissue and help strengthen capillaries in the body. Anthocyanosides are also associated with improving capillary and venous blood flow.

RECOMMENDED USE Standardized extract containing 25 percent anthocyanoside—240 to 480 milligrams in two to three divided dosages

SIDE EFFECTS At therapeutic dosages, there are no known side effects with bilberry extracts.

SAFETY ISSUES There are no known interactions with commonly prescribed drugs. Use of bilberry during pregnancy or lactation is not contraindicated.

LIKE other plants high in bioflavonoids, bilberry has received much attention in medical circles over the past few years. Bioflavonoids are extremely efficient antioxidants and assist the body in counteracting the effect of potentially harmful free radicals.[1,2] Many plants high in bioflavonoids target different tissues and organs of the body. Examples include milk thistle for the liver as well as hawthorn for the cardiovascular system.

Bilberry, with its high content of a bioflavonoid complex known as anthocyanosides, exerts positive effects on the eyes and vision. It is commonly used for a wide array of eye conditions ranging from night blindness to diabetic retinopathy. Bilberry extract has also emerged as a useful supplement to promote healthy circulation throughout the body.

PLANT FACTS

A close relative of the American blueberry, bilberry grows in the woods and forest meadows of northern Europe and in sandy areas of Canada and the United States. A member of the Ericaceae family, it is a shrub-like perennial that grows to about 1 foot in height. The plant flowers in May or June and the ripe fruits are normally collected between July and September.[3] Modern medicinal extracts use only the ripe fruit of the plant.

HISTORY

As a food, bilberries and blueberries have a long history of use that extends to the present. Medically, dried berry and leaf preparations have been used to treat everything under the sun. Bilberry was recommended for scurvy, urinary tract infections, kidney stones, diabetes, and to stop milk flow in a nursing mother.

Perhaps the most sound historical recommendation for bilberries and blueberries is for the treatment of diarrhea. The dried berries were crushed and boiled in water, then strained; the patient was then given the tea to drink. The *astringent* effect (see Part 4) speeded recovery and soothed the irritated intestinal tract following diarrhea.[4]

Modern medical research on the use of bilberry began during the Second World War. Back then bombers didn't have computerized screens; if you wanted to bomb something, you had to *see* it. British Royal Air Force (RAF) pilots noted that their night vision improved when they consumed bilberry jam prior to night bombing raids. These anecdotal reports of improved night vision led to French and Italian research on the medical use of bilberry for a variety of visual disturbances.

MEDICALLY ACTIVE CONSTITUENTS

Research over the past two decades has pointed very clearly to the flavonoids in bilberry as the medically active constituents. In particular, the anthocyanosides have received attention.[5] Bilberry contains more than fifteen types of naturally occurring anthocyanoside. Closely related plants, such as blueberries, black currants, and grapes, also contain these flavonoid complexes.

Research into the medical potential of anthocyanosides has led to the development of a standardized bilberry extract with a highly concentrated amount of anthocyanosides. The most frequently prescribed form has 25 percent anthocyanoside content.[6] The magnitude of this concentration is perhaps best reflected in the fact that the fresh fruit contains only 0.1–0.25 percent anthocyanoside content!

Bilberry is a classic example of the advantage of a modern herbal extract compared to more traditional preparations like tea. First, extracts allow a greater dosage of the medically active component. Also, the measured amount of anthocyanosides in an extract allows more consistent dosing and therapeutic activity.[7]

HOW BILBERRY WORKS

Support for Normal Vision

Following the reports of those wild and crazy RAF pilots, initial research centered on bilberry's effects on the eyes and vision. Studies performed in animals revealed that the anthocyanosides actually speeded the regeneration of rhodopsin (visual purple) in the retina of the eye.[8]

The retina, which lies at the back of the eye, is the part of your eye that "sees," that is, responds to light. It does so by way of specialized cells called cones and rods. The cones are used for detailed vision (e.g., reading) and color perception. The rods are involved in night vision and adaptation to light.[9] Rhodopsin is a purple pigment that is critical for the proper functioning of the rods.

By speeding up the regeneration of rhodopsin, bilberry allows better adaptation to both dark and light.

Support for Normal Circulation

Anthocyanosides strengthen the body's small blood vessels, known as capillaries. When capillaries become fragile (a condition that is not uncommon with aging), bruising occurs more often. Capillary fragility can also have harmful effects on other areas of the body. In the eyes, it can lead to areas of microhemorrhaging known as retinopathy. This is a common complication of diabetes. Weak capillaries also lead to poor blood supply to connective tissues in the body, which can hinder healing of tissue in cases of trauma and inflammatory conditions such as arthritis.

Anthocyanosides strengthen capillaries very efficiently. Owing to their antioxidant capabilities, they protect the capillary from free radical damage.[10] Anthocyanosides also help build stronger capillaries by stimulating the formation of healthy connective tissue.[11] Finally, anthocyanosides are also associated with the formation of new, healthy capillaries.[12]

Anthocyanosides also improve circulation through larger blood vessels. Studies indicate that blood vessel tone is improved in both arteries and veins after exposure to anthocyanosides.[13] Anthocyanosides have been shown to reduce the stickiness of platelets (also known as platelet aggregation)—an effect that is associated with reducing the risk of atherosclerosis.[14] These combined effects have made anthocyanosides popular in the management of such circulatory conditions as varicose veins and hemorrhoids. It also points to these and other bioflavonoids as valuable aids in the long-term maintenance of a healthy circulatory system.

Support for Normal Connective Tissue

As is the case with many bioflavonoids, anthocyanosides also enhance the formation of normal connective tissue throughout the body. They do this by promoting the normal cross-linking of collagen—the backbone of healthy connective tissue.[15]

Anthocyanosides are particularly useful for the protection of connective tissue from damage secondary to inflammation.[16] They also assist in the regeneration of healthy connective tissue following injury.

HEALTH CARE APPLICATIONS

Eye Conditions

Bilberry extract has become the leading herbal prescription for the maintenance of healthy vision and for the treatment of many eye diseases. In the 1960s, French researchers discovered that bilberry extracts improved night vision and a person's ability to adjust visually to bright light.[17]

This has led to the wide use of bilberry extracts for persons with night blindness and/or poor ability to visually adapt to bright light.[18] I also regularly recommend bilberry for eye strain—particularly for those of us sitting behind a computer for long stretches of time! Long-term use may also help improve the vision of near-sighted people.[19]

Bilberry can help diabetics diagnosed with retinopathy. Diabetic retinopathy is the leading cause of blindness among diabetics and is characterized by damage to the capillaries in the retina. One study indicates that daily use of bilberry extract leads to a reduction in capillary fragility and hemorrhaging.[20] Note, however, that the results of this study are based on the reactions of only a small number of patients. Long-term use is optimal for treatment of retinopathy.

Many herbal prescriptions—including gingko and evening primrose oil—help reduce the risk of some of the complications of diabetes, including retinopathy and neuropathy. Perhaps most notable is the fact that these herbal preparations also address healthy circulation in the diabetic patient and are not associated with causing problems with regulation of blood sugar control (see the discussion on diabetes in Part 6, "Endocrine System").

Circulation Problems

Because bilberry extract improves large vessel and small vessel circulation, it is a useful supplement for elderly people with poor circulation to the extremities.[21] It is most commonly prescribed for conditions associated with the veins—namely, varicose veins and hemorrhoids. It should also be considered useful for improving circulation and subsequent healing in persons who have had surgery.

One notable area of use for bilberry extracts is in the prevention and treatment of varicose veins and hemorrhoids during pregnancy. These occur frequently among women in their third trimester, when the weight of the fetus and gravity combine to pull blood toward the point of least resistance. Using bilberry extract both during and after pregnancy reduces symptoms and even the possible onset of these conditions.[22] The Grismond study marks bilberry extract as an herbal prescription that deserves the "safe during pregnancy" seal of approval.

Owing to bilberry's ability to strengthen capillaries, it is also a practical recommendation for people who bruise easily. I frequently recommend it with vitamin C. This combination also benefits children with frequent nosebleeds.

RECOMMENDED USE AND SAFETY ISSUES

For use in diagnosed eye conditions, such as diabetic retinopathy and circulatory disorders, bilberry extract standardized to 25 percent anthocyanoside content is recommended at a daily dose of 480 milligrams in two to three divided dosages. Following improvement, this may be reduced to a maintenance dose of 240 milligrams daily. The lower dose may be used by persons interested in the prevention of eye or circulation disorders.

There are no known side effects to bilberry at the therapeutic or maintenance dosages listed above. Bilberry is not known to interact with drugs commonly prescribed for the eyes or circulation. There are no contraindications to the use of bilberry during pregnancy and lactation. Night bombing raids, with or without bilberry, are contraindicated for the health of the planet!

RELATED CONDITIONS DISCUSSED IN PART 6

- Atherosclerosis
- Bruising
- Cataracts
- Diabetic retinopathy
- Macular degeneration
- Poor night vision
- Varicose veins

Chamomile

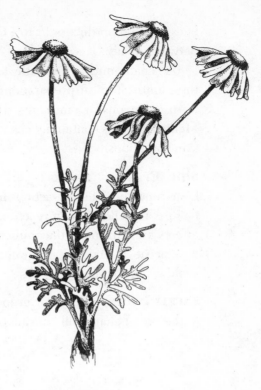

COMMON NAME   German chamomile

BOTANICAL NAME   *Matricaria recutita*

PART USED   Dried flowers

COMMON USES

INTERNAL USES

- Infant colic
- Peptic ulcers
- Irritable bowel syndrome and inflammatory bowel conditions
- Restlessness or sleeplessness in infants (especially with teething) and young children

EXTERNAL USES

- Inflammatory skin conditions (such as eczema)
- Mouthwash for canker sores and other irritations of the mouth and gums

ACTIVE CONSTITUENTS   Volatile oil components: $(-)$-α-bisabolol, $(-)$-α-bisabolol oxides A and B, and matricin, as well as flavonoids including apigenin and luteolin

HOW IT WORKS   Chamomile exerts both an antiinflammatory and an antispasmodic effect in the gastrointestinal tract. Topically, it also has antiinflammatory properties. It promotes wound healing and has mild antibacterial properties.

RECOMMENDED USE   Chamomile is typically taken in tea form. Boiling water is poured over a heaping tablespoon of dried flowers and covered. After 5 to 10 minutes the water is passed through a tea strainer. A cup of freshly brewed tea is drunk three to four times daily, between meals.

Alternatively, you could mix a dried, encapsulated product or alcohol-based tincture with hot water. The dosage should be 2 to 3 grams of the encapsulated product or $\frac{1}{2}$ to 1 teaspoon of the tincture three times daily, between meals.

Use chamomile as a mouthwash for irritations and minor infections in the mouth. Topical preparations for use on the skin are usually in the form of creams or ointments that contain 3 to 10 percent chamomile. Medicinal baths containing chamomile can also be used for inflammatory skin conditions.

SIDE EFFECTS Although rare, allergic reactions to chamomile have been reported. These reactions include bronchial constriction with internal use and allergic skin reactions following topical use. While such side effects are extremely uncommon, people with allergies to plants of the Asteraceae family (e.g., ragweed, asters, and chrysanthemums) should avoid using chamomile.

SAFETY ISSUES Current European monographs list no contraindication to the use of chamomile during pregnancy or lactation.

I am sorry to say that Peter was not very well during the evening. His mother put him to bed and made some chamomile tea; and she gave a dose to Peter! One tablespoon to be taken at bedtime.
BEATRIX POTTER, *THE TALE OF PETER RABBIT*

CHAMOMILE is as popular in German herbal medicine as ginseng is in Chinese herbal medicine. Used historically as a folk remedy for digestive complaints and inflammatory skin conditions, chamomile continues to be a cornerstone of European and American herbal medicine today. With 4,000 tons of chamomile produced annually, the herb has become important worldwide both medically and economically.[1]

PLANT FACTS

Since the intent of this book is to transform you into a responsible herbal consumer, not a botanist, I won't burden you with the confusion surrounding different forms of chamomile. Two major forms are used worldwide—German and Roman chamomile. With the exception of Great Britain, where Roman chamomile is preferred, German chamomile (previously referred to in older literature as *Matricaria chamomilla*) is the most commonly used and best researched form of chamomile.[2] Since it's also the most frequently used in the United States, we'll limit our discussion in this chapter to the German form.

Chamomile is a member of the daisy family and is native to Europe and western Asia. An annual, it grows from 1 to 2 feet high and forms distinctive yellow flowers with white rays. The flowers typically bloom in late July or early August.[3] Traditional and modern medical preparations of chamomile use the flower heads just prior to blooming.

HISTORY

German and Roman chamomile have been used for centuries as medicinal plants. The Egyptians believed the plant was a treatment for "ague," or malarial fever. The origin of the name *chamomile* comes from the Greek *kamai* (on the ground) and *melon* (an apple). This name referred to the freshly harvested plant, which carries the scent of apples. During the Middle Ages, the plant was cultivated for use as an aromatic stewing herb.[4]

In Europe, the herb became something of a cure-all. Germans use the phrase *alles zutraut* ("capable of anything") to describe chamomile. The plant reached its pinnacle of popularity in 1987, when the Germans named it "plant of the year" (a kind of Academy Award of plants, I guess).[5]

Today, the chamomile industry is huge in Europe. Chamomile is found in liquid and dried preparations for internal use, ointments, creams, bath products, cosmetics, and even hair dyes. In Germany alone, more than 90 licensed products contain chamomile.

MEDICALLY ACTIVE CONSTITUENTS

The flowers of chamomile contain volatile oil, anywhere from 1 to 2 percent. Key constituents in the volatile oil are α-bisabolol, α-bisabolol oxides A and B, and matricin. Matricin is usually converted to chamazulene during the extraction process. German chamomile extracts are often produced to contain an established amount of chamazulene and α-bisabolol.

Also among chamomile's active constituents are bioflavonoids. These include apigenin, luteolin, and quercetin.[6]

The medical benefits of chamomile result from a complex interplay of these two groups. The primary antiinflammatory activity was originally attributed to the essential oil constituents[7,8]; however, more recent studies with flavonoids indicate that they also possess significant antiinflammatory activity.[9]

Both components also contribute to the antispasmodic, or muscle-relaxing, effect of chamomile. This effect is particularly noteworthy in the smooth muscles of the gastrointestinal tract.[10]

HEALTH CARE APPLICATIONS

Americans have relegated chamomile to the status of a "calming" herb. This is largely because of its use in commercial teas suggesting a calming or sleep-inducing effect. But the clinical applications of chamomile are more wide ranging than this. For example, homeopathic chamomile products are available for teething and colic in young children. Rudolf Fritz Weiss (see Part 2) advocates the use of chamomile for intestinal ailments and skin conditions. He suggests chamomile as a gentle, long-term alternative to aggressive, short-term therapies such as atropine and cortisone.[11]

Varo Tyler, a respected advocate for the rational use of herbal medicine in the United States, gets right to the point when he calls chamomile "perhaps the best example of the wide chasm separating medicinal practice in Western Europe and the United States."[12]

Gastrointestinal Tract Spasms and Irritation
Peter Rabbit's mother was an insightful herbalist. Along with peppermint, chamomile is probably the perfect embodiment of the term *carminative* (see "Carminatives" in Part 4). The major advantage of chamomile

is its noted antiinflammatory action. This makes it valuable for a wide range of gastrointestinal (GI) tract disorders.

While I'm attempting to be specific here, keep in mind that chamomile's broad-spectrum approach to the GI tract leaves room for you to use it to treat a variety of conditions, and even for mild, soothing effects. It should be considered whenever the GI tract is either cramping or irritated due to anxiety or stress. Chamomile also heals and calms the GI tract following a bout of diarrhea.

Use chamomile to treat the following conditions:[13]

Irritable bowel syndrome
Indigestion
Infant colic
Gastritis
Peptic ulcer disease
Cramping secondary to diarrhea
Spastic colon

Remember that inflammatory conditions of the GI tract, such as ulcers, Crohn's disease, and ulcerative colitis, can also lead to bleeding and possible anemia. While chamomile may help in the long-term management of these serious conditions, it should not be thought of as a substitute for proper medical monitoring and more aggressive short-term therapies.

Chamomile can be used as part of a program to keep your GI tract well. In addition to helping maintain normal GI tone, it also stimulates normal digestion.[14]

Mouth Irritations and Gum Disease

Because of its soothing effect on mucous membranes (the area lining the inside of your mouth and GI tract), and healing properties, chamomile is also useful for the treatment of canker sores and other irritations or sores inside the mouth.[15]

The added benefit of antibacterial activity by the essential oil constituents makes it valuable in the treatment and prevention of gum diseases such as gingivitis.[16] The best approach here is to gargle with a strong tea several times daily.

Topical application to the gums is also useful for infants during teething. I usually recommend that parents apply a strong tea or liquid extract directly to the gums every 2 to 3 hours. Chamomile will help your child's gums feel better and will also exert a calming effect that will help them sleep.

Skin Irritations

Chamomile is widely used in Europe for the treatment of skin irritations.[17] Topical chamomile creams and ointments are used to treat eczema, insect bites, and poison ivy or poison oak rashes. I find it extremely useful in combination with calendula (marigold) ointment or cream for the treatment of diaper rash in infants.

Owing to the above-mentioned wound-healing and antibacterial effects, Europeans often apply chamomile in wound dressings.[18] Studies of chamomile in combination with corticosteroids and antihistamines have shown excellent results in the treatment of stasis ulcers in elderly, bed-ridden patients.[19] *Note:* Please use chamomile as a wound-healing treatment only under the supervision of a health care professional.

Mild Sedative

Chamomile does appear to have mild sedating properties.[20] While not as strong as herbal sedatives such as valerian and passion flower, it can be considered an option for treatment of mild sleep disorders in children, especially for sleeplessness caused by teething or colic.

HOW TO USE CHAMOMILE

The German Commission E monograph[21] gives the following instructions for the preparation and use of chamomile tea for medicinal purposes:

> Pour hot water (150 ml) over a heaped tablespoonful of matricaria flowers (approx. 3 grams), covered, and after 5–10 minutes, pass through a tea strainer. Unless otherwise prescribed,

for gastrointestinal complaints a cup of the freshly prepared tea is drunk three or four times a day between meals. For inflammation of the mucous membranes of the mouth and throat, the freshly prepared tea is used as a wash or gargle.

If you don't want to prepare your own chamomile tea, take a short-cut: use either a powdered, encapsulated herb preparation or an alcohol-based tincture. The dosage of the powdered herb is 2 to 3 grams, two to three times daily between meals. Tinctures are usually dosed at ½ to 1 teaspoon three times daily. I'm a big proponent of placing these delivery forms in hot water and drinking them like a tea. European extracts, which are usually liquid based, are much stronger than our commercial chamomile products. They would be a welcome addition to herbal product offerings in the United States.

For infants and young children, I recommend one-half the adult dosage. Chamomile tea is unique among the many herbs discussed in this book because it actually tastes good. This makes it a bit easier to give directly to infants.

Topically, European creams and ointments are usually made with a 3 to 10 percent concentration of chamomile. A similar concentration is also used for medicinal baths and poultices.

Side effects are extremely rare with either internal or external use of chamomile tea. The big red flag that's been waved in the faces of herb users is the risk of an allergic reaction. Bronchial tightness and shortness of breath, as well as a skin rash, have been reported. How common has this been? Between the years 1887 and 1982, fifty allergic reactions resulting from chamomile use have been reported. Only five could be attributed to German chamomile![22]

Concern about allergies is primarily limited to those with allergies to members of the daisy family. If you're allergic to ragweed, asters, or chrysanthemums, you're probably better off avoiding chamomile.

European monographs list no contraindication to the use of chamomile during pregnancy and lactation. No interactions with commonly prescribed medications have been reported.

Related Conditions Discussed in Part 6

- Blocked tear duct
- Canker sores
- Colic
- Diarrhea
- Eczema
- Heartburn
- Insomnia
- Irritable bowel syndrome

Cranberry

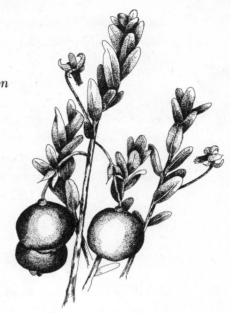

BOTANICAL NAME   *Vaccinium macrocarpon*
PART USED   The ripe fruit

COMMON USES
- Recurrent urinary tract infections
- Prevention of urinary tract infections

HOW IT WORKS   Cranberry inhibits the adherence of *Escherichia coli* (*E. coli*) bacteria to the cells lining the wall of the bladder. These bacteria are responsible for the large majority of recurrent urinary tract infections.

RECOMMENDED USE   Take one capsule (300 to 400 milligrams) of a concentrated cranberry juice extract in the morning and one capsule in the evening. Ample intake of fluids throughout the day is also recommended. Several glasses of a high-quality cranberry juice (not the cocktail!) daily will approximate the effect of the encapsulated concentrate.

SIDE EFFECTS   None known

SAFETY ISSUES   There are no known contraindications to the use of cranberry during pregnancy or lactation. There are no known interactions with antibiotics or other drugs. Cranberry should not be used as a substitute for antibiotics during an acute urinary tract infection.

CRANBERRY is the perfect example of the Hippocrates adage, "Let your food be your medicine." Regularly recommended by health care professionals and widely used by consumers for the prevention of urinary tract infections, cranberry is one of those herbal medicines that has enjoyed acceptance in modern medical circles for quite some time. New research is clarifying the way cranberry works to protect the urinary tract.

This has served to validate its historical use and to expand the use of this common food in the future.

PLANT FACTS

A close relative of American blueberry and European bilberry, cranberry has been used for centuries in cooking and as a garnish. More recently, it has become a major cash crop due to the commercial sales of cranberry juice cocktail. Cranberry is cultivated extensively in natural and artificial bogs throughout the United States, especially in Massachusetts and Washington.

HISTORY

The Pilgrims learned about cranberries from American Indians. Use of the berry spread, both as a food and in some medical applications. Historically, cranberry was used to prevent kidney stones and "bladder gravel." It was also believed to remove blood "toxins" from the body.

Since the early part of the twentieth century, however, most of the focus on cranberry has been related to the urinary tract, especially for the prevention of urinary tract infections. In 1923, American scientists showed that the urine of individuals consuming large amounts of cranberries became more acidic.[1]

Part of this acidifying process included an increase in hippuric acid, a chemical that can have a potent antibiotic effect in the urinary tract.[2] Because the bacteria (*E. coli*) causing most urinary tract infections (UTIs) prefer an alkaline pH, cranberry became a common recommendation among physicians for prevention of UTIs and treatment of women with recurrent UTIs.[3,4]

FACTS ABOUT URINARY TRACT INFECTIONS

Women suffering from UTIs account for approximately 5.2 million visits to physicians' offices each year. One of five women in the United States will suffer a UTI at some time in their lives. If you've been treated for an acute urinary tract infection, your risk of recurrence is 20 percent! Recurring UTIs increase the risk of kidney infections and may result in scarring of the bladder wall.[5]

That nasty bug *E. coli* causes 90 percent of first-time UTIs in women (by the way, they don't contract it by eating hamburgers). Among women it is also the leading cause of recurrent UTIs. *Escherichia coli* causes UTIs by adhering to the wall of the bladder and causing inflammation. It is interesting to note that among women with recurrent UTIs, *E. coli* seems to adhere more easily to the cells lining the bladder. Thus, their risk of recurrent UTIs goes up dramatically.[6]

How Cranberry Works

In 1984, A. E. Sobota of Youngstown State University (Youngstown, Ohio), disproved the acidifying theory of cranberry.[7] He demonstrated that cranberry does not acidify the urine sufficiently to produce an antibacterial effect. Instead, he showed that cranberry prevented *E. coli* from adhering to the cells lining the bladder wall.[8] If *E. coli* can't adhere, it can't cause an infection. His work altered thinking about the way cranberry prevents UTIs and has actually strengthened the rationale for using it to prevent recurrent UTIs—especially when long-term antibiotic therapy has failed.

Sobota's work has been expanded by a group of researchers in Israel. Their work has focused on the most virulent strains of *E. coli* and shows that cranberry powerfully deters the adhesion of these strains in the bladder.[9] Their work also indicates that other members of the *Vaccinium* genus (e.g., blueberry and bilberry) also possess antiadherence properties.[10]

Health Care Applications

Recurrent Urinary Tract Infections
As noted earlier, the primary group suffering from recurrent UTIs is younger women. Ironically, no clinical studies have been completed to demonstrate the use of cranberry in this group.

However, with the introduction of concentrated cranberry juice extracts in capsules, consumers have a powerful tool at their disposal for lowering their risk of recurring UTIs. A daily dosage as low as 300 to 400 milligrams safely and effectively reduces UTI recurrence and also clears *E. coli* bacteria from the urine. Equally important, it lowers the need for recurrent use of antibiotics and the risk of yeast infections that often follow.

Prevention of Urinary Tract Infections

Two recent studies[11,12] indicate that cranberry may also protect elderly individuals from *E. coli* in the urinary tract. The first study, involving 153 women (average age 78.5 years), found that cranberry juice (300 milliliters daily) reduced the amount of bacteria in their urine. While the study used a very weak cranberry preparation (they sweetened it with saccharin!), it does demonstrate the ability to lower the risk of UTI in this population.[11]

The importance of this study lies in the reduction of bacteria in the urinary tract. People over the age of 65 years are more likely to have higher urinary levels of *E. coli*. It's important to note that these higher levels, presaging a UTI, may not produce any noticeable signs or symptoms; but such people are nevertheless at greater risk of a UTI. A higher risk of kidney infection is also a possibility.

A second, smaller study found that 4 to 6 ounces of cranberry juice administered daily to twenty-eight nursing home patients resulted in an absence of UTIs in nineteen of the patients. The same researchers later administered an encapsulated cranberry juice extract to twenty-one patients for varying lengths of time. Although the results were observational, twenty of these patients reported no UTIs while taking cranberry.[12]

How to Use Cranberry

Take one capsule (300 to 400 milligrams of concentrated, cranberry juice extract) in the morning and one capsule in the evening. Make sure you drink plenty of water throughout the day. Several glasses of a good-quality cranberry juice can be used as an alternative to the capsules. Don't rely on commercial cranberry cocktail, which contains sweeteners and only a small amount of actual cranberry juice.

Encapsulated cranberry juice extract seems to offer more consistent antiadherence activity and is certainly lower in sugar than cranberry juice cocktail. It's a good alternative for those of you who don't like the taste of cranberry and aren't willing to drink several glasses daily.

For those of you with recurrent UTIs, proper medical diagnosis is essential. Remember, improperly treated UTIs can lead to serious kidney infections. Cranberry is not a substitute for antibiotics in the treatment of UTIs!

RELATED CONDITIONS DISCUSSED IN PART 6

- Urinary tract infections (recurrent)

Echinacea

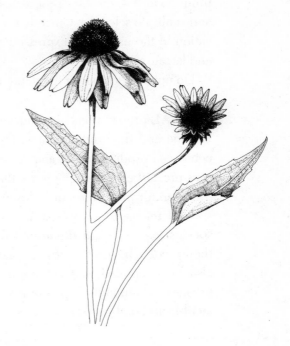

COMMON NAME   Purple coneflower

BOTANICAL NAMES   *Echinacea purpurea, Echinacea angustifolia, Echinacea pallida*

PARTS USED   The best-researched form of echinacea is a juice made from the above-ground portion of *E. purpurea* (including leaves and flowers). Herbal preparations made from the roots of *E. purpurea* and *E. angustifolia* are also sold.

COMMON USES

- Prevention and treatment of colds and flu
- Supportive treatment of recurrent infections of the ears, respiratory tract, and urinary tract
- Recurrent vaginal yeast infections

HOW IT WORKS   Stimulates the immune system

RECOMMENDED USE   Use either the expressed (i.e., squeezed) juice of the E. purpurea herb or the encapsulated dried juice. For short-term use, take 40 drops of the juice or two capsules initially; then 40 drops of the juice or one capsule every 2 hours throughout the day for 48 hours or until symptom relief is noted.

For long-term use, take 40 drops of the juice three times daily or one capsule of the dried juice three to four times daily. Echinacea should not be taken for more than 8 weeks continuously. A 2-week break is recommended before resuming.

SIDE EFFECTS   None known

SAFETY ISSUES   Echinacea is contraindicated in individuals with auto-immune illness, or other progressive systemic disease such as tuberculosis and multiple sclerosis. Current European monographs list no contraindication to the use of the expressed juice of *E. purpurea* during pregnancy and lactation.

Do not use echinacea if you are allergic to flowers of the daisy family.

HERBAL preparations of echinacea are among the most popular in both Europe and the United States. On the German market more than 300 echinacea products are available. In 1994, German doctors and pharmacists prescribed echinacea more than 2.5 million times![1] The primary use has been for prevention or treatment of colds and flu.

To date, medicinal preparations of *E. purpurea* and other echinacea species (e.g., *E. angustifolia* and *E. pallida*) have 200 journal articles to their credit.[2] In addition to its general use for colds and flu, echinacea has also been applied to treat recurrent vaginal yeast infections, chronic prostate inflammation (prostatitis), and bronchitis. In Europe, both injectible and oral forms are used.

PLANT FACTS

Echinacea is a native American wildflower belonging to the sunflower family. It is commonly referred to as "purple coneflower" because of the flower's distinctive shape and color. Of the nine species native to the United States and Canada, three are used medicinally: *E. purpurea, E. angustifolia,* and *E. pallida.* Although echinacea can be found growing in the wild, most medicinal preparations are harvested from cultivated plants in either the United States or Europe.[3]

HISTORY

The history of echinacea's medicinal use begins in American and Western herbal lore. It was used by American Indians for a variety of ailments, including treatment of venomous bites and external wounds. Echinacea was first introduced into U.S. medical practice by John King in 1887. Also recommended by John Uri Lloyd (a pharmacist of Cincinnati, Ohio), echinacea was very popular among medical professionals in the late nineteenth century. By the early part of the twentieth century, however, echinacea had largely disappeared from U.S. medicine.[4]

Echinacea was rediscovered in the 1930s by Dr. Gerhard Madaus of Germany. Madaus, the founder of the pharmaceutical manufacturing firm Madaus AG of Cologne, Germany, came to the United States in search of *E. angustifolia* seeds. This species of echinacea was the most widely used medicinally at that time. Perhaps fooled by some tricky U.S. herbalist, Madaus returned to Germany with seeds of *E. purpurea* instead of *E. angustifolia*. By default, *E. purpurea* became the subject of Madaus' pharmacological studies. The result was the development of a product called Echinacin, an expressed juice prepared from the aboveground part of the plant. This preparation has become the most extensively researched and frequently prescribed echinacea preparation worldwide.

MEDICALLY ACTIVE CONSTITUENTS

Studies show that echinacea boosts the activity of the immune system. Most of echinacea's immune-enhancing properties are attributed to complex sugar molecules known as polysaccharides.[5] One of echinacea's polysaccharides, arabinogalactan, has shown significant ability to stimulate the immune system.[6] Other components of echinacea influence immune system activity as well.

HOW ECHINACEA WORKS

Simply put, echinacea activates the immune system. The polysaccharides, as well as other constituents in echinacea, stimulate the cells of the immune system. These include white blood cells, such as lymphocytes and macrophages. Echinacea also supports the production of interferon, an important part of our immune response to viral infections causing colds and flu.[7-9] The end result is a better defense against infections.

Colds and Flu

Echinacea has emerged as one of the most effective herbal prescriptions for the prevention and treatment of colds and flu and has become a leading herbal treatment prescribed by health care practitioners in both Europe and the United States. Two recent studies[10,11] verify its usefulness in this area.

One study examined the effect of an *E. purpurea* liquid preparation on the length of time and severity of colds in 108 patients. Half the group received echinacea and the other half received a placebo (inactive) preparation. After treatment for 8 weeks, people taking echinacea stayed healthy longer, that is, a longer period of time elapsed between infections. When they did get sick, the echinacea group experienced symptoms of less severity than those of the others, and recovered far more quickly.[10]

A second study looked at the effect of an echinacea preparation on people afflicted by the flu. One hundred and eighty volunteers (age range, 18 to 60 years) with the flu were assigned to one of three groups: (1) placebo; (2) 450 milligrams of echinacea daily; and (3) 900 milligrams of echinacea daily. Those receiving 900 milligrams daily showed a significant reduction in flu symptoms, such as weakness/low energy, chills/sweating, sore throat, muscle/joint aches, and headaches. Results were not favorable at the lower dosage of 450 milligrams daily.[11]

These studies, which reflect vast clinical experience, suggest echinacea belongs in your medicine cabinet during the cold and flu season. It not only prevents these threats to your health but dramatically curtails their troublesome symptoms once they've begun.

Recurrent Infections

Echinacea is also an excellent supportive therapy for people with recurring infections. I commonly recommend echinacea for my pediatric patients with recurring ear infections. It's particularly useful when antibiotic therapy is failing. While echinacea should not be considered a substitute for antibiotics, it may stimulate a "sluggish" immune system to resist infection more effectively.

Others likely to benefit from echinacea are women with recurring vaginal yeast infections. Recurrence even with topical antifungal medications exceeds 60 percent! This is another indication that killing the bug doesn't address the underlying problem: an immune system that's not mounting a strong enough defense.

The positive effect of *E. purpurea* was illustrated in a study of 203 women suffering from recurrent vaginal yeast infections.[12] All of these women were being treated with a topical econazole nitrate cream (a commonly prescribed antifungal/antiyeast medication).

Women using the econazole nitrate alone experienced a 60.5 percent recurrence rate. Women taking echinacea orally lowered this recurrence rate to 16.7 percent! Researchers also noted a normalization of immune function (as measured by skin test) in all of the women receiving echinacea.

HOW TO USE ECHINACEA

Take echinacea at the onset of a cold or flu for a period of 10 to 14 days, without interruption. For long-term use, namely, for individuals with recurrent infections or for those wishing to add some extra defense before flu season, use echinacea for 6 to 8 weeks continuously. Breaks of several days should follow these 6- to 8-week stretches, as echinacea's immune-enhancing effect may weaken if used for more than 8 weeks.

While the dosage recommended for the expressed juice of *E. purpurea* and its dried, powdered equivalent have been the best researched, root preparations of both *E. purpurea* and *E. angustifolia* are sometimes recommended. Daily dosage of these preparations is in the range of 900 milligrams daily for adults.

Don't take echinacea if you have an autoimmune illness such as lupus, or other progressive systemic disease, including tuberculosis and multiple sclerosis. Avoid taking echinacea if you are allergic to flowers of the daisy family. The current German Commission E monograph (see discussion of Commission E monographs in Part 2) lists no contraindications to the use of the expressed juice of *E. purpurea* herb during pregnancy and lactation.[13]

Related Conditions Discussed in Part 6

- Canker sores
- Colds and flu
- Cold sores
- Recurrent ear infections
- Periodontal disease
- Recurrent sinus infections
- Sore throat
- Recurrent urinary tract infections
- Vaginal yeast infections

Eleuthero

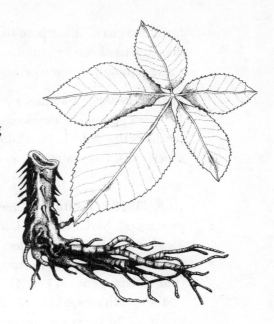

BOTANICAL NAMES *Eleutherococcus senticosus, Acanthopanax senticosus*
OTHER COMMON NAME Siberian ginseng
PART USED The root

COMMON USES
- Fatigue and declining work ability
- Support during exercise and physical exertion
- Support for the body during times of stress
- Prevention of colds and flu
- Supportive use during radiation or chemotherapy
- Chronic fatigue syndrome
- Human immunodeficiency virus (HIV) infection

ACTIVE CONSTITUENTS A complex group of glycosides known as eleutherosides

HOW IT WORKS Eleuthero is notable for its ability to support and enhance adrenal function. Optimal adrenal function is associated with greater energy and better reaction to stress. Eleuthero also supports and strengthens the immune system. In addition, it maximizes the utilization of oxygen by working muscles, keeping them in an aerobic state for a longer period of time.

RECOMMENDED USE Dry extract of the root, 2 to 3 grams daily in two or three divided dosages; concentrated solid extract standardized for eleutherosides B and E, 300 to 400 milligrams daily; alcohol-based extract, 8 to 10 milliliters in two to three divided dosages. Historically, eleuthero is taken continuously for 6 to 8 weeks, followed by a 1- to 2-week break before resuming.

SIDE EFFECTS   Eleuthero has few reported side effects. Mild, transient diarrhea has been reported by a small number of users. Eleuthero may cause insomnia in some people if taken too close to bedtime.

SAFETY ISSUES   Eleuthero can be used during pregnancy or lactation. However, pregnant or lactating women using eleuthero should avoid products that have been adulterated with *Panax ginseng* or other related species that are contraindicated.

ELEUTHERO, often referred to as Siberian ginseng, is a frequently prescribed herbal tonic. Used for hundreds of years in Asian and Eastern European countries, eleuthero is an *adaptogen*—a substance that can increase our resistance to a wide variety of negative influences (see "Adaptogens" in Part 4).

Today, athletes often use eleuthero to enhance performance. It is a major ally in stress management. This is because eleuthero supports the normal functioning of the adrenal glands. Clinical research also points to eleuthero as a promising supplement in the long-term management of conditions such as chronic fatigue syndrome and HIV infection.

PLANT FACTS

Eleuthero belongs to the Araliaceae family and is a distant relative of Asian ginseng (*Panax ginseng*). Also known commonly as touch-me-not and devil's shrub, eleuthero has been most frequently nicknamed Siberian ginseng in the United States. The common botanical name for the plant is *Eleutherococcus senticosus,* although some oriental textbooks also refer to it as *Acanthopanax senticosus.*

Eleutherococcus senticosus is a slender, thorny shrub that grows to a height of 3 to 15 feet. It is native to the taiga forests of the Far East (southeastern part of Russia, northern China, Korea, and Japan). Medicinal preparations of the plant are made largely from the root. The largest share of raw herb used for extracts in the United States comes from Russia.[1]

HISTORY

Although not as popular as *Panax ginseng*, eleuthero dates back 2,000 years in the records of Chinese medicine. Referred to as *Ciwuju* in Chinese medicine, it was used to prevent respiratory tract infections, as well as colds and flu. The Chinese also believed eleuthero provided energy and vitality.[2]

In Russia, eleuthero was originally used by people in the Siberian taiga to increase performance and quality of life and decrease infections. In 1856, the Russian botanists Franz J. Ruprecht and Karl Johann Maximowicz named the plant *Hedra sentocosa*. Maximowicz later changed the name to *Eleutherococcus senticosus*.

MODERN DEVELOPMENT

The modern history of eleuthero began with I. I. Brekhman and colleagues in the 1940s. During a search for a more economical herbal alternative to Asian (Chinese or Korean) ginseng, Brekhman discovered that eleuthero offered many of the same benefits as the famous Asian tonic. Having already investigated the actions of *Panax ginseng* (and coining the term "adaptogen" to describe them), Brekhman shifted his attention to eleuthero.[3] Eleuthero became the center of extensive clinical research over the next 3 decades.

In Russia, eleuthero's ability to increase stamina and endurance was so well regarded that the cosmonauts used it instead of the amphetamines taken by American astronauts. Soviet Olympic athletes used it to enhance their training and then went on to dominate many of the endurance sports. Explorers, divers, sailors, and miners used eleuthero to prevent stress-related illness.[4] After the Chernobyl accident, many Russian citizens were given eleuthero to counteract the effects of radiation.

Today, more than 1,000 papers have been published on eleuthero (primarily in Russian). Approximately 6 million people in Russia are believed to use eleuthero on a daily basis.

MEDICALLY ACTIVE CONSTITUENTS

The constituents in eleuthero that have received the most attention are the *eleutherosides*. Predominantly glycosides, these constituents are thought to contribute to the adaptogenic actions of eleuthero.[5] Seven primary eleutherosides have been identified, with the most research focusing on eleutherosides B and E.[6] These substances are not the same as ginseng's active constituents, known as *ginsenosides*.

Eleuthero also contains complex polysaccharides (a kind of super sugar molecule).[7] These constituents play a critical role in eleuthero's ability to support immune function.

HOW ELEUTHERO WORKS

I can't think of an herbal medicine that better fits the definition of an adaptogen. Acting on a wide range of body functions, eleuthero has a remarkable ability to increase the body's resistance to stress and provide an impetus to move toward a state of balance.

Stress Reduction

Stress takes its toll on our bodies daily. Psychological stress due to deadlines, emotional distress, and existential dilemmas has been shown to affect the body. More easily measured are the physical stresses such as physical labor, strenuous exercise, poor diets, and environmental pollution. While stress can eventually wreak havoc on a number of body systems, its initial target is the adrenal glands. Chronic stress can overwhelm the adrenals and lead to chronic fatigue, poor immune function, and improper blood sugar metabolism.[8]

As an adaptogen, eleuthero helps us adapt to stress. It does this by providing fuel to the adrenal glands, allowing them to function optimally when challenged by stress.[9] This means eleuthero should be considered as a daily supplement for anyone experiencing stress on a regular basis. I firmly believe that many of the chronic conditions unique to our modern society could be reduced significantly with stress reduction and better care for our adrenal glands.

Enhanced Mental Performance

The most common response to mental fatigue in our society is to grab a cup of coffee. You can even buy herbal supplements that are high in caffeine to increase mental alertness. Eleuthero has been shown to enhance mental acuity without the letdown that comes with caffeinated products.[10]

This effect again is due to eleuthero's ability to support adrenal function as well as the optimal functioning of the hypothalamus–pituitary–adrenal axis. My Chinese medical colleagues continually remind me that it's a cooperation of the three and to quit focusing on just the adrenals.[11]

Enhanced Physical Performance

Owing to the extensive use of eleuthero by Russian and East German athletes, research has accumulated on its ability to enhance physical performance. A 1986 study[12] conducted at the Institute of Health and Sport Sciences at the University of Tsukba in Japan demonstrated that eleuthero improves the use of oxygen by the exercising muscle.

Twelve male athletes were given either eleuthero or a placebo. Athletes taking eleuthero showed a 23.3 percent increase in total exercise duration and stamina compared to only 7.5 percent in those taking the placebo.

Eleuthero has become a favorite of endurance athletes. As is the case with ginseng, athletes taking eleuthero notice improved performance and quicker recovery time following competition or workouts.[13] The ability of eleuthero to increase physical performance extends beyond the boundaries of athletics. Research indicates eleuthero enhances the stamina of airline personnel and people engaged in physical labor.[14]

Antitoxin Actions

Eleuthero also reduces bodily stress by combating harmful toxins. In animal studies the herb has exerted a protective effect against such chemicals as ethanol, sodium barbital, tetanus toxoid, and chemotherapeutic agents.[15] Eleuthero also reduces the side effects of radiation exposure.[16]

These actions have led to the specific use of eleuthero in alcohol rehabilitation centers. It is also used extensively as a supportive treatment for cancer patients receiving radiation or chemotherapy.

Immune Enhancing Actions

Evidence is also mounting that eleuthero enhances and supports the immune response. Russian studies have found eleuthero useful as a preventive measure during cold and flu season. Recent evidence suggests that eleuthero may prove valuable in the long-term management of various diseases of the immune system, including HIV (human immunodeficiency virus) infection, chronic fatigue syndrome, and autoimmune illnesses such as lupus.

Research in Germany shows that eleuthero increases important components of the immune system known as lymphocytes.[17] Lymphocytes act as the body's primary defense against viral infection and have become the focus of study, particularly with regard to HIV infection. Recent research has focused on agents that possess the ability to enhance certain subsets of lymphocytes. These agents have been coined "immunomodulators" (see the discussion of herbal immunomodulators in Part 4).

Eleuthero increases the activity and number of T lymphocytes. The most significant increase is in the subset of T lymphocytes known as helper/inducer or CD4 cells. Without proper CD4 cell activity, the rest of the immune system cannot function properly. CD4 cells are a major target of HIV and decrease in number significantly following HIV infection and the progression to AIDS (acquired immunodeficiency syndrome).

HEALTH CARE APPLICATIONS

Optimizing Wellness

Unlike the situation with ginkgo or milk thistle, it's difficult to zero in on conditions specifically requiring eleuthero. Many of its actions fall into the preventive category, hence the use of eleuthero should address the goal of optimizing wellness. Eleuthero often forms the centerpiece of my daily supplement recommendations for many patients.

I highly recommend it for patients under stress, as it helps with adrenal function. Eleuthero often becomes a cornerstone of treatment for patients dealing with chronic viral illnesses and autoimmune conditions.

Prevention of Colds and Flu

I like to think of eleuthero as long-term insurance against colds and flu, whereas echinacea takes care of short-term needs. Several studies in Russia suggest that it greatly reduces the incidence of influenza, colds, and pharyngitis.

A Russian auto plant gave each of more than 13,000 employees 2 milliliters of eleuthero daily during November and December. Colds, flu, and other infections dropped an average of 40 percent compared to previous winters. In another study, 1,000 employees of a mining/smelting plant enjoyed a more than twofold reduction in acute respiratory diseases and influenza with daily use of eleuthero.[18]

M. P. Zykov and S. F. Protasova of the Research Institute of Influenza in Leningrad have suggested that eleuthero be used either in combination with influenza vaccinations or by itself in the prevention of influenza—particularly in high-risk populations. Their research indicates that it protects against postvaccination reactions.[19]

Supportive Use for Cancer Patients

Eleuthero is a valuable supplement for persons receiving treatment for cancer. Oncology clinics in Russia and Germany have reported success in improving the general health of cancer patients by adding eleuthero to their treatment regimen; immune function also improved. Also noted was a reduction in the number and intensity of side effects commonly encountered with radiation and chemotherapy.[20]

The Institute of Oncology (Georgia, Russia) examined the effects of daily supplementation of 2 milliliters of a liquid eleuthero extract in women being treated for breast cancer.[21] A group of eighty patients was chosen, all of whom had gone through surgery for cancer and were receiving both chemotherapy and radiation treatment.

Half of the women were given eleuthero while the other group received no additional treatment. The patients in the eleuthero group showed a significant reduction in side effects caused by radiation and chemotherapeutic treatment (i.e., nausea, dizziness, and loss of appetite).

Adaptogens such as eleuthero and astragalus have been shown to help the bone marrow bounce back more quickly following chemotherapy.

This means that patients can begin producing infection-fighting white blood cells (i.e., lymphocytes and macrophages) more quickly. Eleuthero also appears to improve appetite, promote weight gain, and increase lymphocyte activity in cancer patients.[22]

Other Potential Applications

The following lists potential health care applications for eleuthero:

HIV infection	Chronic fatigue syndrome
Chronic hepatitis	Lupus
Recovering alcoholics	Recovery following long-term steroid use

Eleuthero, in combination with a polypeptide extract from spleen, is being studied in the United States and Africa for potential use against HIV infection. Preliminary results indicate that this combination may slow the progression of the disease. It has also shown some promise in reversing some of the weight loss noticed in AIDS patients with wasting syndrome.[23]

Chronic fatigue syndrome (CFS) is emerging both as a disease of the immune system and as the outward manifestation of sluggish adrenal glands. Eleuthero has become a cornerstone of my treatment recommendations for CFS.

HOW TO USE ELEUTHERO

The most extensively researched form of eleuthero is an alcohol extract made from the root. The recommended daily dosage is 8 to 10 milliliters in two to three divided dosages. Encapsulated, dried root supplements are recommended at a dosage of 2 to 3 grams daily in two or three divided dosages. Concentrated solid extracts, standardized for eleutherosides B and E, have recently been introduced. The dosage of this form is 300 to 400 milligrams daily. Eleuthero should be taken continuously for 6 to 8 weeks followed by a 1- to 2-week break before resuming.

Reported side effects have been minimal. Mild, transient diarrhea has been reported by a very small number of users. Eleuthero is less likely to cause the overstimulation reported by some individuals taking Asian ginseng. However, the final dose of the day should not be taken too close to bedtime or it may keep you up beyond the "Late Show." Eleuthero is not associated with any masculinizing effect in women and will not interfere with a normal menstrual cycle (these effects have been reported anecdotally by women using Asian ginseng).

Current European monographs list no contraindications during pregnancy or lactation. However, pregnant or lactating women should avoid products that may be adulterated with Asian ginseng or other related species.

RELATED CONDITIONS DISCUSSED IN PART 6

- Alcohol-related liver disease
- Attention deficit disorder
- Chronic fatigue syndrome
- Depression
- Diabetes
- HIV infection/AIDS
- Stress and fatigue

Evening Primrose

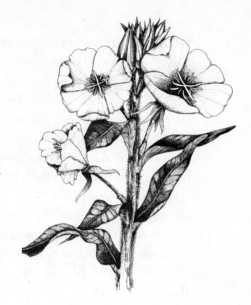

BOTANICAL NAME   *Oenothera biennis*
PART USED   Oil extracted from the seed

COMMON USES

- Eczema
- Diabetic neuropathy
- Rheumatoid arthritis
- Premenstrual syndrome and cyclical breast pain

ACTIVE CONSTITUENTS   The essential fatty acid gamma-linolenic acid (GLA) and the triglyceride structure to which it is attached (also known as "enotherol")

HOW IT WORKS   Evening primrose oil provides a highly available source of GLA to the body. This is particularly useful for persons with conditions that are associated with a poor conversion of dietary oils to GLA and other important essential fatty acid metabolites. Providing GLA allows for more efficient incorporation of important essential fatty acids into the membranes of cells. Higher levels of GLA in the body also tend to decrease inflammation and smooth muscle cramping.

RECOMMENDED USE   Oil of evening primrose—3 to 6 grams daily taken with meals

SIDE EFFECTS   Side effects are rare with the use of a high-quality, extracted evening primrose oil (EPO). At the recommended dosages, vague abdominal discomfort, nausea, and headache have been reported by less than 2 percent of people taking EPO long-term.

SAFETY ISSUES   Evening primrose oil is not known to interact with commonly prescribed medications. There are no known contraindications to the use of EPO during pregnancy or lactation.

DIETARY fats have become a rallying point for nutritional educators in our country. We know that consuming diets high in saturated fats from animal sources (beef, cow's milk, and cheese) and fried foods is associated with an increased risk of cardiovascular disease. High saturated fat consumption is also linked to increased risk of cancer of the prostate, breast, and colon.[1]

The public health message has been to urge reduction of these fats in the diet and increase the "good" fats—largely those coming under the heading of polyunsaturated. Vegetable and fish oils have received most of the good press and are being consumed in greater quantities by health-conscious individuals. In the case of vegetables, the combination of healthy oils, fiber, and antioxidant nutrients make these one of nature's most powerful deterrents to many diseases common in our culture.

While diet should be the cornerstone of any plan for optimal health, three decades of research also indicate that concentrated amounts of beneficial oils are useful in the treatment of certain diseases. Use of fish oil to lower cholesterol and treat psoriasis is one example. In this chapter, we'll look at the use of oil extracted from the seeds of evening primrose and its use in the treatment of conditions such as eczema, premenstrual syndrome (PMS), and diabetic neuropathy. Before exploring medical applications for evening primrose oil (EPO), let's take a little detour and discuss essential fatty acids (EFAs).

ESSENTIAL FATTY ACIDS: HOW YOUR BODY USES THEM

Fatty acids are the building blocks that make up the fats and oils we consume in our diet. Adding the designation "essential" implies that the fatty acid is required by our body but can't be produced by it. Essential fatty acids can be obtained only from our diets. Note also that EFAs are polyunsaturated (although not all polyunsaturated fats are EFAs). Polyunsaturated fats (PUFAs) contain two or more special double bonds, described as "cis," between carbon atoms. Polyunsaturated fats can readily become saturated, that is, the healthy cis bonds can be converted to unhealthy "trans" bonds, by heat, rancidity, and food processing.

The two primary categories of EFAs are the omega-6 EFAs and the omega-3 EFAs. The "6" and "3" designations refer to the position of the first carbon double bond (there will be a chemistry quiz at the end of the chapter!) when counting from a designated end of the fatty acid.[2] Seed oils such as flax, sunflower, pumpkin, and walnut contain both omega-6 and omega-3 EFAs, with one category often predominant (e.g., flax seed oil is 58 percent omega-3 and safflower is 65 percent omega-6).

When we consume EFAs, our bodies go through a complex series of steps to convert an EFA to a form that can be used by the body. This is accomplished largely through the actions of enzymes. One of these enzymes is delta-6-desaturase (see Figure 5.1, which outlines the steps in

FIG. 5.1. OUTLINE OF THE PATHWAYS OF OMEGA 6 (n-6) AND OMEGA-3 (n-3) ESSENTIAL FATTY ACID METABOLISM

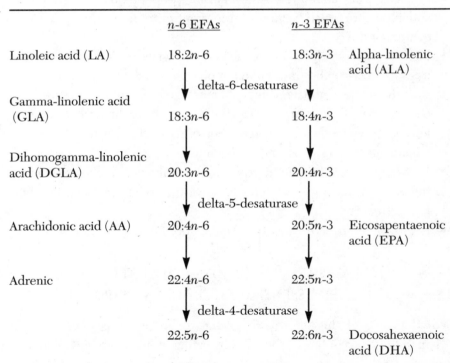

	n-6 EFAs	n-3 EFAs	
Linoleic acid (LA)	18:2n-6	18:3n-3	Alpha-linolenic acid (ALA)
	delta-6-desaturase		
Gamma-linolenic acid (GLA)	18:3n-6	18:4n-3	
Dihomogamma-linolenic acid (DGLA)	20:3n-6	20:4n-3	
	delta-5-desaturase		
Arachidonic acid (AA)	20:4n-6	20:5n-3	Eicosapentaenoic acid (EPA)
Adrenic	22:4n-6	22:5n-3	
	delta-4-desaturase		
	22:5n-6	22:6n-3	Docosahexaenoic acid (DHA)

the metabolism of EFAs). Delta-6-desaturase performs the first step in the metabolism of dietary EFAs.

Dietary oils such as flaxseed oil and safflower oil contribute linoleic acid (an omega-6 EFA) and alpha-linolenic acid (an omega-3 EFA), which enter at the beginning of this cascade of steps. Other oils, such as fish oil and evening primrose oil, provide the body with omega-6 and omega-3 EFAs that actually bypass some of the initial steps of metabolism (including delta-6-desaturase). This has made these oils valuable for persons who have difficulty converting the more common dietary oils into the important EFA metabolites so essential to the health of the body.

Essential fatty acids contribute to a variety of mechanisms essential to the normal, healthy functioning of the body.[3] Major roles of EFAs in the body include the following:

- EFAs are required for the normal structure of all cell membranes in the body. They confer a fluid and flexible property on cell membranes and allow for normal passage of important nutrients to the operating centers of the cells.
- EFAs are essential for the formation of prostaglandins. These hormone-like substances orchestrate a number of actions in the body, including smooth muscle contraction and inflammation. Buildup (i.e., an excess) of certain types of prostaglandins can be detrimental to the health. Essential fatty acids can modulate the production of prostaglandins so as to reduce inflammation and smooth muscle cramping.
- EFAs are involved in the transport and metabolism of cholesterol in the body. EFAs are associated with lowering cholesterol levels in the bloodstream.
- EFAs are required to keep the skin healthy.

DISEASES AND CONDITIONS ASSOCIATED WITH IMPROPER ESSENTIAL FATTY ACID METABOLISM

On the basis of this information, what to do seems perfectly simple: change the types of fats in your diet by eating more vegetables, vegetable oils, and fish, and be healthier. If you were taking odds, you'd be right most of the time. However, some people don't seem able to convert EFAs properly at the step involving the enzyme delta-6-desaturase. What results is a build-up of dietary EFAs such as linoleic acid and alpha-linolenic acid without conversion to a form that is useful to the body (see Figure 5.1). This seems to apply particularly to the production of gamma-linolenic acid (GLA) from linoleic acid.[4]

Certain conditions are associated with improper conversion of EFAs at the delta-6-desaturase step:

Nutritional deficiencies (e.g., zinc, magnesium, vitamin B_6)
Aging
Diabetes
Alcoholism
Viral infections
Cancer
Eczema
Premenstrual syndrome
Cyclical breast pain

Most research has linked these conditions to a defect in the normal activity of delta-6-desaturase. In the case of diabetics, there also appears to be some malfunctioning in the activity of delta-5-desaturase.[5]

You should know that EFAs such as GLA, dihomogamma-linolenic acid (DGLA), and arachidonic acid are important components of human breast milk.[6] These preformed omega-6 metabolites are used by infants for the development of many body tissues—most notably the brain. Infant formulas, which are high in linoleic acid, don't provide the same levels of these metabolites. This creates obvious concerns for the developing nervous system in very young infants. Later, we'll explore the use of supplemental GLA, in the form of EPO, in the nurturing of both formula-fed infants and infants whose mothers may be producing low amounts of breast milk GLA.

EVENING PRIMROSE OIL: A THERAPEUTIC ESSENTIAL FATTY ACID

Science has pointed to the therapeutic use of EFAs that bypass the delta-6-desaturase step. As mentioned earlier, fish oil is one common example.

Fish oil from cold-water species such as salmon is a source of the omega-3 EFAs eicosapentaenoic acid (EPA) and docosahexaenoic acid (DHA) (see Figure 5.1). Fish oil supplements high in these two metabolites are frequently recommended for the treatment of psoriasis and ulcerative colitis.

The most widely researched plant source of omega-6 EFAs is the evening primrose. Evening primrose is noted for its large and delicate flower, which blooms and lasts for only one evening. The small seeds of the plant are high in GLA as well as linoleic acid. Cross-breeding has led to the cultivation of plants whose seeds consistently yield 7 to 10 percent GLA.[7]

Years of research have pointed to EPO as the most reliable source of GLA. This is due to its very simple structure, which allows for greater absorption of GLA without interference from other fats. More complex plant sources of GLA, including borage oil and black currant oil, contain higher concentrations of GLA compared to EPO, but they also have a number of competing fatty acids (including saturated fats in the case of borage oil). This leads to inferior GLA absorption and utilization in the body. Borage and black currant oils, being less researched, may also contain other, toxic substances. In fact, the long-term use of either of these oils may be associated with an increased risk of overaggregation of platelets in the bloodstream—an event associated with an increased risk of atherosclerosis.[8,9]

What this means is that a person taking EPO will be assured of a balanced increase in omega-6 metabolites such as DGLA and also (to a lesser extent) arachidonic acid. This leads to a more efficient production of prostaglandins of the "1" series (see the previous discussion on prostaglandins). These prostaglandins (along with those of the "3" series produced from omega-3 EFA metabolites) have a tendency to discourage inflammation, smooth muscle cramping, and even overaggregation of platelets in the bloodstream.[10]

A remarkable body of medical research has been conducted on EPO. This has led to EPO becoming one of the most widely prescribed plant-derived medicines in the world.

Eczema

Eczema is an allergy-based skin disease with a clear hereditary link. One of the things that seems to be inherited in children with eczema is a difficulty in converting EFAs such as linoleic and alpha-linolenic acids to GLA.[11] This has led to the use of EPO, alone or in combination with fish oil, in the treatment of children and adults with eczema.

Before jumping into a review of some of the clinical results concerning EPO treatment for eczema, let's look a little more closely at young children with the condition. First, we know that breast feeding lowers the risk of eczema, whereas early introduction of cow's milk formulas boosts the risk.[12] Breast milk is high in preformed GLA and DGLA, whereas formula is not.

However, another variable comes into play when mom also has eczema. Research shows that mothers with a history of eczema, or who have children with recently developed eczema, have higher levels of linoleic acid and lower levels of GLA and DGLA in their breast milk.[13] This means that they are not properly converting EFAs. As a result, their breast milk does not transfer any protection from eczema to their infant.

One solution that has proven helpful to both mother and child is dietary EPO supplementation. Studies have indicated that maternal consumption of EPO is effective in raising breast milk levels of omega-6 EFA metabolites.[14] In Japan, many infant formulas actually contain added GLA.

So, what about using EPO to treat eczema? This has become a leading area for use of EPO in the clinical setting. In fact, EPO (sold under the trade name "Epogam") is recognized by the governments of Great Britain, Germany, Denmark, Ireland, Spain, Greece, South Africa, Australia, and New Zealand as a treatment for eczema. The typical dosage for adults is 4 to 6 grams daily; for children it is 2 to 4 grams daily. Remember that evening primrose oil is a long-term therapy—immediate results should not be expected.

Studies on EPO as a treatment for eczema indicate that, when successful, patients benefit after 3 to 4 months of use. The most notable benefit: relief from itching.[15] This is significant, because it means patients can decrease and sometimes stop using topical steroid creams. Patients have also noted a decrease in skin roughness.

Studies indicate that the best candidates for EPO treatment are younger children with eczema.[16] Adult patients with severe eczema who have been on steroids for long periods of time will probably see only minor results.[17,18] Evening primrose oil is clearly best when started before eczema becomes too serious.

Recent investigations in England suggest that a combination of EPO and fish oil may be superior to EPO alone in the treatment of some eczema patients. A combination known as "Efamol Marine," containing 80 percent EPO and 20 percent fish oil, has shown promising results and may become the EFA treatment of choice for eczema in the future.[19]

Diabetic Neuropathy

Evening primrose oil, like other herbal medicines and nutritional supplements (e.g., *Ginkgo biloba* and bilberry), offers a safe and nontoxic way to slow many of the complications of diabetes. Evening primrose oil has emerged as a promising long-term therapy to delay the onset and slow the progression of diabetic neuropathy.[20]

As we will note in our discussion of diabetes in Part 6, neuropathy is an extremely common complication that affects approximately 30 percent of all diabetics. This progressive disorder of the nerves leads to an initial "pins and needles" sensation in the soles of the feet and palms of the hands. Later, it advances to such a point that the ability to differentiate temperature and pressure changes in the extremities is impaired.

A 1990 study conducted at the University of Glasgow in Scotland[21] examined the effect of 4 grams of EPO daily versus placebo in diabetic patients with confirmed diabetic neuropathy. The study lasted for 6 months and found that patients taking EPO experienced an improvement in sensing cold, heat, and pain. Numbness and weakness also were diminished with EPO. A key finding was the fact that EPO supplementation did not disrupt control of blood sugar.

A follow-up study[22] of 111 diabetic patients with mild neuropathy confirmed the results of the Glasgow study. In a comparison of EPO and placebo (6 grams of EPO daily or placebo for 1 year), seven different medical centers found that administration of EPO resulted in an improvement in nerve conduction, sensation in the extremities, and other signs and symptoms associated with neuropathy. The authors noted that clinical outcomes were better in those patients with better blood sugar control. As in the Glasgow study, EPO did not result in any loss of control of blood sugar.

Again, early intervention is preferable when considering EPO as a treatment for diabetic neuropathy.

PMS and Breast Pain

One of the most popular uses for EPO has been for PMS and for breast pain—particularly pain associated with a woman's period. Research indicates that EFA metabolism is often impaired in women with PMS and cyclical breast pain.[23,24] Correcting EFA metabolism may benefit women with these conditions.

Clinical studies of EPO treatments for these conditions (which often appear together) indicate that the most notable relief provided by EPO is for breast pain and tenderness. Using EPO at a dosage of 3 grams daily for 4 to 6 months has resulted in a notable reduction in cyclical breast pain and cyst formation about 40 to 50 percent of the time.[25]

Perhaps most notable is the fact that EPO compares favorably to commonly used drug therapies for cyclical breast pain. These include bromocriptine and danazol. Two large clinical reports[26,27] indicate that EPO matches symptom relief. What makes EPO superior, particularly as an initial therapeutic choice, is that it has virtually no side effects. The two drugs mentioned above result in side effects in almost one-third of the women using them. Evening primrose oil has become a front-line treatment in Great Britain for the initial treatment of cyclical breast pain and fibrocystic breast disease.[28]

The results of clinical trials of EPO for women suffering from PMS are less convincing.[29,30] It is essential with any treatment for PMS that therapy be monitored for at least three to four cycles to determine success. Evening primrose oil appears to be fairly slow in its actions and probably requires at least four to six cycles before an accurate assessment of results can be made.

Evening primrose oil should be considered as one part of a comprehensive treatment approach to PMS. See the section on PMS in "Female Health Conditions" in Part 6.

Other Clinical Applications

Many other conditions have been treated successfully with EPO:

Rheumatoid arthritis
Dry eyes associated with Sjögren's syndrome
Endometriosis
Raynaud's disease
Chronic fatigue syndrome

Notable among these conditions is rheumatoid arthritis, and dry eyes associated with Sjögren's syndrome (an autoimmune illness). Like eczema, rheumatoid arthritis may benefit from the EPO and fish oil combination mentioned earlier.

HOW TO USE EVENING PRIMROSE OIL

The recommended daily dose of EPO varies according to the condition. If you're using EPO for eczema, diabetic neuropathy, or rheumatoid arthritis, take 4 to 6 grams daily. Women with PMS and cyclical breast pain can use 3 grams daily. Children with eczema should take 2 to 4 grams daily. Because it is an oil, EPO should be taken with meals for proper absorption.

I highly recommend taking any EFA supplement with some vitamin E. The amount contained in most good-quality multiple vitamin/mineral supplements is probably fine. Vitamin E is a natural antioxidant for EFAs and will protect them from free radical damage. Taking a good daily multiple also provides nutritional cofactors (such as zinc, vitamin B_6, biotin, and magnesium) needed for proper EFA metabolism.

Evening primrose oil is virtually devoid of side effects. In clinical studies, a handful of people (less than 2 percent) sometimes experienced bloating and mild abdominal discomfort. Mild headache was also reported, but the frequency of occurrence of this side effect was about the same as for the people taking placebo.

There are no known contraindications to the use of EPO with prescription medications. Some have speculated that steroids and nonsteroidal antiinflammatory medicines may interfere with proper metabolism of GLA.[31] Research has yet to test this theory. There are no known contraindications to the use of EPO during pregnancy or lactation.

RELATED CONDITIONS DISCUSSED IN PART 6

- Atherosclerosis
- Attention-deficit hyperactivity disorder
- Chronic fatigue syndrome
- Diabetic neuropathy
- Dry eyes associated with Sjögren's syndrome (sicca syndrome)
- Eczema
- Fibrocystic breast disease
- Premenstrual syndrome
- Rheumatoid arthritis
- Raynaud's disease

Feverfew

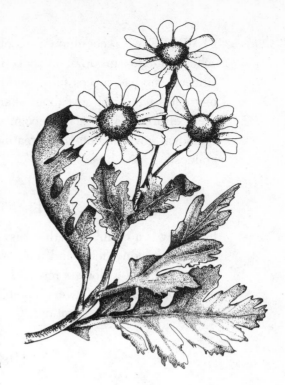

BOTANICAL NAME *Tanacetum parthenium*

PART USED Dried leaves

COMMON USE

- Long-term treatment and prevention of migraine headaches

ACTIVE CONSTITUENTS The sesquiterpene lactones—particularly parthenolide

HOW IT WORKS Feverfew blocks the overaggregation of platelets as well as the release of serotonin from platelets. It also blocks the formation and action of proinflammatory mediators released from cells.

RECOMMENDED USE Feverfew extract with a standardized parthenolide content of at least 250 micrograms per daily dose; continuous use is recommended for the treatment and prevention of migraine headaches

SIDE EFFECTS No studies have been conducted on the long-term toxicity of feverfew. Studies using standardized feverfew tablets have demonstrated minimal side effects. These have been minor (i.e., nervousness and mild gastrointestinal upset). Chewing the leaves of feverfew has resulted in mouth ulceration and swelling of the tongue and mouth in about 10 percent of cases.

SAFETY ISSUES Feverfew is not recommended during pregnancy or lactation. Children under the age of 2 years should not use feverfew.

FEVERFEW'S recognition as an effective treatment for migraine head-aches is due to a group of outspoken health care consumers. Some British citizens who had successfully used feverfew leaves for treatment of their migraines were not shy about sharing their success stories. Thanks to their efforts, feverfew is recognized today by both the British and Canadian governments as a treatment and preventive measure for mi-graines.

PLANT FACTS

Feverfew is a member of the daisy family. It is a short, bushy perennial that grows along fields and roadsides all over Europe. Its yellow-green leaves and yellow flowers resemble those of chamomile, with which it is often confused. The flowers bloom from July to October. The leaves are used in medicinal preparations.[1]

HISTORY

The name *feverfew* is derived from the Latin for "chase away fevers." It once enjoyed wide use by British herbalists in the treatment of fevers and as a pain reliever, but later faded into obscurity. Only in the past two decades has feverfew experienced a revival, owing primarily to its use in the treatment of migraine headaches.[2]

MEDICALLY ACTIVE CONSTITUENTS

Feverfew contains compounds known as *sesquiterpene lactones* (STLs). The most important of these compounds is parthenolide. First identified in 1960, parthenolide represents about 85 percent of the STL content in feverfew and is the portion of the leaf responsible for feverfew's anti-migraine activity.[3]

A critical consideration in commercial feverfew products has been the highly variable content of parthenolide. An analysis of commercial fever-few products in Canada found about half to be virtually devoid of this compound.[4] The Health Protection Branch of the Health and Welfare

Department of the Canadian government (try saying that three times with a mouthful of bagel!), has proposed that feverfew preparations should contain at least 0.2 percent parthenolide content. If you want to use feverfew to treat your migraines, seek out products that guarantee a stable parthenolide content.

HOW FEVERFEW WORKS

Migraine headaches are, for the most part, a mystery; medical research and drug development are currently focused on the role of platelets. Platelets, which are a normal part of the blood and are involved in clotting, appear to act abnormally in migraine sufferers. During a migraine attack, platelets not only tend to overcongregate (aggregate), but also to release the substance *serotonin*. Serotonin and inflammatory substances released from platelets are widely believed to be the primary chemical triggers of migraine headaches.[5]

Feverfew, and specifically parthenolide, counters overaggregation of platelets and the release of serotonin.[6,7] The result is a reduction in the severity, duration, and frequency of migraine headaches and an improvement in blood vessel tone.

Feverfew also discourages the formation of certain inflammatory substances released from platelets and other cells.[8,9] While this is another plus for migraine sufferers, it may also explain its historical use for inflammatory conditions such as arthritis. Modern clinical studies have not shown favorable results for arthritis patients using feverfew.[10]

HEALTH CARE APPLICATIONS

Feverfew is the premier herbal therapy for migraine sufferers. By prescribing feverfew along with stress reduction, dietary modifications, and magnesium supplements, I have witnessed a major drop in the severity, duration, and frequency of migraine headaches in many of my patients (see my recommendations for migraines in "Nervous System" in Part 6).

Modern interest in feverfew arose in Great Britain because of its use by a group of people determined to treat their migraines successfully.

Their results, published in *Prevention* magazine in 1978, gained widespread attention. The story related the success of a certain Mrs. Jenkins, who used feverfew for her migraines. A migraine sufferer for more than 50 years, Mrs. Jenkins found relief after self-administering feverfew leaves daily for 10 months. She became an outspoken advocate for feverfew treatment of migraines and her experience prompted the Migraine Trust of the United Kingdom to start medical studies.

The initial clinical study[11] involved migraine patients who had been using feverfew for several years. Seventeen patients were enrolled and given either feverfew (50 milligrams per day) or placebo. Eight patients, who had the good fortune to stay on feverfew, experienced continued relief from migraines over a 6-month period. The nine receiving placebo suffered an almost three-fold increase in migraines!

A second study[12] enrolled 72 migraine sufferers. They received either 82 milligrams of feverfew (containing approximately 500 micrograms of parthenolide) daily or placebo. After 4 months with feverfew treatment, fewer migraines occurred, and those that did were less severe. Feverfew also led to fewer vomiting attacks and fewer visual disturbances during migraines.

How to Use Feverfew

Remember to check the parthenolide content! Put a bit more technically, Canada's Health Protection Branch recommends a daily dosage of 125 milligrams of a dried feverfew leaf preparation, from authentic *Tanacetum parthenium* containing at least 0.2 percent parthenolide for the treatment and prevention of migraines. This equates to approximately 250 micrograms of parthenolide daily.

Feverfew is a long-term treatment, not an immediate cure for a migraine attack. The recommended daily dose of a standardized feverfew extract should ensure delivery of at least 250 micrograms of parthenolide. Clinical experience suggests that 4 to 6 weeks are usually required to note an initial response. However, average duration of use will vary among migraine patients. Success should be measured by decreased frequency, severity, and duration of migraine attacks.

Don't use feverfew if you are pregnant or lactating. Parents should not give feverfew to children under the age of 2 years. If you're taking prescription medications for migraines, consult a health care professional before using feverfew.

RELATED CONDITION DISCUSSED IN PART 6

- Migraine headache

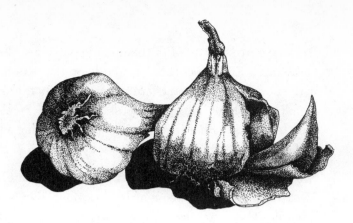

Garlic

BOTANICAL NAME   *Allium sativum*

PART USED   The bulb

COMMON USES

- Reduction of high cholesterol and triglyceride levels
- Lowering of mildly elevated blood pressure
- Improvement of poor circulation, including intermittent claudication
- Prevention of colds and flu
- Prevention of chronic yeast infections
- Cancer prevention

ACTIVE CONSTITUENTS   The sulfur compound allicin, which is produced with crushing or chewing of the fresh bulb. Allicin in turn produces other sulfur compounds, including allyl sulfides, ajoene, and the vinyldithiins. These compounds are found only in garlic oil products produced by maceration (not in steam-distilled garlic oils).

HOW IT WORKS   Garlic lowers serum cholesterol and triglycerides while raising "good" HDL-cholesterol (lipoproteins that help transport cholesterol from various parts of the body to the liver). Garlic also reduces the "stickiness" of platelets, making blood circulation more efficient. It causes a mild reduction in blood pressure. Garlic is antibacterial, antiviral, antifungal, and antiparasitic, and exerts action against organisms causing yeast infections. Regular consumption of garlic is also associated with lowered risk of stomach and colon cancer.

RECOMMENDED USE   For therapeutic purposes, chew one fresh clove of garlic daily. For those averse to the odor, odor-controlled, enteric-coated garlic powder supplements are the next best bet. For therapeutic use, the supplement should provide at least 5,000 micrograms of allicin daily. One-half the dose of either fresh garlic or garlic powder supplement is probably sufficient for those using garlic as part of a wellness program.

SIDE EFFECTS   Consumption at these doses rarely poses health risks. Heartburn and flatulence may be experienced by some persons sensitive to garlic. There are rare reports of allergic reactions to garlic.

SAFETY ISSUES   People undergoing anticoagulant drug therapy should use garlic with caution. There are no known contraindications to the use of garlic during pregnancy and lactation.

> *The Professor's actions were certainly odd and not to be found in any pharmacopoeia that I ever heard of. First he fastened up the windows and latched them securely; next, taking a handful of the flowers, he rubbed them all over the sashes, as though to ensure that every whiff of air that might get in would be laden with garlic smell.*
>
> BRAM STOKER, DRACULA

GARLIC may be the best example of the continuum between plants as food and plants as medicine. One of the most ancient remedies known to humanity, garlic is a staple in the diets of an incredibly diverse number of cultures. Most of these cultures use garlic for medicinal purposes.

But let's not dwell on the past! Garlic has enjoyed a surge in popularity over the last decade. The star of more than 1,000 research publications, garlic is noted for promoting cardiovascular health and preventing some forms of cancer. Not only obnoxious to vampires, garlic also seems to be the bane of nasty little beasts like bacteria, viruses, and yeast.

Has this research made an impression on the public? Fresh garlic sales in the United States are growing by about 8 percent yearly. Even more noteworthy, garlic supplement sales rose by approximately 163 percent during 1991–1992![1]

PLANT FACTS

Garlic is a member of the lily family and belongs to the genus *Allium*, which also includes onions. *Allium* is the Latin name for garlic and derives from a Celtic word meaning "hot" or "burning." The word *sativum* means that the plant is cultivated (i.e., planted). Garlic in its present form is not found in the wild, having evolved to its present form after thousands of years of cultivation.[2]

Garlic bulbs are typically harvested in the early summer. The largest commercial production of garlic is in central California, which harvests about 250 million pounds of garlic every year. I won't burden you with stories of a young college student hallucinating about pesto while hurtling through the garlic-saturated air of Gilroy, California. China is also a supplier of commercial garlic.

HISTORY

Talk about stories to tell! Garlic has seen the rise and fall of the pharaohs in Egypt. The Book of Numbers in the Bible reports of dissent among the Israelites as they fled Egypt, owing to a lack of garlic in their travel provisions. Apparently manna without a little babaghanoush really is unacceptable! Even more racy is the fact that the Talmud encourages the consumption of garlic to encourage matrimonial love making![3]

Garlic has been cultivated in the Middle East for more than 5,000 years. It was a common crop and dietary staple in Mesopotamia. It was also a common trade commodity in Babylon.

Greek and Roman physicians such as Hippocrates, Galen, Pliny the Elder, and Dioscorides recommended garlic for a dizzying array of conditions. Among these were parasites, respiratory problems, weight loss, poor digestion, and low energy.

Garlic has also been an important part of traditional Chinese medical history. Known as *da-suan* in China, medicinal use of garlic is first mentioned in Tao Hong-jing's *Ming Yi Bie Lu* (*Miscellaneous Records of Famous Physicians*), written in 510 A.D. Garlic was administered for digestive difficulties, diarrhea, dysentery, colds, and tuberculosis. It was also used externally in the treatment of pinworms, snake bites, and fungal infections of the skin.[4]

Garlic did not escape the scientific eye of Louis Pasteur. In 1858, the father of pasteurization engaged in studies to confirm the antibacterial activity of garlic. Albert Schweitzer used garlic to treat amebic dysentery during his sojourn in Africa.

MEDICALLY ACTIVE CONSTITUENTS

Garlic's medicinal effects in the body depend on a series of chemical reactions. Figure 5.2 shows what happens when you crush or chew a garlic clove. Garlic cloves, before they are crushed or chewed, are high in an odorless, sulfur-containing amino acid known as alliin. With crushing or chewing, alliin comes into contact with the enzyme alliinase. Alliinase very rapidly (in less than 6 seconds) transforms alliin into allicin, which is the source of the familiar garlic odor.

Allicin is not very stable. Depending on the conditions, it breaks down into a number of other sulfur compounds, including ajoene, vinyldithiins, and diallyl disulfide and trisulfide.[5] These compounds are found only in macerated garlic oil products—not in garlic powder supplements.

Allicin and its fellow sulfur compounds fuel many of garlic's actions in the body. Allicin is known to have extensive antimicrobial activity. It inhibits the growth of many bacteria and fungi (including *Candida albicans*). Ajoene also has weak antifungal effects and can reduce the "stickiness" of platelets.[6] Some of the other sulfur compounds have antitumor activity.

All of this rambling about alliin and allicin is based on what happens when you eat *raw* garlic. With chewing, allicin forms quickly in the mouth. Allicin does not form in the stomach, because alliinase is inactivated by stomach acid.[7] Once you've chopped up garlic and dried it or cooked it, a good amount of the allicin is lost. Raw garlic is clearly the best source of allicin.

Research suggests that the best garlic supplements closely approximate the eating of raw garlic. Carefully prepared garlic powder will yield allicin almost as efficiently as raw garlic (only 4 percent less). Aged garlic

FIGURE 5.2. TRANSFORMATION OF GARLIC'S ACTIVE INGREDIENTS

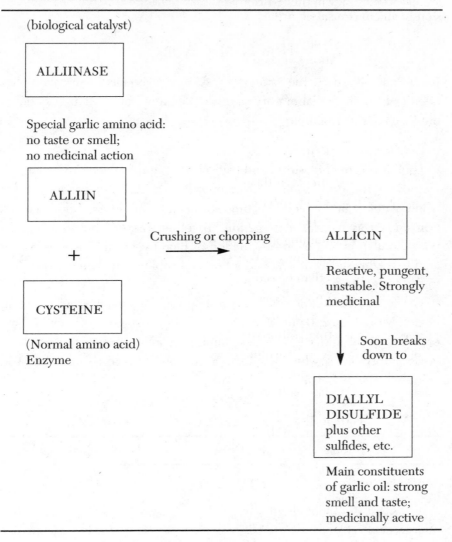

(biological catalyst)

ALLIINASE

Special garlic amino acid:
no taste or smell;
no medicinal action

ALLIIN

+

CYSTEINE

(Normal amino acid)
Enzyme

Crushing or chopping →

ALLICIN

Reactive, pungent,
unstable. Strongly
medicinal

↓ Soon breaks
down to

DIALLYL
DISULFIDE
plus other
sulfides, etc.

Main constituents
of garlic oil: strong
smell and taste;
medicinally active

products don't make the grade, since they yield no allicin and only about 10 percent of the other sulfur compounds present in garlic. Allicin is not present in garlic oil macerates.

Stomach acid inhibits allicin formation. The best way to counter this is to purchase garlic tablets that are enteric coated. Enteric coating allows safe passage through the intensely acidic environment of the stomach and refuge in the more alkaline pH of the small intestine. There the conversion to allicin can safely occur.[8]

HOW GARLIC WORKS

In the past 40 years, the "stinking rose" (as garlic has been called) has been as busy in the laboratory as in the kitchen. Table 5.1 breaks down the focus of this research.

Cardiovascular Effects

High levels of cholesterol and triglycerides in the blood are major risk factors for the development of atherosclerosis. Another concern arises when platelets in the blood become sticky and clump together—a condition known as *platelet aggregation*. Together, these conditions lead to poor circulation and even obstruction of blood vessels. This in turn can lead to angina, heart attack, and a host of problems involving blood flow to the extremities.

Garlic is a full-service herbal prescription for cardiovascular system health. More than 250 publications have shown that garlic effectively lowers cholesterol and triglycerides, inhibits platelet aggregation, and increases fibrinolysis, which results in a slowing of blood coagulation. Add

Table 5.1
GARLIC RESEARCH PUBLICATIONS (1950–1992)*

Topic	Number of publications
Antibiotic effect	171
Cardiovascular (including cholesterol-lowering) effect	258
Anticancer effect	154
Effect on blood sugar level	13
Effectiveness as heavy metal antidote	14
Potential alleviation of intestinal problems	8
Other biological effects	150
Chemical studies	320
Total	1088

*Reprinted by permission from L. D. Lawson *Human Medicinal Agents from Plants*, ACS, Washington, D.C., 1993.

to this a mild antihypertensive effect as well as antioxidant activity, and garlic emerges as one of nature's most potent weapons against cardiovascular disease.[9,10]

Garlic interferes with the creation of cholesterol in the liver.[11] This means that less cholesterol is released into the bloodstream. Allicin appears to be the sulfur compound in garlic responsible for this action.[12] Also, garlic helps to package the remaining cholesterol as high-density lipoprotein (HDL)-cholesterol. This form of cholesterol is associated with decreased risk of cardiovascular disease because it's transported to the liver and broken down.[13]

Garlic also reduces platelet stickiness and excessive blood clotting—two factors associated with blockage of blood vessels and sluggish circulation. In one study,[14] ten "healthy" volunteers were given 900 milligrams of garlic powder daily; 2 to 4 hours after garlic ingestion, platelet stickiness was found to be reduced. The fibrinolytic, or anticlotting, activity took several days to be noted. Ajoene, which is present only in garlic oil macerates, also appears to help reduce platelet stickiness.[15]

By the way, the anticlotting effect of garlic won't cause you to bleed excessively if you're cut. It keeps *excess* clotting in check, a benefit for persons at risk for cardiovascular disease. *Note:* This is not meant to suggest that garlic can effectively replace stronger anticlotting drugs; its primary value is as a preventive. Garlic is useful in the early stages of cardiovascular disease that involves poor circulation due to atherosclerosis (e.g., angina and intermittent claudication). Data from Spain and Italy, where garlic consumption is high and atherosclerosis low, add weight to the argument that garlic should be a part of any supplement program for cardiovascular health.[16]

Antimicrobial Actions

Another benefit of garlic is the creation of an environment that is inhospitable to a wide variety of microorganisms bent on wreaking havoc in our bodies. Garlic exerts antibacterial, antiviral, and antifungal activity. It has even been shown to chase away intestinal worms!

As mentioned earlier, garlic's antibacterial effect was first noted by Louis Pasteur in 1858. The strength of garlic appears to be about 1 percent that of penicillin in killing certain types of bacteria. This means it's not a substitute for antibiotics, but should be considered as a defense against bacterial infections—particularly by those of you with recurrent infections.[17]

One of the more intriguing uses of garlic is for the prevention of tuberculosis (TB). Garlic has noted anti-TB activity and was actually used for this purpose during the 1800s. As described further on, individuals infected with the human immunodeficiency virus (HIV), particularly those with AIDS-related complex (ARC) or acquired immunodeficiency syndrome (AIDS), may find some added benefit by taking garlic to increase resistance to secondary infections from bacteria and yeast.

In test tube studies, garlic and some of its sulfur compounds are emerging as promising antiviral substances. These studies show that garlic inhibits the herpes simplex virus type 1 (HSV-1), cytomegalovirus (which can cause eye and lung problems in immunocompromised individuals), and also HIV.[18-20]

The anti-HIV activity is associated with isolated ajoene and allyl disulfide, which are found only in garlic oil macerates, not garlic powder products. We don't know whether real-life use of garlic can match these results.

A final area of antimicrobial action for garlic is in the treatment of yeast infections. Growth of *Candida albicans*, the organism most widely responsible for intestinal, vaginal, and oral yeast infections, is inhibited by garlic.[21] Many health care professionals use garlic to treat recurrent, chronic yeast infections. This should be limited to localized yeast infections. Systemic yeast infections can be dangerous and should be treated with stronger drugs.

Once again, I'd like to emphasize that the best protection against a wide variety of microorganisms is going to come from raw garlic, or garlic supplements that approximate the allicin potential of raw garlic. Studies have shown conclusively that allicin exerts the most broad-spectrum antimicrobial activity of any sulfur compound in garlic.[22]

Anticancer Actions

Human population studies show that regular garlic intake reduces the risk of esophageal, stomach, and colon cancer. This is partly due to garlic's ability to reduce the formation of N-nitroso compounds such as ni-trosamine.[23] A major source of nitrosamines is the charcoal broiling of fats. You'd be better off getting rid of flame-broiled hamburgers altogether, but if that's the break you need, at least take some garlic along for the ride.

Animal and test tube studies also show that garlic and its sulfur compounds inhibit the growth of different types of cancer. Notable among them are breast cancer and skin tumors.[24,25] More research is needed to determine whether garlic will actually aid persons with cancer. The evidence does argue for a protective/preventive effect of regular garlic intake.

HEALTH CARE APPLICATIONS

High Cholesterol and Triglycerides

Since 1975, more than thirty-two human studies have been done on the cholesterol- and triglyceride-lowering (lipid-lowering) effects of garlic.[25] Of these, the majority were performed with garlic powder tablets standardized for allicin potential. The dosages ranged from 600 to 900 milligrams daily and the lengths of the studies ranged from 4 to 16 weeks. Patients with either high cholesterol, high triglycerides, or both were studied. Table 5.2 summarizes the results of three studies. [26–28]

Table 5.2
EFFECTS OF GARLIC POWDER WITH STANDARDIZED
ALLICIN POTENTIAL ON ELEVATED CHOLESTEROL AND
TRIGLYCERIDES: THREE HUMAN STUDIES

Number of patients	Daily dose	Length of study	Decrease in cholesterol	Decrease in triglycerides	Study
261	800 mg	16 weeks	12%	17%	Mader, 1990 (Ref. 26)
40	900 mg	16 weeks	21%	24%	Vorberg and Schneider, 1990 (Ref. 27)
42	900 mg	12 weeks	6%	11%	Jain et al., 1993 (Ref. 28)

Other reports[29,30] have analyzed the results of all studies performed to date on the cholesterol/triglyceride-lowering effects of garlic powder. They indicate that over a 1- to 3-month period, the administration of garlic powder tablets (dosage, 600 to 900 mg daily) results in an average reduction in total serum cholesterol of 9 to 12 percent (range, 6 to 21 percent); triglyceride levels fell from 8 to 27 percent.

One study[31] compared garlic with bezafibrate (similar to the U.S. drug clofibrate). Ninety-eight patients with high cholesterol and triglycerides received one of two treatments—garlic at 900 mg/day or bezafibrate at 600 mg/day. At the end of the 12-week study, reduction in cholesterol and low-density lipoprotein (LDL)-cholesterol ("bad" cholesterol) was almost identical for both treatments, as was the rise in HDL-cholesterol ("good" cholesterol).

Although garlic does not lower serum cholesterol and triglycerides as aggressively as drugs such as Mevacor, it is far safer for long-term use. I highly recommend speaking with your doctor about a 4-month trial with garlic before jumping on the drug bandwagon. Garlic is also a useful follow-up for those who do require the quick drop in cholesterol and triglycerides afforded by Mevacor.

High Blood Pressure

Garlic exerts a mild blood pressure lowering effect.[32] This is probably due to its ability to make circulation more efficient (see earlier comments). You should consider garlic as only one part of an overall program for lowering mildly elevated blood pressure, and not a substitute for stronger blood pressure medications.

Intermittent Claudication

Most common in the elderly, intermittent claudication involves severe cramping of the muscles in the back of the lower legs during walking or running. It is caused by poor blood flow to the muscles.

While the best herbal prescription for this condition is ginkgo (see the chapter on *Gingko biloba*), one study has shown that garlic offers promise.[33] This 12-week study found that garlic powder tablets (800 mg daily) led to a significant increase in pain-free walking distance.

Increasing Resistance to Infection

Garlic helps your body resist infection. As we discussed earlier, this is partly due to its wide-spectrum antimicrobial properties. Garlic assists in the prevention of colds and flu and aids people suffering from chronic or recurrent infections. I heartily endorse using it for the treatment of recurrent yeast infections.

Topically applied (usually in an oil base), it can be used to treat both yeast and fungal infections (e.g., athlete's foot). It has even been applied in the treatment of children with pinworms.

While I don't have any solid clinical research data to back my beliefs, I'm a big proponent of making garlic part of the regular supplement regimen for HIV-infected individuals. Although it probably doesn't have much direct effect on HIV, garlic may deter organisms and viruses that are responsible for secondary (opportunistic) infections that characterize the more advanced stages of the illness. These include cytomegalovirus (CMV), *Mycobacterium avium* (the cause of tuberculosis in AIDS patients), and *Cryptococcus*, the fungus responsible for intestinal infections as well as meningitis in AIDS patients.[34,35]

Again, we're talking prevention and stronger defenses here. If you're HIV positive and have any of these infections, drug intervention is critical. In the meantime, however, grab an FDA representative and, with your strongest garlic breath, demand more research dollars for nontoxic herbal medicines.

Cancer Prevention

The medical establishment has finally gotten smart and realized that diet can be a powerful preventive tool against many forms of cancer. Mainstream research has discovered antioxidants and fiber, and how more of them means less cancer. Garlic should be at the top of the list.

As mentioned previously, garlic appears to have its greatest benefit in the prevention of esophageal, stomach, and colon cancer. An Iowa study[36] examining the diets of women (ranging in age from 55 to 69 years old) found that consumption of garlic was a greater deterrent to colon cancer than dietary fiber and vegetables. The risk of colon cancer dropped by 35 percent with one or more servings of garlic weekly! This reached 50 percent with even greater consumption.

Population studies in China and Italy have shown that consumption of garlic also reduces the risk of esophageal and stomach cancer.[37]

HOW TO USE GARLIC

For you bold souls, take about one whole clove of raw garlic daily. If you dislike the smell and the social ramifications, try an odor-controlled, enteric-coated garlic powder tablet with standardized allicin potential. The daily dose should be 900 milligrams (about 5,000 micrograms of allicin) taken in two or three divided doses. *Remember:* The critical measure is allicin. You can estimate the amount of allicin by reading the "allicin potential" on the label. For health maintenance, you'll enjoy benefits with one-half the therapeutic dose.

Consumption of garlic at these doses does not pose health risks for most people. Heartburn and flatulence may be experienced by those who are sensitive to garlic. A garlicky taste can sometimes be noticed even with so-called "deodorized" garlic products. There are rare reports of allergic reactions to garlic.

Because of the mild anticlotting properties of garlic, persons undergoing anticoagulant drug therapy should use garlic with caution. There are no known contraindications to the use of garlic during pregnancy and lactation.

An interesting study[38] has disproved the popular belief that mothers who consume garlic while nursing cause their infants to shun the garlic-laden breast milk. They actually found that infants breast fed longer when mom ate garlic! Of course, pasta with a garlic-laden red sauce was in high demand when solid foods were introduced.

RELATED CONDITIONS DISCUSSED IN PART 6

- Atherosclerosis
- Colds and flu
- HIV infection/AIDS
- Hypercholesterolemia (high cholesterol)
- Intermittent claudication
- Interviews with vampires
- Sore throat
- Vaginal yeast infections (recurrent)

Ginger

BOTANICAL NAME   *Zingiber officinale*
PART USED   The rhizome (the underground stem)

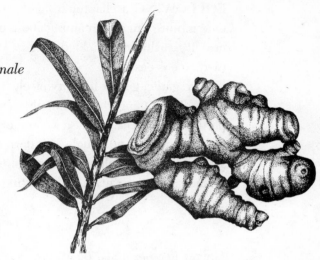

COMMON USES
- Promotes normal digestion
- Alleviates motion sickness
- Reduces nausea and vomiting of pregnancy
- Counteracts postanesthesia nausea following surgery

ACTIVE CONSTITUENTS   Volatile oil components, including gingerols and shogaols

HOW IT WORKS   Ginger acts as a bitter and carminative herb. It helps stimulate digestion and also improves the tone of intestinal muscles. It also soothes upset stomachs. The gingerols and shogaols in the essential oil counter nausea and vomiting. Ginger also reduces platelet "stickiness" in the blood, aiding circulation. It also exerts mild antiinflammatory actions.

RECOMMENDED USE   Two to 4 grams daily of the dried rhizome powder, in two to three divided doses. For treatment of nausea, use single doses of at least 1 gram. For prevention of motion sickness, begin taking ginger two days before the trip begins.

SIDE EFFECTS   No side effects have been noted with the use of ginger at these doses.

SAFETY ISSUES   The German Commission E monograph suggests that people with gallstones consult a physician before using ginger. Short-term use of ginger to treat nausea and vomiting associated with pregnancy appears to pose no safety problems. Long-term use during pregnancy is not recommended. Use of ginger before surgery to counteract possible postanesthesia nausea should be done only with the approval of your physician.

FOLLOWING a chapter on garlic with one on ginger is pure torture! One minute I'm daydreaming about calamari with roasted garlic, and the next it's sushi with pickled ginger. Who said writing a book on herbal medicine is easy?

Like garlic, ginger fits very nicely into the classification of food or spice as medicine. Ginger is commonly used in the cooking of many cultures—particularly in Asia. It is also a common household remedy for digestive disorders, nausea, and coughs. Modern research has established ginger as a safe and effective alternative in the treatment of two conditions: motion sickness, and the nausea and vomiting associated with pregnancy.

PLANT FACTS

Ginger is a perennial plant, growing from 1 to 3 feet in height. The underground stem of the plant, known as the *rhizome*, is light brown or tan on the outside, and yellow on the inside. Most of the ginger in the U.S. market arrives with its outer, barklike layer scraped off, giving it a pale appearance. The branches off the rhizome are irregularly shaped and are sometimes referred to as hands or fingers.[1]

The annual world production of ginger is estimated at 100,000 tons. Major exporting countries include India, Fiji, Nigeria, Mexico, and China. During the 1980s, the United States imported more than 4,000 metric tons of ginger per year.[2]

HISTORY

Cultivated for thousands of years in China and India, ginger was sold to the ancient Greeks and Romans by Arabian traders. It was actually subject to Roman taxes in the second century A.D. (the money paid for that new luxury stadium). Tariff duties on ginger appear in the records of Barcelona in 1221, Marseilles in 1228, and Paris in 1296. About 1280, Marco Polo reported ginger production in China and India.[3]

Traditional Chinese medicine has recommended ginger for more than 2,500 years. Chinese herbalists prescribe it for abdominal distension, coughing, vomiting, diarrhea, and rheumatism. They view fresh ginger and dried ginger as having different medicinal properties.[4] Ginger is also an important part of the traditional healing systems of Nigeria, the West Indies, and India.

MEDICALLY ACTIVE CONSTITUENTS

The dried rhizome of ginger contains about 1 to 4 percent volatile oils. These oils are responsible for ginger's characteristic odor and taste, and contain the medically active constituents. The aromatic principals include the sesquiterpene hydrocarbons zingiberene and bisabolene. The pungent counterparts, known as gingerols and shogaols, have received most of the research attention in the last few years.[5] They give ginger its characteristic taste and are credited with its antinausea and antivomiting effect.

While most of the clinical research over the past two decades has focused on the powdered rhizome, ginger products produced in the last 5 years have concentrated the volatile oils and established a standardized content of gingerols and shogaols.

HOW GINGER WORKS

Digestive System Actions

Ginger is a classic tonic for the digestive tract. Classified as an "aromatic bitter," it stimulates digestion and benefits those with sluggish digestion. By keeping the intestinal muscles "toned,"[6] ginger also eases the transport of substances through the digestive tract, lessening irritation to the intestinal walls.[7] Ginger improves the production and secretion of bile from the liver and gallbladder. This aids digestion of fats and helps lower the amount of cholesterol in the bloodstream.[8]

Ginger also qualifies as a carminative herb (see Part 4 for more on carminatives). If you're having problems with flatulence, intestinal spasms, or irritation, you'll benefit from the use of ginger.

An animal study conducted in Saudi Arabia[9] showed that ginger protects the stomach from the damaging effects of nonsteroidal anti-inflammatory drugs (e.g., ibuprofen) and alcohol. This means ginger may be another plant medicine that offers help against ulcers.

Antinausea/Antivomiting Actions

Ever wonder what to do when your pet frog starts vomiting? Well, another one of those wonderful animal studies has your answer!

A Japanese study conducted on frogs[10] found that shogaols and gingerols isolated from ginger prevented vomiting induced by chemicals. What is particularly interesting about their findings is that at least part of ginger's action may occur in the central nervous system (CNS), and not just in the gastrointestinal tract. This supports an earlier study in mice indicating that gingerol and shogaol activity was partially centered in the CNS.[11]

Studies with humans, on the other hand, have led us to believe that the antinausea and antivomiting actions of ginger are limited to the gastrointestinal tract.[12] But these studies looked only at ginger powder and not at the isolated gingerols and shogaols. Whether ginger extracts with concentrated amounts of these constituents would also exert a CNS effect in humans remains to be proven.

Circulatory Effects

Ginger also improves the health of the cardiovascular system. Like garlic, ginger makes platelets less "sticky," that is, less likely to aggregate. This action reduces a major risk factor for atherosclerosis. Ginger does this by raising levels of a substance known as prostacyclin. Prostacyclin inhibits the action of thromboxane, a substance associated with increasing platelet aggregation.[13]

A study involving twenty healthy males[14] explored the effect of ginger on platelet aggregation when large amounts of fat were consumed. The men in this study were fed 100 grams of butter daily for 7 days. Not surprisingly, their platelet aggregation went up significantly. However, the addition of 2.5 grams of ginger twice daily led to a significant drop in platelet aggregation. Add ginger to your list of herbs and foods that reduce the risk of cardiovascular disease.

Antiinflammatory and Analgesic Effects

The Ayurvedic system of medicine offers ginger in the treatment of in-flammatory joint diseases, including arthritis. Ginger counters the formation of proinflammatory substances such as leukotrienes and certain prostaglandins. The gingerols seem to be the most effective constituents in this activity.[15]

Studies with experimental animals also suggest ginger acts as a mild pain reliever. In fact, the shogaols may act very much like capsaicin, the hot and pungent portion of cayenne pepper.[16] Capsaicin is widely used in topical creams for arthritis and the treatment of pain following a shingles outbreak.

HEALTH CARE APPLICATIONS

Motion Sickness

Ginger has been widely studied as a treatment for motion sickness. In 1982, Daniel Mowrey of Brigham Young University (Provo, Utah) and Dennis Clayson of Mount Union College (Alliance, Ohio) found that ginger was superior to dimenhydrinate (Dramamine) for reducing motion sickness (caused by rotating a chair). The dose of ginger was 940 milligrams and it was consumed 20 to 25 minutes before the test.[17]

A handful of studies since have both agreed and disagreed with Mowrey and Clayson's results. A study that I love because of its subtitle, "A controlled trial on the open sea," tested ginger against seasickness in eighty Danish naval cadets unaccustomed to sailing in heavy seas.[18] One gram of ginger reduced vomiting and cold sweating. In addition, fewer symptoms of nausea and vertigo were reported. Reduced seasickness allowed them more free time to engage in useful activities, such as watching reruns of *Sea Hunt* or reading *Mutiny on the Bounty*.

A study completed at Louisiana State University (Baton Rouge, Louisiana) and funded by the National Aeronautics and Space Administration (NASA) is more skeptical.[19] Because motion sickness is common among astronauts, the researchers compared the anti-motion sickness activity of ginger and scopolamine (commonly used as a topical patch in the treatment of motion sickness). Using the old rotating chair test, they found that scopolamine was effective in reducing motion sickness, whereas 1 gram of either fresh or dried ginger was not.

I have a few problems with this study. First, in their discussion of the results, the authors note that the incidence of vomiting and sweating (but not nausea and vertigo) in the ginger group decreased noticeably—so there was some clinical effect!

Second, the comparison substance, scopolamine, is one of the most potent antinausea drugs. While astronauts may require the "strong stuff," are we to believe that ginger should be written off for car sickness, sea sickness, and even air sickness in planes? The comparison doesn't seem fair. A more compelling comparison would involve a ginger extract with highly concentrated amounts of gingerols and shogaols.

I find that ginger works best when taken ahead of a planned excursion. I instruct patients to take 1 gram of ginger root daily, in two divided doses, beginning two days before their trip. This dosage is continued during the trip. Judging from patient feedback, the results have been on a par with milder anti-motion sickness drugs such as Dramamine, but without drowsiness and other side effects. Ginger is a particularly good alternative for children as well as pet frogs!

Nausea and Vomiting Associated with Pregnancy

Ginger is often recommended by practitioners of herbal medicine for the morning sickness that afflicts many women during the first trimester of pregnancy. Ginger is usually recommended as a tea and should be used only for short periods of time.

The nausea and vomiting associated with pregnancy can sometimes become much more than just morning sickness. Severe vomiting can lead to hospitalization in some cases. This condition is known as *hyperemesis gravidarum*. Fortunately, this occurs in only 0.3 percent of pregnancies.

A Danish study[20] found that 1 gram of ginger daily (in four divided doses) was extremely effective against hyperemesis gravidarum. In nineteen of twenty-seven women taking ginger, nausea and vomiting became less frequent within the first 4 days of treatment. No side effects appeared.

Ginger should be used only for short periods of time during pregnancy and should not exceed 1 gram of powder daily. Treatment of hyperemesis gravidarum should be undertaken with your doctor or midwife's supervision.

Nausea and Vomiting following Surgery

Many people experience nausea and vomiting after surgery—especially when anesthesia is involved (I always thought it was the slop that passes for food in the hospital). Even with the advent of new antinausea drugs, the incidence still hovers around 30 percent. Two studies[21,22] have found that ginger may be the most consistently effective and safe treatment for this condition.

The application of 1 gram of ginger before anesthesia cut the rate of postsurgical nausea and vomiting by more than half in women undergoing laparoscopic surgery.[21] Positive results were also seen in sixty women undergoing major gynecological surgery.[22]

If you decide to use ginger before surgery, check with your doctor first. There is concern that ginger may cause excessive bleeding. However, this was not reported in either of the postsurgical nausea studies.

Other Potential Uses

As mentioned earlier, ginger possesses mild antiinflammatory and analgesic properties. Published case reports indicate that ginger may help people with rheumatoid arthritis, osteoarthritis, and muscular pain. The daily doses employed in these reports ranged from 3 to 7 grams. The length of treatment varied from 3 months to 2.5 years. Three-quarters of the patients with arthritis enjoyed, to varying degrees, relief from pain and swelling.[23]

Ginger may also offer promise for migraine sufferers. Unfortunately, the only published paper on the topic is mostly theoretical and involves only one case study.[24] More research is needed before ginger can reach the same level of clinical assurance enjoyed by feverfew.

HOW TO USE GINGER

The German Commission E monograph recommends 2 to 4 grams of dried rhizome powder daily in two to three divided doses.[25] For prevention of motion sickness, the nausea and vomiting of pregnancy, or postsurgical nausea and vomiting, 1 gram daily seems to be sufficient.

Those of you using it to prevent motion sickness should begin taking ginger a couple of days before your excursion and throughout the trip.

Side effects are rare with ginger consumption. Some people may be sensitive to the taste and report some heartburn. The German Commission E monograph suggests that people with gallstones consult a physician before using ginger. Short-term use of ginger to treat the nausea and vomiting of pregnancy appears to pose no safety problems. Long-term use during pregnancy is not recommended.

RELATED CONDITIONS DISCUSSED IN PART 6

- Atherosclerosis
- Migraine headache
- Morning sickness associated with pregnancy
- Nausea associated with motion sickness
- Rheumatoid arthritis

Ginkgo biloba

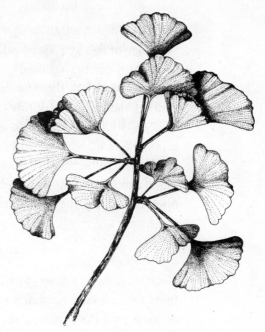

PART USED   The leaves of younger trees

COMMON USES
- Memory loss associated with aging
- Early stages of Alzheimer's disease
- Poor circulation to the extremities; intermittent claudication
- Long-term recovery from a stroke
- Tinnitus (ringing in the ears) and hearing loss

ACTIVE CONSTITUENTS   Ginkgo flavone glycosides (bioflavonoids) and terpene lactones—ginkgolides and bilobalide

HOW IT WORKS   Ginkgo extract increases blood flow to the brain and central nervous system. It also increases peripheral circulation. Ginkgo is a powerful antioxidant for the brain and central nervous system and also exerts a protective effect on the cells of the nervous system.

RECOMMENDED USE   Standardized extract containing 24 percent ginkgo flavone glycosides and 6 percent terpene lactones—120 to 240 milligrams daily in two or three divided doses

SIDE EFFECTS   Side effects are rare with use of the standardized extract. Mild gastrointestinal upset occurs in less than 1 percent of patients in clinical studies. Some patients with poor blood flow to the brain (i.e., cerebrovascular insufficiency) may experience a mild, transient headache for the first one or two days of use.

SAFETY ISSUES   There are no known interactions with commonly prescribed drugs. The current German Commission E monograph lists no contraindications to the use of ginkgo during pregnancy or lactation.

WHEN I think of an herbal medicine that is a perfect example of the marriage of folklore and modern science, *Ginkgo biloba* invariably comes to mind. Few herbal medicines better typify the vast potential of plant medicines within the standards of modern medicine. Ginkgo is prescribed daily by thousands of doctors and used by millions of people around the world. It is not only the most commonly prescribed herbal medicine in Germany and France but also ranks among the top five most frequently prescribed medicines in those countries. Perhaps most exciting is the continuing research on this herbal medicine that continues to open new doors for human use.

PLANT FACTS

Ginkgo biloba is a living fossil. The world's oldest living species of tree, its fossil records date back more than 200 million years. The ginkgo tree lives as long as 1,000 years and may grow to a height of 100 to 122 feet. Because of its amazing ability to resist temperature extremes, pollution, and insects, it is commonly grown in urban centers as an ornamental tree. Ginkgo has characteristic fan-shaped, bilobed leaves. Ginkgo is occasionally referred to as the "maidenhair tree." Modern herbal preparations (extracts) of ginkgo employ the leaves of cultivated trees.

HISTORY

If I tried to cover all the details of ginkgo's history, you'd need some ginkgo just to remember half of it. Ginkgo, which originally grew in North America and Europe, was destroyed in many parts of the world during the Ice Age. It did survive in parts of Asia and was later cultivated in China as a sacred tree.

Use of ginkgo medicinally can be traced back almost 5,000 years, to the origins of Chinese herbal medicine. Ginkgo was first introduced by Chen Noung (2767–2687 B.C.) in the first pharmacopoeia, *Chen Noung Pen T'sao*. Ginkgo was recommended for respiratory tract ailments as well as memory loss in the elderly.

In 1771 the Swedish botanist Linnaeus christened the tree *Ginkgo biloba*, on the basis of an early description by Dr. Englebert Kaempfer and the bilobed structure of the leaf. Ginkgo made its grand return to America in 1784, when it was planted on the estate of William Hamilton near Philadelphia.[1]

MODERN DEVELOPMENT

Spearheaded by the Dr. Willmar Schwabe Company of Germany, pharmacological research into the active constituents and activity of ginkgo leaves began in the late 1950s. Twenty years of research resulted in a standardized, concentrated extract of ginkgo leaves. Using leaves from cultivated trees, the twenty-seven-step extraction process takes up to 2 weeks to complete, and requires approximately 50 pounds of ginkgo leaves to create 1 pound of extract. Most importantly, the active constituents are measured at various points throughout this process to assure an optimal product (and optimal medical benefits).[2]

Ginkgo biloba extract (GBE) is one of the best researched herbal medicines in the world, with more than 400 published studies and reports and several books to its credit. Ginkgo is among the most frequently prescribed herbal medicines.

MEDICALLY ACTIVE CONSTITUENTS

The medical benefits of GBE rely on the proper balance of two groups of active components—the ginkgo flavone glycosides and the terpene lactones. The 24 percent ginkgo flavone glycoside designation on GBE labels indicates a carefully measured balance of bioflavonoids, including quercetin, kaempferol, and isorhamnetin. These bioflavonoids are primarily responsible for GBE's antioxidant activity and ability to inhibit platelet aggregation ("stickiness"). These two actions are critical in the prevention of circulatory diseases such as atherosclerosis, and also contribute to GBE's benefits for the brain and central nervous system.[3]

While most plants contain bioflavonoids, none possess the unique terpene lactone components found in GBE. Conveniently known as ginkgolides and bilobalide, these components give GBE its ability to increase circulation to the brain and other parts of the body as well as exert a protective effect on nerve cells.

Ginkgolides improve circulation and inhibit the actions of platelet-activating factor (PAF) (see the section "Nerve Protection and Platelet-Activating Factor Inhibition"). These constituents, particularly ginkgolide B, have been widely researched and compose the subject of two textbooks.[4,5]

Bilobalide protects the cells of the nervous system. Recent animal studies indicate that bilobalide may help regenerate damaged nerve cells.[6,7]

How Ginkgo Works

Ginkgo biloba Extract and Circulation

Ginkgo biloba extract increases circulation—both to the brain and the extremities. In addition to inhibiting platelet stickiness, GBE regulates the tone and elasticity of blood vessels.[8] In other words, it makes circulation more efficient. This improvement in circulation efficiency extends to both the large vessels (arteries) and smaller vessels (capillaries) of the circulatory system. One study[9] dramatically illustrated increased blood flow through the capillaries: an hour after administration of GBE to healthy adults, there was a 57 percent increase in blood flow measured through the nail-fold capillaries!

This positive effect on circulation extends to the brain. *Ginkgo biloba* extract's ability to increase circulation to the brain and central nervous system (CNS) is well documented and has led to its use against depression and memory loss in the elderly.[10] These positive effects on circulation—both to the extremities and the CNS—have made GBE the herbal treatment of choice in both the prevention and management of circulatory disorders in the elderly.

Antioxidant Properties

As we will note throughout this book, many herbs have antioxidant capabilities. This means that, like vitamin E, selenium, and vitamin C, some herbal medicines protect parts of the body susceptible to damage by free radicals. This may help combat many age-related diseases of the CNS and cardiovascular system.[11]

Numerous studies demonstrate that GBE exerts antioxidant activity in the brain, retina, and cardiovascular system. Its antioxidant activity in the brain and CNS make it an extremely promising herbal for prevention of age-related declines in brain function. It may also prove useful in the prevention and early treatment of Alzheimer's disease and strokes. *Ginkgo biloba* extract also has therapeutic potential in the prevention of eye disorders such as senile cataracts, macular degeneration, and diabetic retinopathy.[12]

Ginkgo biloba extract's antioxidant activity in the brain is of particular interest. The brain and CNS are particularly susceptible to free radical attack. Free radical damage in the brain is widely accepted as being a major factor in many disorders associated with aging, such as Alzheimer's disease.[13] The use of antioxidants to prevent these disorders has been the subject of many clinical studies.

Nerve Protection and Platelet-Activating Factor Inhibition

The terpene lactones in GBE take center stage in nerve protection and platelet-activating factor (PAF) inhibition. At the 1992 Congress for Phytotherapy held in Munich, Germany, GBE's primary benefit to the brain was attributed to its terpene lactone constituents. Protection afforded by ginkgolides arose primarily from their ability to inhibit PAF. Three ginkgolides, A, B, and C, have demonstrated PAF inhibition, with ginkgolide B being the most active.[14]

When platelet-activating factor is released from cells, it causes platelets to aggregate (clump together). High amounts of PAF are associated with damage to nerve cells, poor blood flow to the central nervous system (CNS), inflammatory conditions, and bronchial constriction.[15] Much like the free radicals we discussed earlier, higher PAF levels are associated with aging.[16] Thus, in addition to its antioxidant properties, GBE eases another concern of aging.

Ginkgolides A and B, as well as bilobalide, protect nerve cells in the CNS from damage during periods of ischemia (lack of blood flow to body tissues).[17] This makes GBE particularly attractive for use by people who have suffered a stroke. It should also be considered in the treatment of transient ischemic attacks (TIAs), which can be a warning sign of an impending, full-blown stroke.

The combined PAF-inhibiting and antioxidant activity of GBE are being researched for use in recovery from brain trauma and injury.[18]

HEALTH CARE APPLICATIONS

Ginkgo biloba extract has become popular in Europe and worldwide because of its ability to aid circulatory problems in the elderly, especially cerebrovascular insufficiency (poor blood flow to the brain) and intermittent claudication (poor circulation to the lower legs).[19] As we will note, both of these conditions are successfully treated with GBE.

Ginkgo biloba extract also protects against hearing loss, tinnitus (ringing in the ears), vertigo, and degenerative eye conditions such as macular degeneration. Research is also exploring GBE's potential in the treatment of degenerative nerve diseases such as multiple sclerosis, male impotence, and bronchial asthma.

Cerebrovascular Insufficiency

Isn't modern medicine amazing? Sophisticated terms are used to describe conditions that my eight-year-old daughter could define more simply and clearly. Cerebrovascular insufficiency is a case in point. If my seventy-year-old patient George suddenly begins forgetting things and appears depressed, I don't say, "Geez, George, you seem to be getting a bit less blood up to the ol' noggin." Instead, with medical etiquette intact, I inform George that he may be suffering from cerebrovascular insufficiency. He may not feel terrific to get that news but his insurance company seems to be more willing to pay for the visit!

Well, cerebrovascular insufficiency implies a diminished amount of blood flow to the brain. A reduction in blood flow to the brain leads to symptoms such as depression, memory loss, and disorientation. This is commonly associated with the mental decline experienced by some elderly people.

Ginkgo biloba extract is the best treatment known to medicine for the treatment of cerebrovascular insufficiency. Combined with its antioxidant and PAF-inhibiting actions, GBE's ability to increase blood flow to the brain makes it an excellent therapeutic option for depressed elderly individuals who are not responding to antidepressants, and also for those in the early stages of Alzheimer's disease.

Clinical studies show that daily doses of 120 to 240 milligrams of GBE (taken in two to three divided doses) lead to an improvement in the symptoms associated with cerebrovascular insufficiency, such as memory loss, depression, and tinnitus within 8 to 12 weeks.[20,21] These results have been extended to include individuals with poor blood flow stemming from arteriosclerosis (hardening of the arteries).[22]

Resistant Depression

Another thing I love about modern medical diagnosis is the labeling of someone as "resistant" when drug therapy fails. Such is the case with many elderly individuals who are being pumped full of antidepressants when, in fact, they aren't getting sufficient blood flow to their brain. Reduction in blood flow to the brain has been clearly established in many depressed individuals over the age of 50 years.[23]

Using a daily dose of 240 milligrams of GBE, a recent study[24] succeeded in reversing depression among elderly patients. The researchers simply added GBE to the daily regimen of the patients. Significant differences in mood, motivation, and memory were noted after only 4 weeks! The results were even more notable at the end of the 8-week study.

Alzheimer's Disease

While I certainly don't think GBE is a cure for this serious condition, it is emerging as a potential tool to slow the progression in the early stages. A 1994 study involving forty patients in the early stages of Alzheimer's disease found that the use of 240 milligrams of GBE daily for 3 months resulted in an improvement in memory, attention, and mood. Improvements were noted at 1 month and became progressively better over the 3-month study.[25]

The results of a 6-month study with 217 early-stage Alzheimer's patients were presented at the Sixth Congress of the International Psychogeriatric

Association.[26] The authors found that patients treated daily with 240 milligrams of GBE or placebo, for 6 months, showed similar levels of improvement. These studies set the stage for even longer-range studies. For more on Alzheimer's disease, see "Nervous System" in Part 6.

On the basis of current evidence, GBE may be one of the few "smart drugs" that actually lives up to its billing.

POOR CIRCULATION TO THE EXTREMITIES

Ginkgo biloba extract is also a leading treatment for intermittent claudication. The condition, which involves severe cramping and pain in the lower legs during walking or exercise, affects primarily the elderly population. It is frequently debilitating and can severely curtail physical activity. Intermittent claudication is clearly linked to poor circulation (see "Cardiovascular System" in Part 6).

Numerous clinical studies have shown that 120 to 160 milligrams of GBE daily for 3 to 6 months is successful in the treatment of intermittent claudication.[27,28] People using GBE typically experience an increase in pain-free walking distance and an increase in blood flow to the affected leg(s) after about 4 to 6 weeks of treatment.

I also recommend GBE to diabetics, to assist circulation and nerve conduction. I've also administered GBE in the treatment of Raynaud's disease and scleroderma, to help with circulation to the hands.

HOW TO USE GINKGO

As a preventive measure and for circulation problems to the extremities, GBE standardized to contain 6 percent terpene lactones and 24 percent ginkgo flavone glycosides is recommended at a daily dose of 120 to 160 milligrams in two or three divided doses. Daily dosages of 240 milligrams daily may be required in some cases of cerebrovascular insufficiency, early-stage Alzheimer's disease, resistant depression, and minor head injury. I usually recommend an initial 6- to 8-week period to ascertain effectiveness of GBE.

Using Ginkgo for Head Injury or Trauma: A Case Study

Effective treatment is lacking for patients who have experienced head injuries and are suffering from long-term side effects, including memory loss, dizziness, and mood alterations. I recommend GBE for patients suffering from the long-term effects of mild to moderate head injuries. Here's a case study from my clinical practice.

N.G., a 36-year-old female, reported to my office with a 9-month history of sleep disturbance, dizziness with exercise, headaches, and short-term memory loss, following a blow to the back of her head. She had slipped and fallen backward on the kitchen floor. N.G. told me that her symptoms included frequent disorientation—especially while driving.

She held an important managerial position at a local university and was forced to take a leave of absence due to her inability to work without making numerous mistakes. She had been to several neurologists. No improvement was reported. As a matter of fact, her exasperated physician had actually put her on an antidepressant drug (presumably, to help with sleep).

We decided to try her on 120 milligrams of GBE daily in three divided doses. N.G. called back in 10 days to tell me she had been able to stop the antidepressant and was sleeping fine. At a 4-week follow-up visit N.G. reported significant improvement in most of her major complaints. She reported a great deal more mental clarity, improved short-term memory, and was able to exercise 20 to 30 minutes daily with no dizziness or discomfort. She had returned to work half-time and planned to increase this over the next 2 months.

An 8-week follow-up found N.G. back at work full-time with none of the problems reported at our initial visit! She discontinued GBE after 9 months. Two years later, she continues to live a normal life with no work or activity-related problems.

Note: I now recommend 240 milligrams daily for patients with head injury or trauma.

Ginkgo biloba extract is essentially devoid of any serious side effects. In less than 1 percent of persons studied,[29] use of GBE resulted in mild gastrointestinal upset. Persons with cerebrovascular insufficiency may sometimes experience a temporary, mild headache with GBE use. Ironically, this may signal that the extract is working and usually ceases within 48 hours. There are no known drug interactions with GBE. The current German Commission E monograph lists no contraindications to the use of GBE by pregnant and lactating women.[30]

It is important to remember that circulatory conditions in the elderly can involve serious disease. Seek proper medical care and accurate medical diagnosis prior to self-prescribing GBE or other herbal medications.

RELATED CONDITIONS DISCUSSED IN PART 6

- Alzheimer's disease
- Asthma
- Atherosclerosis
- Cerebrovascular insufficiency
- Depression
- Neuropathy (diabetic)
- Diabetic retinopathy
- Impotence
- Intermittent claudication
- Macular degeneration
- Migraine headache
- Raynaud's disease
- Uveitis

Asian Ginseng

BOTANICAL NAME *Panax ginseng* C.A. Meyer
PART USED The root

COMMON USES

- Revitalizes those experiencing fatigue and debility with declining concentration and physical endurance
- Supports the adrenals of those under stress
- Assists in recovery following surgery or a long convalescence
- Supports those undergoing radiation or chemotherapy
- Forms part of the training program for endurance athletes and body builders

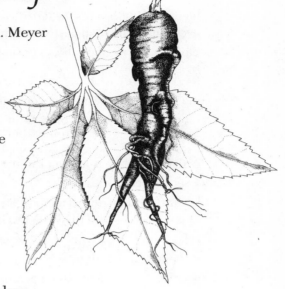

ACTIVE CONSTITUENTS Asian ginseng is a complex mixture of many different constituents—the most important, according to research, are the ginsenosides

HOW IT WORKS Ginseng is notable for its ability to support and enhance adrenal function. This allows for more consistent energy and better reaction to stress. Ginseng sharpens mental acuity and concentration. It maximizes the use of oxygen and glycogen by working muscles, allowing them to function in an aerobic state for longer periods of time. Ginseng also helps the body maintain normal blood sugar and cholesterol levels.

RECOMMENDED USE The best researched form of ginseng is extracts supplying approximately 4 to 7 percent ginsenosides. The recommended dosage is 100 milligrams once or twice daily. Crude, nonstandardized extracts require a higher daily dose of 1 to 2 grams. Ginseng is usually used for 2 to 3 weeks continuously, followed by a 1- to 2-week "rest" period before resuming.

SIDE EFFECTS   Used at the recommended dosage, ginseng is generally safe. In rare instances, it may cause overstimulation and possibly insomnia. Consuming caffeine with ginseng boosts the risk of experiencing overstimulation and gastrointestinal upset. People with uncontrolled high blood pressure should use ginseng with caution.

SAFETY ISSUES   Long-term use of ginseng may cause menstrual abnormalities and breast tenderness in some women. Ginseng is not recommended for pregnant or lactating women.

ASIAN ginseng is among the most popular herbal medicines worldwide. Used for centuries in the Orient as a "tonic" herb, it is the perfect embodiment of an herbal adaptogen (see the discussion in Part 4). Hundreds of studies have confirmed its benefit to a variety of body systems. These effects on the body include increased energy, mental alertness, and physical endurance. Along with eleuthero (Siberian ginseng), it is a major ally against stress and offers long-term support of adrenal function. With antioxidant nutrients and herbal medicines such as ginkgo, it is also a premier "antiaging" compound.

PLANT FACTS

Asian ginseng is a member of the Araliaceae family, which also includes American ginseng (*Panax quinquefolius*) and Siberian ginseng (*Eleutherococcus senticosus*). It is a perennial herb that reaches heights of 2 feet and produces pale yellowish-green flowers that give way to small, red, berry-like fruit. Because of its long taproots, the harvested root has a look suggestive of a human form.[1]

Asian ginseng commonly grows on mountain slopes in the northeastern provinces of China, adjacent Korea, and also Russia. Ginseng is usually harvested in the fall after the fifth year of growth, when the active ginsenosides are most highly concentrated.[2]

The sheer number of products manufactured from the root of Asian ginseng has led to some confusion; a good example is "white" versus "red" ginseng. There's actually nothing mystical about either. White ginseng is simply the dried, unprocessed root or root powder. Red ginseng is created when the root is steamed for a period of several hours and then dried over a low fire or in the sun. Some sources cite mild differences between the two, the most notable being the slightly greater antioxidant activity attributed to the red version.[3]

In Asia, wild-harvested ginseng is revered—and rare. Take a walk through an Asian herb shop some time and price wild ginseng root. In Hong Kong, the mecca of ginseng trade, a wild-harvested root has been known to sell for as much as $20,000!

HISTORY

Asian ginseng has been a part of Chinese medicine for more than 2,000 years. I defer to my friend Steven Foster when it comes to accurate and heart-felt history. I highly recommend his book (cowritten with Yue Chongxi) *Herbal Emissaries: Bringing Chinese Herbs to the West*. The book, which offers a concise and understandable guide to Chinese herbal medicines, explores ginseng's long and illustrious history in the Orient.

The first reference to Asian ginseng is found in the *Shen Nong Ben Cao Jing*, written around the first century A.D. This work is thought to be the earliest listing of traditional Chinese medicines. S. Y. Hu, in her translation of the text, states that "it is used for repairing the five viscera, quieting the spirit, curbing the emotion, stopping agitation, removing noxious influence, brightening the eyes, enlightening the mind and increasing wisdom. Continuous use leads one to longevity with light weight."[4]

Ginseng acquired the status of "superior" in the Chinese classification of herbs. Reference to ginseng's medical use is listed in the classic Chinese materia medica, *Ben Cao Gang Mu*, written in 1596 by Li Shizhen. Small amounts were noted for improving vitality and again for keeping one slim and trim![5] Ginseng was commonly used by elderly persons in the Orient to enhance energy and to improve memory.

Petrus Jartoux, a Jesuit missionary, is credited with the introduction of Asian ginseng to the West. In 1711, his observations of the plant and its use in China were published.

MODERN DEVELOPMENT

Since the 1940s, ginseng has been one of the most highly researched herbs in the world. Hundreds of scientific studies have attempted to discover what makes this ancient tonic work and what effect it has on the body. Steven Foster and Yue Chongxi have the following to say about the approach to ginseng research in Asia: "Chinese researchers, as is the case with medicinal plants in general, have focused on how ginseng works, whereas Western researchers focus on if it works. This reflects a fundamental difference between the East and West. In Asia, the efficacy of an herb is already established in a cultural context. In the West, we presuppose that traditional or folk uses have no rational scientific basis."[6]

Ginseng's actions make it applicable to a vast array of conditions and also for optimizing health.

Modern research shows that ginseng protects the body from a wide range of harmful influences, including pollution, radiation, and even alcohol. Ginseng protects nerve cells, lowers cholesterol, and is an antioxidant.[7] Its antifatigue and endurance-enhancing actions make it a favorite supplement for athletes.

MEDICALLY ACTIVE CONSTITUENTS

Ginseng's actions in the body are due to a complex interplay of constituents. The primary group consists of ginsenosides. Thirteen ginsenosides have been identified in Asian ginseng. Ginsenosides Rg1 and Rb1 have received the most attention.[8]

The interplay of Rg1 and Rb1 offers a glimpse of the unique synergism that exists among the constituents in ginseng. Rg1 mildly stimulates brain and central nervous system activity. It increases energy, counters fatigue, and enhances intellectual and physical performance.

Rb1, on the other hand, relaxes the activity of the brain and is associated with lowering blood pressure.[9] This balancing effect allows ginseng to adjust various body functions and encourage their return to a healthy, normal function.

Other components beside ginsenosides are also important. A group of constituents known as panaxans help lower blood sugar. Polysaccharides (complex sugar molecules) support immune function.[10]

HOW GINSENG WORKS AND HEALTH CARE APPLICATIONS

Ginseng is the granddaddy of adaptogenic herbs. I. I. Brekhman, the Russian researcher responsible for coining the umbrella term *adaptogen* to describe certain herbs, began with ginseng as his original model (see Part 4 for more information on adaptogens).[11]

Ginseng and other adaptogens work on the premise that the body is in a state of dynamic flux. Wellness depends on the balanced functioning of a number of control centers in the body, including the nervous and endocrine systems. Optimal health depends on keeping these systems in balance.

That's why I've combined the "How It Works" and "Health Care Applications" sections in this chapter, unlike for the other herbs; breaking down ginseng's potential health care applications into nice, convenient categories is difficult because of ginseng's multifaceted actions in the body. *Some* of ginseng's potential uses are as follows:

Chronic fatigue syndrome
Mental and physical fatigue
Anxiety
Depression
Memory loss in the elderly
Diabetes
High cholesterol
Drug and alcohol withdrawal
Adjunctive use during radiation or chemotherapy

Another reason why it is hard to categorize ginseng is because of the way ginseng's effects overlap: antifatigue, improved mental activity, antioxidant activity, and improved cholesterol metabolism are all important considerations for optimizing health.

Antifatigue/Antistress Actions

Most of my patients with chronic fatigue have run-down adrenal glands. The adrenals, which sit atop your kidneys, resemble rechargeable batteries. Highly efficient at helping our bodies react and adapt to stressful situations, the adrenals can become run down if the body is constantly stressed. This stress can come from the daily commute on the Nimitz Freeway, working for Prima Publishing and dealing with authors like me, or chronic illness.

Ginseng supports the adrenals through a unique action. Instead of directly stimulating adrenal action, ginseng influences the control centers that regulate adrenal function—the hypothalamus and pituitary.[12] In traditional Chinese medicine, the hypothalamus–pituitary–adrenal axis is not thought of as three separately functioning entities, but rather as one cohesive unit. Ginseng treats the unit as a whole.[13]

This model of indirect support of adrenal function helps us understand ginseng's antifatigue actions. By supporting the function of the hypothalamus–pituitary–adrenal axis, ginseng allows the body to adapt more efficiently to stress and thus ease the burden on other systems in the body, including the heart and brain.[14] It also aids in the recovery of physical and mental balance following stress.

Enhanced Mental Performance

Ginseng improves and sharpens mental concentration and performance. One of my favorite nonhuman studies exploring ginseng's effect on memory is a Bulgarian study with rats.[15] According to this study, rats given ginseng showed improved learning and memory. This was in contrast to rats receiving no ginseng. How did they decide the ginseng-taking rats were smarter? My personal image is of the ginseng rats huddled together over afternoon cocktails discussing the works of Sartre while the other rats are drinking Bud Lite and watching arena football!

Human studies show that ginseng improves attention, performance, and memory. One test with sixteen volunteers who took ginseng showed improvement on a wide battery of tests, including arithmetic.[16] Another study found that concentration and performance improved in radio operators and proofreaders taking ginseng.[17]

Ginseng is commonly used in Asia by older individuals showing signs of memory loss. While not as thoroughly researched as ginkgo for this condition, studies have shown that ginseng effectively improves memory and also counters depression in the elderly.[18] In fact, some European phytomedicine supplements have begun to combine ginseng and ginkgo.

Enhanced Physical Performance

A favorite among endurance athletes and body builders, ginseng increases physical endurance and speeds up recovery time following a work-out.[19] Ginseng also builds muscle mass in body builders without the side effects associated with steroids.[20]

Ginseng improves athletic performance through a number of related actions. First, it increases the uptake of oxygen by the body.[21] It also lowers the maximum exercise heart rate—an indication that the work load on the heart during exercise is less than before treatment. Last, and perhaps most notable, it enables exercising muscles to maintain glycogen stores more efficiently.[22] Glycogen, a type of sugar, is the primary source of fuel to the exercising muscle. With ginseng use, muscles stay in an aerobic (nonexhausted) state longer before reaching exhaustion.

Effects on Blood Sugar

Ginseng is commonly used in traditional Chinese medicine to treat diabetes. Animal studies show that ginseng enhances the release of insulin from the pancreas and increases the number of insulin receptors.[23,24] It also has a direct blood sugar-lowering (hypoglycemic) effect.[25]

It is also interesting to note that insulin is needed for the breakdown of fat. This should steer people to the use of ginseng for weight-loss programs.

Antitoxin and Antioxidant Actions

Ginseng helps remove harmful chemicals and toxins from the body. Ginseng also protects cells from the damaging effects of radiation, including workplace sources and radiation from medical treatment.[26]

An intriguing area of application for ginseng is in drug-withdrawal programs. A study with mice indicates that ginseng significantly inhibits morphine dependence. This could make ginseng useful for persons trying to withdraw from morphine or similar pain medications.[27]

Ginseng also fights the damaging activity of free radicals in the body.[28] Its antioxidant activities help protect the cardiovascular system, liver, and lungs.[29]

Cholesterol-lowering Effects

Ginseng helps the body metabolize and break down cholesterol more efficiently. Ginseng reduces total cholesterol and triglycerides while raising the levels of the "good" high-density lipoprotein (HDL)-cholesterol. Ginseng also reduces platelet stickiness.[30] High levels of HDL-cholesterol and decreased aggregation of platelets are actions that lower the risk of atherosclerosis and cardiovascular disease.

Anticancer and Immune System-supporting Actions

A Korean study[31] indicates that regular intake of ginseng may also reduce the risk of cancer. A survey of more than 1,800 patients at a hospital in Seoul found that people without cancer were more likely to consume ginseng regularly compared to those who had developed cancer. The protective effect applied to men and women equally. Ginseng extracts and powders scored better than freshly sliced ginseng.

Animal studies show ginseng and some of its constituents inhibit the growth of ovarian cancer cells, lung tumors, and liver tumors (treatment of the latter included a chemotherapeutic drug).[32,33] These results have not been tested in humans.

Evidence is mounting that ginseng's anticancer activity stems from immune system support.[34] Ginseng increases the levels of T lymphocytes and natural killer cells (sounds like a Sylvester Stallone movie), two key components of the immune system's ability to combat viral infections. Particularly noteworthy is ginseng's ability to raise the levels of helper T lymphocytes (also known as CD4 cells) and influence the ratio of these cells to suppressor T lymphocytes (also known as CD8 cells).[35] Fewer CD4 cells and a decreased CD4/CD8 ratio are features of human immunodeficiency virus (HIV) infection and progression to acquired immunodeficiency syndrome (AIDS). Low natural killer cell activity is common among people with chronic fatigue syndrome.

This evidence points to using ginseng as a supportive supplement for cancer patients. Much like astragalus and eleuthero (Siberian ginseng), it supports immune function and also helps the bone marrow bounce back and begin producing white blood cells following chemotherapy. This is extremely valuable for those undergoing treatment for cancer.

I lean toward using eleuthero and astragalus for HIV infection, because of the greater research and clinical evidence for these adaptogens.

How to Use Ginseng

Most research has been expended on ginseng extracts that supply approximately 4 to 7 percent ginsenosides. The recommended dosage is 100 milligrams once or twice daily. Crude, nonstandardized extracts require a higher daily dose of 1 to 2 grams. I am not a fan of highly extracted ginseng products. Products containing ginsenoside concentrations that exceed 4 to 7 percent often lack other important constituents that contribute to immune support and regulation of blood sugar.

Use ginseng for 2 to 3 weeks without interruption, followed by a 1- to 2-week "rest" period before resuming. At the recommended dosage, ginseng is generally safe. In rare instances, it may cause overstimulation and possibly insomnia. Consuming caffeine with ginseng, particularly on an empty stomach, increases the possibility of overstimulation and gastrointestinal upset. People with uncontrolled high blood pressure should not use ginseng.

In 1979, the *Journal of the American Medical Association* published a report citing a "ginseng abuse syndrome" caused by long-term consumption of ginseng. Symptoms included high blood pressure, nervousness, insomnia, and morning diarrhea.[36] This report has largely been discredited, because it did not provide information on what type of ginseng was being ingested; furthermore, the amounts of ginseng begin consumed (more than 15 grams per day) greatly exceeded what is recommended.[37]

Contrary to the German Commission E monograph on ginseng, I do not recommend its use during pregnancy or lactation. I also urge women of menstruating age to use ginseng with caution, because abnormal periods and cyclical breast pain may occur. Eleuthero (Siberian ginseng) is a good alternative. On the other hand, menopausal women will benefit greatly by adding ginseng to their supplement regimen.

RELATED CONDITIONS DISCUSSED IN PART 6

- Alzheimer's disease
- Atherosclerosis
- Chronic fatigue syndrome
- Diabetes
- Impotence
- Stress and fatigue

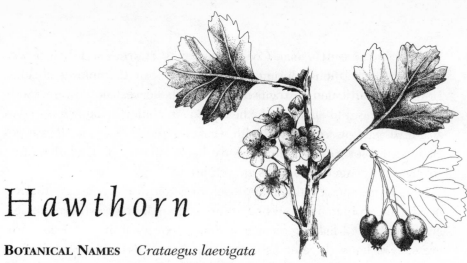

Hawthorn

BOTANICAL NAMES *Crataegus laevigata*
(synonym: *Crataegus oxyacantha*) and *Crataegus monogyna*

PARTS USED Modern European extracts use the leaves and flowers. Traditional preparations use the ripe fruit.

COMMON USES

- Early stages of congestive heart failure
- Stable angina pectoris
- Long-term recovery from a heart attack

ACTIVE CONSTITUENTS Oligomeric procyanidins and other flavonoids

HOW IT WORKS Hawthorn extract improves the efficiency of the heart by increasing blood supply to the heart muscle. As a result, the heart is able to pump more blood to the body. Hawthorn also lowers the resistance to blood flow in the peripheral vessels.

RECOMMENDED USE Hawthorn extracts standardized on oligomeric procyanidin content—160 milligrams daily in two divided doses. A higher dose of 160 milligrams three times daily is recommended for individuals requiring more intensive treatment. Traditional berry preparations—4 to 5 grams daily.

SIDE EFFECTS None are currently known

SAFETY ISSUES There are no known interactions with other cardiac medications. European monographs list no contraindication to the use of hawthorn during pregnancy or lactation.

WHEN one considers the dizzying array of heart drugs and their potential side effects, the need for gentler and less toxic therapies is obvious. Hawthorn, particularly extracts made from the leaves and flowers, exerts a gentle, measured effect on the heart and circulation, making it useful as an initial therapy for persons with weakened heart function. It is especially useful for early-stage congestive heart failure—particularly before stronger drugs such as digitalis are required.

This represents a rational approach to cardiovascular disease that we need to incorporate into our health care system. Using hawthorn not only gives the heart a fighting chance at some recovery, it may also slow progression of heart disease. As is true with other herbs that slow disease progression, this also equates to incredible savings in medical costs!

PLANT FACTS

Hawthorn is a small, shrublike tree with sharp thorns, often found in woodlands. It is a member of the Rosaceae family. Hawthorn is the popular name given to the plant genus *Crataegus*, which includes more than 100 species. *Crataegus* species are commonly found in Europe, western Asia, and North Africa. The two species most frequently used for medicinal purposes in Europe are *Crataegus laevigata* (often referred to as *Crataegus oxyacantha*) and *Crataegus monogyna*.[1]

Hawthorn has small white or pink flowers that develop a bright, red fruit. Until recently, herbal preparations were made largely from the fruit. In the past decade, standardized extracts from Europe have used primarily the leaves and flowers.[2] These portions of the plant are higher in medically active constituents.

HISTORY

That wild and crazy Greek herbalist, Dioscorides, was using hawthorn medicinally in the first century A.D. Otherwise, the early literature on hawthorn centers on the religious and political symbolism attributed to the plant, and details little about its medicinal benefits.

Early medical uses attributed to the plant weren't exactly narrow in scope. Everything from stomach ailments to dropsy were mentioned. Throughout history, however, the heart continued to be the target of use. In *A Modern Herbal*, Grieve mentions the use of the dried fruits (known as "haws") as a tonic for chronic heart ailments.[3]

MODERN USE OF HAWTHORN

Modern herbal development of hawthorn extracts began with the discovery of certain compounds in the leaves, flowers, and berries that were responsible for the cardiac actions attributed to the plant. The first among these was a flavonoid-like complex of oligomeric procyanidins; other compounds included the flavonoids vitexin, quercetin, and hyperoside.[4]

The leaves and flowers appear to contain concentrated amounts of these constituents—especially the oligomeric procyanidins.[5] The action of these compounds on the cardiovascular system has led to the development of European hawthorn extracts, which are widely used in general medical and cardiology practices.[6]

HOW HAWTHORN WORKS

The actions of hawthorn extract[7-11] on the cardiovascular system include the following:

- Improves blood flow through the blood vessels supplying the heart muscle (coronary arteries)
- Improves the contractions of the heart muscle, making it more efficient in pumping blood out to the body
- Improves circulation to the extremities by lowering resistance in the arteries. This is partly due to hawthorn's ability to inhibit a substance in the body known as angiotensin-converting enzyme (ACE). ACE is

associated with leading to the creation of angiotensin II, a potent constrictor of blood vessels.

- Combats free radicals by way of its potent antioxidant properties. Because of its high bioflavonoid content, hawthorn is very adept at counteracting the damaging effects of free radicals on the cardiovascular system.

In addition, hawthorn extracts are mildly effective in lowering blood pressure. However, medicinal preparations of hawthorn are rarely used as the primary means by which to treat high blood pressure. European physicians will incorporate hawthorn into the management of mild high blood pressure and cardiac arrhythmia in elderly patients.

Put simply, hawthorn and its active flavonoid compounds make the heart a more efficient pump. It achieves this partly by increasing blood supply to the heart muscle. It also increases the output of blood from the heart and decreases the resistance of blood vessels to the normal flow of blood. What we're left with is stronger and healthier heart function, as well as better flow of blood throughout the body.

The best news is hawthorn's safety. As opposed to digitalis and other cardiac glycoside drugs that can become very toxic, hawthorn can be used long term without side effects.[12,13]

HEALTH CARE APPLICATIONS

Congestive Heart Failure

In the last decade, hawthorn extracts have been used successfully to treat the early stages of congestive heart failure (CHF).

People in the early stages of CHF usually do not require stronger heart medications such as digitalis. They are perfect candidates for nontoxic natural medicines such as hawthorn. Because of its ability to strengthen weakened heart muscle and improve blood flow, those with early-stage CHF are able to be more active and enjoy life more. Equally important, hawthorn may slow the progression to more advanced stages of CHF and stave off the need for stronger cardiac medications.

A simple way to see if a medication is helping people in early-stage CHF is to measure their endurance on a stationary bicycle. Thirty early-stage CHF patients, ranging in age from 50 to 70 years, participated in an 8-week study that required them to exercise on a stationary bicycle. Blood pressure and heart rate were measured, along with exercise tolerance and endurance. Patients were given either a hawthorn extract prepared from leaves and flowers (standardized to contain 18.75 percent oligomeric procyanidins) or placebo. The daily dose of the hawthorn extract was 160 milligrams. After 8 weeks, the patients taking the hawthorn extract were able to perform aerobic exercise longer (relative to the control patients) before reaching exhaustion. They also reported increased endurance and feelings of well-being.[14]

Other studies with early-stage CHF patients have used daily doses ranging from 160 to 900 milligrams. As before, exercise tolerance improved while shortness of breath and postexercise fatigue lessened. These studies have also shown improved heart function, as measured by electrocardiogram (ECG).[15–17] Finally, hawthorn extract compares favorably with the cardiac drug Captopril in the treatment of early-stage CHF patients.[18] This drug is used to reduce the resistance to blood flow in peripheral arteries. Hawthorn does this equally well, with the added benefit of working on the heart.

Angina Pectoris

Hawthorn combats angina, another heart condition that is rampant in western culture. Often caused by atherosclerosis, angina results from insufficient blood flow reaching the heart muscle. Without enough oxygen, the heart muscle spasms.

Physical exertion or stress often triggers angina attacks. A 1983 study[19] demonstrated the usefulness of hawthorn extract in the treatment of patients with stable angina pectoris. Sixty angina patients were given either 180 milligrams of hawthorn extract or placebo daily for 3 weeks. The patients taking hawthorn exercised for longer periods of time without an angina attack. Their ECG measures improved, and blood flow and oxygen delivery to the heart muscle rose.

Heart Attacks and the Recovery Process

Heart failure patients often have a history of one or more heart attacks. Studies performed on rat hearts indicate that hawthorn extract protects heart muscle during times of oxygen loss.[20] This protection comes primarily in the form of antioxidant activity, which prevents free radical damage to the heart.[21] However, hawthorn's other effects (mentioned earlier) make it useful in recovery of strength in the heart muscle following a heart attack.

How to Use Hawthorn

The extracts used most commonly today are those made from the leaves and flowers. These extracts are standardized for oligomeric procyanidin and the daily recommended dose is currently set at 160 milligrams in two divided doses. Persons requiring more intensive treatment should initially use 160 milligrams three times daily. If you choose to use one of the traditional hawthorn berry preparations available in the United States, the dosage should be at least 4 to 5 grams daily. Hawthorn usually takes 1 to 2 months to provide a maximum effect and should be considered long-term therapy.

As is true of other plant medicines high in bioflavonoids, hawthorn is extremely safe for long-term use. There are no known interactions with prescription cardiac drugs. There are no known contraindications to use of hawthorn during pregnancy and lactation.

Related Conditions Discussed in Part 6

- Atherosclerosis
- Angina
- Congestive heart failure

Kava-Kava

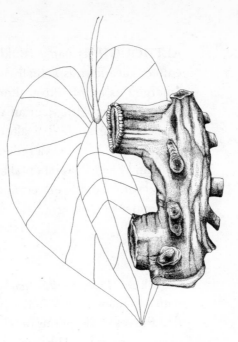

BOTANICAL NAME *Piper methysticum*

PART USED The rhizome

COMMON USES

- Anxiety and conditions of tension and restlessness

ACTIVE CONSTITUENTS Kava lactones (also known as kava α-pyrones)

HOW IT WORKS Kava exerts a relaxing effect on the central nervous system. Kava is noted for promoting relaxation without loss of mental sharpness. This makes it particularly useful for daytime management of anxiety. Kava also promotes normal, restful sleep, and exerts a mild, relaxing effect on skeletal muscles.

RECOMMENDED USE Standardized extract containing 70 percent kava lactones, 100 milligrams two to three times daily (equivalent to 140 to 210 milligrams of kava lactones daily).

SIDE EFFECTS At the therapeutic dosage just given, the only reported side effects are mild gastrointestinal disturbances. Long-term consumption may turn the skin yellow temporarily. If this occurs, you should stop taking kava. In rare cases, an allergic skin reaction (rash) may occur.

The intake of large quantities of nonstandardized kava liquid preparations can lead to a dry, scaly skin rash known as "kava dermopathy." Problems with equilibrium (body balance) have also been reported. Risk of this rash or equilibrium problems occurs only at kava lactone dosages in excess of several grams daily.

SAFETY ISSUES Kava is not recommended for use by pregnant or lactating women. The German Commission E monograph on kava also warns against using it with barbiturates, antidepressants, or other substances that may act on the central nervous system.

ALTHOUGH its name could easily be mistaken for a brand of instant coffee, kava-kava is actually a Polynesian and Melanesian herb that has emerged as an effective alternative to drugs commonly prescribed for anxiety. Along with valerian root extracts, kava root extracts in Europe have become an herbal alternative to antianxiety medications such as Xanax and Valium. Kava reduces anxiety and promotes a relaxed, sociable state and heightened mental acuity. Best of all, kava extracts are not associated with the side effects and addictive properties common to prescription antianxiety drugs.

PLANT FACTS

Kava-kava (*Piper methysticum*) is a member of the pepper family, and is native to many islands of the Pacific. The plant is a robust perennial shrub that thrives at elevations of 500 to 1,000 feet above sea level. It grows best in stony ground and likes good sun exposure. Although it can reach heights of 20 feet, it is usually harvested at about 7 to 8 feet.[1] Modern herbal preparations of kava primarily use the rhizome or root stock for extraction.

The plant appears to have originated in Papua New Guinea–Indonesia and then spread to other islands through trade and by explorers.[2] For a complete overview of plant origins, traditional use of kava, and its chemical constituents, I highly recommend a book by Vincent Lebot, Mark Merlin, and Lamont Lindstrom entitled *Kava: The Pacific Drug* (Yale University Press, 1992).

HISTORY (CHEWIN', SPITTIN', DRINKIN', AND CHILLIN')

The incredible history of kava and its use in traditional ceremonies of the Pacific islands have been the subject of many lengthy anthropological reports and textbooks.

Introduction of kava to the modern world is attributed to a botanist and artist who accompanied Captain James Cook on his first voyage in the *Endeavor* (1768–1771). Daniel Scholander and Sydney Parkinson are given credit for being the first to describe the plant and its use as an intoxicating drink. The actual botanical name, *Piper methysticum,* was coined by Johann Georg Forster to describe an intoxicating pepper drink.[3]

A nonalcoholic drink made from the root of kava played an important role in a variety of ceremonies in the Pacific islands. The kava ceremonies were a key event to welcome visiting royalty or highly honored guests. It was also a part of smaller meetings among village elders. Less formal kava drinking was a common part of many social gatherings.

The manner of preparation of the kava beverage probably horrified a few of the European explorers. After the root is scraped, designated "chewers" chew cut pieces of the root and spit the macerated root into a bowl. Coconut milk was then added and the mixture strained and decanted to another bowl.[4]

Today, the traditional chewing has largely been replaced by pounding or grating of the root. Special bowls and utensils are used in the ceremony. The kava beverage is placed in a cup by a designated person who, in turn, delivers it to the special guest. The whole cup must be chugged without stopping! The audience claps three times and shouts *maca* ("It is empty"). Others can then be served.

Although the ceremony has been altered and even outlawed on some islands, it continues elsewhere today. Rumor has it that Hillary Clinton took part in a kava ceremony held in her honor by a Samoan community on the Hawaiian island of Oahu.[5] Whether she's continued the ceremony during meetings with Newt Gingrich and his mother is open to speculation.

So, how do people feel when they drink kava? The drink initially causes the mouth to numb. This is followed by a mellow and tranquil state that encourages socializing. As long as the mixture is not too strong, the kava drinker usually attains a state of contentment and often enjoys a greater sense of well-being. Along with relaxation, many people experience sharper mental acuity, improved memory, and heightened sense awareness.[6]

Excessive consumption can lead to muscle weakness and dizziness. As we'll note later, long-term, excessive use can also lead to a skin rash that will leave one feeling anything but sociable.

MEDICALLY ACTIVE CONSTITUENTS

The search for kava's active constituents spans 130 years. The initial monograph on the chemical components and pharmacological activity of kava was written and published by the pharmacologist Louis Lewin in 1886.

Repeating work that had originally been published in 1860 and 1861, Lewin traced the relaxing properties of kava to a group of constituents in the root and rhizome.[7] These and other compounds discovered later would eventually be called *kava lactones*. The collective action of these constituents is responsible for kava's antianxiety effects.[8]

The kava lactones, sometimes referred to as kava pyrones, have become the focal point of modern kava extracts. These compounds are found in the fat-soluble portion of the root and rhizome. Good-quality kava rhizome contains between 5.5 and 8.3 percent kava lactones.[9] The standard phytopharmaceutical preparation used in clinical research in Europe contains 70 percent kava lactones.

HOW KAVA WORKS

In animal studies, kava lactones have shown antianxiety, analgesic (pain-relieving), muscle-relaxing, and anticonvulsant effects.[10] Kava's mode of action on the nervous system appears to differ from that of many sedative and muscle relaxants. Benzodiazepine-based drugs such as Xanax and Valium act by binding to or "turning on" specific receptors in the brain known as GABA receptors. By binding these receptors, these drugs promote sedation. Valerian root weakly binds similar receptors, partially explaining its actions as a sedative and antianxiety herbal medicine.

Kava lactones appear to be less selective.[11] Studies suggest that kava directly influences the limbic system—the ancient part of the brain associated with emotions and other brain activities.[12] This may partly explain why kava's antianxiety effects seem to extend beyond psychological processes to include muscle relaxation as well. Animal studies also indicate that kava has pain-reducing capabilities.[13]

Kava does not reduce pain by the same pathway as that used by opiate analgesics. Kava is rarely prescribed by modern herbalists to reduce pain, but it has been used extensively for this purpose by native medicine men of the Pacific islands. Kava lactones also have anticonvulsive properties and seem to protect the brain during times of ischemia (reduced blood flow leading to low oxygen supply).[14,15] A major focus of current research on kava lactones is in the treatment of epilepsy. While this certainly has exciting ramifications, it is too early to begin recommending kava extracts for the primary treatment of epilepsy.

HEALTH CARE APPLICATIONS

One of the primary uses for kava is in the treatment of anxiety and nervous tension. It creates changes in brain activity (as measured by electroencephalogram, or EEG) typical of antianxiety drugs but without their sedative and hypnotic effects.[16,17] Paradoxically, people taking kava show increased attentiveness and concentration while feeling relaxed! This is a remarkable effect for an antianxiety treatment to possess and really places kava in a class all its own.

In head-to-head studies with benzodiazepine-based drugs, kava has fared wonderfully. One study[18] showed that volunteers improved in terms of reaction time and performance on a word recognition test while taking kava. Volunteers taking oxazepam (Serax), a benzodiazepine drug, did not do as well as those taking kava.

How about the treatment of anxiety? One study measured the effect of 100 milligrams of a kava extract (containing 70 percent kava lactones) administered three times daily for 4 weeks against placebo. Fifty-eight patients suffering from anxiety and tension took part in the study, with half the group getting kava and the other half placebo. Less anxiety was already noted in the kava group after 1 week. By 4 weeks, the difference between the two groups was striking. Patients taking kava had an improved sense of well-being and marked reduction in nervousness and tension. No side effects were noted.[19]

The same extract and dosage were used in a study with women suffering from anxiety associated with menopause.[20] Again, compared to placebo, use of kava led to less anxiety and enhanced well-being. Treatment with kava was well tolerated.

Two earlier clinical trials[21,22] demonstrated that an isolated kava lactone, D,L-kavain, reduced anxiety without side effects. One study compared kava directly with oxazepam and found it to be equally effective in reducing anxiety over a 4-week period.[22] Because of the synergistic actions of the combined kava lactones, the preferred delivery form combines all these constituents.

HOW TO USE KAVA

A kava extract containing 70 percent kava lactones is the current standard. The daily dose is 100 milligrams taken two to three times daily (this is equivalent to 140 to 210 milligrams of kava lactones daily). Evaluate its antianxiety effects over a 4- to 8-week period.

At this therapeutic dosage the only reported side effects are mild gastrointestinal disturbances. Long-term consumption may turn the skin yellow temporarily. If this occurs, you should stop taking kava. In rare cases, an allergic skin reaction (rash) may occur.

The intake of large quantities of nonstandardized kava liquid preparations can led to a dry, scaly skin rash known as "kava dermopathy." Problems with equilibrium (body balance) have also been reported. Risk of this rash or equilibrium problems occurs only at kava lactone dosages in excess of several grams daily.

Kava is not recommended for use by pregnant or lactating women. I also would not recommend it for young children. The German Commission E monograph on kava also warns against using it with other substances that may act on the central nervous system, such as alcohol, barbiturates, and antidepressants.[23] However, a recent study did not find any negative effects when kava and alcohol were combined.[24]

RELATED CONDITION DISCUSSED IN PART 6

• Anxiety

Milk Thistle

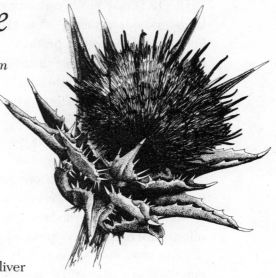

BOTANICAL NAME   *Silybum marianum*

PART USED   The seeds of the dried flower

COMMON USES
- Liver disease associated with alcohol abuse
- Drug-induced liver disease
- Chronic hepatitis
- Liver protection for those working with toxic chemicals, pesticides, and other substances that may harm the liver

ACTIVE CONSTITUENTS   The bioflavonoid silymarin complex and its component known as silibinin

HOW IT WORKS   The silymarin complex, particularly the silibinin component, protects the liver through antioxidant activity and stabilization of cell membranes. It prevents certain toxins from entering liver cells and stimulates regeneration of damaged cells.

RECOMMENDED USE   Concentrated extract standardized to 70 or 80 percent silymarin content—420 milligrams of silymarin daily in three divided doses for 6 to 8 weeks. Once improvement begins, this may be reduced to 280 milligrams of silymarin daily.

SIDE EFFECTS   Milk thistle extract is essentially free of side effects. Because of its stimulating effect on the liver and gallbladder, some people may experience loose stools for the first few days of use.

SAFETY ISSUES   There are no known interactions with commonly prescribed medications. Current monographs list no reasons to avoid milk thistle extract during pregnancy or lactation.

THE DETOXIFYING capabilities of our bodies face an immense challenge in modern society. Auto exhaust, secondary cigarette smoke, alcohol, industrial solvents, pesticides, and even some of the water and food we consume burden the cleansing organs of our body. Positive life-style choices such as exercise and a healthy diet certainly contribute to strengthening these systems. However, when pushed to the limit or even beyond, these organs of detoxification need support.

The liver, one of the body's major "antipollution" organs, removes toxins that can damage other organ systems, including the heart, blood vessels, eyes, and skin. When its actions are impaired by alcohol or diseases such as hepatitis, the negative effects on long-term health can be staggering.

Milk thistle and its active component, known as silymarin, are nature's offering for optimal liver protection. It is the leader among treatments for chronic liver disease caused by alcohol abuse and hepatitis. It is also emerging as an important supplement for those desiring to optimize liver function and maximize the detoxifying potential of this important organ.

PLANT FACTS

Also known by its Latin name *Silybum marianum*, milk thistle is commonly found growing wild in a variety of settings, including roadsides. The name *Silybum* is derived from the name given to edible thistles during the first century by Dioscorides. The name *marianum* comes from the legend that the white mottling of the leaves was caused by a drop of the Virgin Mary's milk. Other common names attributed to the plant include Mary thistle, Marian thistle, Lady's thistle, and Holy thistle. Today, extracts are produced from the seeds of the dried flower.

HISTORY

Medical use of milk thistle can be traced back more than 2,000 years. Pliny the Elder, a first-century Roman naturalist, noted that the juice of the plant mixed with honey was good for "carrying off bile." Culpepper, the well-known eighteenth century herbalist, cited its use for opening "obstructions" of the liver and spleen, and recommended it for the treatment of jaundice.[1] Rademacher, a German physician of the early nineteenth century, gave patients with liver disease a tincture made from the seeds.

Milk thistle was first mentioned in American medical circles in the late nineteenth century. J. U. Lloyd and H. W. Felter, physicians and herbal experts, list the seeds as useful in relieving congestion of the liver, spleen, and kidneys.[2] While liver and onion recipes survived in the United States, milk thistle slowly faded away by the early twentieth century.

MODERN DEVELOPMENT AND MEDICALLY ACTIVE CONSTITUENTS

Leave it to Europe to bring back another valuable plant medicine! Thirty years ago intensive research on the liver-protecting properties of milk thistle seeds began in Germany. In 1968, a bioflavonoid complex in milk thistle seed was identified and isolated. Christened *silymarin*, this complex was found to be responsible for the medical benefits of the plant.[3]

The silymarin complex is made up of three parts: silibinin, silidianin, and silicristin. Silibinin is the most active of the three, and is largely responsible for the benefits attributed to the silymarin complex.[4,5] Extensive research ultimately led to the approval of a standardized milk thistle extract in Germany for the treatment of alcohol-induced liver disease and other chronic diseases of the liver. The extract is standardized to 70 percent silymarin content. To date, more than 200 clinical studies have been completed with this extract.

Note: Throughout the remainder of this chapter, the term "silymarin" will be used interchangeably with "milk thistle extract."

HOW MILK THISTLE WORKS

Milk thistle extract protects liver cells both directly and indirectly. It also possesses the unique ability to regenerate liver cells that have been injured. Let's take a closer look at each of these actions and how they work together to make milk thistle extract a logical choice for persons with liver disease.

Liver Cell Protection

Silymarin, and more specifically silibinin, directly aids liver cells by binding to the outside of the cells and blocking the entrance of certain toxins. This was first noted in experimental studies[6,7] investigating toxins from *Amanita phalloides* (death cap mushroom). Swallowing death cap mushroom causes swift and severe damage to liver cells. Silymarin blocks the receptor sites by which the death cap toxins enter the cells. In addition, toxins that have already penetrated the liver cells are neutralized by silibinin. These actions mean that milk thistle can remain effective even if the initial poisoning occurred several hours earlier. Intravenous preparations of purified silibinin are therefore a mainstay in German hospital emergency rooms for treating death cap mushroom poisoning.

Similar protective effects have been shown against carbon tetrachloride, anticonvulsive drugs such as phenobarbital, as well as some antidepressants.

Antioxidant Activity

Silymarin also protects liver cells by boosting their antioxidant activity. As is true with other nutrient and herbal antioxidants, it accomplishes this by helping the cells produce a powerful antioxidant known as *glutathione*.[8,9] Glutathione is the front-line defense against the ravages of free radicals. Silymarin has been shown to raise the glutathione level in liver cells by as much as 50 percent![10]

Silymarin also increases the activity of another antioxidant, superoxide dismutase, in red blood cells.[11] This effect, combined with the increase in liver cell glutathione, is a major aid for those with a history of alcohol abuse.

Regeneration of Damaged Liver Cells

Alcohol abuse and viral hepatitis can lead to liver cell injury. Under these conditions silymarin actually helps the cell to synthesize new protein, thus enabling it (and ultimately the liver tissue as a whole) to regenerate. This has been clearly demonstrated in studies involving patients with alcoholic liver disease and also chronic hepatitis. Silymarin's protein-regenerating action helps return liver cells to a healthy, functional state.[12,13]

Note: Silymarin's regenerative abilities apply only to normal liver cells. It does not appear to stimulate growth of cancerous cells.[14]

HEALTH CARE APPLICATIONS

A milk thistle extract standardized to 70 percent silymarin content has been extensively studied and recommended in Europe for treatment of a host of liver diseases.

More than 200 experimental and clinical reports involving more than 5,000 patients have been published to date. Conditions for which silymarin is commonly recommended include alcohol-related liver disease, drug-related liver disease, chronic hepatitis, and liver damage caused by toxic chemical exposure. Large clinical trials of silymarin, involving a cross-section of "toxic" liver diseases, have shown phenomenal results in reducing damage to the liver and improving the quality of life of patients.[15]

Alcohol-Related Liver Disease

The leading cause of liver disease in the United States and most western countries is alcohol abuse. While alcohol recovery programs have made progress against alcoholism, many alcoholics continue to go untreated. The legal and emotional costs due to this disease are immense.

Silymarin is often prescribed to treat liver disease caused by alcohol abuse. In studies[16,17] exploring silymarin's effect, the daily dose was 420 milligrams. Alcoholic patients generally must take milk thistle extract for 4 to 8 weeks before seeing any signs of reversal of liver damage. Improvement is measured by blood tests comparing before-and-after liver enzyme levels, as well as by liver biopsy. Successful treatment with silymarin results in a significant lowering of elevated liver enzymes (a lowering of these enzyme levels indicates healing of damaged liver cells) over this period of time. In addition, patients report a reversal in symptoms such as weakness, loss of appetite, and nausea. It should be noted that even with improvement most alcoholic patients will require several months of treatment of milk thistle extract.

Besides correction of liver function in alcoholics, silymarin also appears to improve immune function in these patients.[18] Improving immune function in alcoholic patients is a critical consideration in their long-term recovery.

Collectively, these results make silymarin a key to any alcohol recovery program. It would be nice to see alcohol recovery units begin using silymarin as part of their treatment plan for alcoholic patients—particularly those with compromised liver function.

Liver Cirrhosis

How about patients with advanced liver disease? European studies again point to a role for silymarin in slowing the advancement of liver cirrhosis (a chronic disease characterized by loss of normal liver-cell structure and preceded by fatty infiltration of the liver—particularly in alcoholics). Approximately 20 percent of chronic alcoholics develop cirrhosis, with severe forms often proving fatal. While the liver cell-regenerating capabilities of silymarin do not reverse cirrhosis once it has advanced (cirrhosis appears to be an irreversible process), it improves quality of life and even extends life expectancy in some patients.

One hundred and seventy patients with advanced cirrhosis of the liver participated in a study that compared a daily dose of 420 milligrams of silymarin to placebo (an inactive substance).[19] The average length of treatment was 41 months. The silymarin group showed improvements in liver enzyme measures and liver biopsy results. Most impressive, however, was the fact that most of these patients also lived longer due to silymarin therapy!

Chronic Hepatitis

While I advocate treating an acute case of viral hepatitis with silymarin relatively soon, be sure to see your doctor first and get the appropriate rest needed to alleviate this self-limiting condition.

Silymarin does play a big role in the treatment of chronic viral hepatitis B or C. These chronic viral conditions cause ongoing inflammation and impairment of liver function. They are also linked to an increased risk of liver cancer. Current treatment boils down to either alpha interferon, or watchful waiting. Alpha interferon treatment is successful in some cases of chronic hepatitis B but has been disappointing in the management of hepatitis C.

Silymarin does not directly impact the hepatitis virus. Owing to its protective and regenerating capabilities, however, it is extremely useful for minimizing the damage to liver cells commonly seen in chronic hepatitis. The same 420 milligrams of silymarin daily, used for an average of 9 months, has been shown to reverse liver cell injury effectively (according to biopsy), and led to a decrease in liver enzyme levels. Patients undergoing treatment also noted an increase in appetite and energy.[20,21]

Current research in Europe is focusing on the long-term use of silymarin to treat patients with chronic hepatitis C who have not benefited from alpha interferon treatment.[22]

Liver Support during Drug Therapy

Silymarin also wards off the damage caused by certain prescription drugs, such as antidepressants and anticonvulsive drugs. A recent study showed that adding silymarin to the daily regimen of patients receiving psychotropic drugs reduced the free radical damage to the liver associated with long-term use of these medications.[23] Silymarin can also block the potential liver-damaging effects of anesthesia and is often used both pre- and postsurgery in Germany.

Other Potential Uses

People with multiple chemical sensitivities, and workers encountering toxins on the job, will benefit by adding milk thistle extract to their daily supplement regimen. I've also noted some improvement in psoriasis patients; this observation is based, however, on isolated case histories. The psoriasis in these patients appeared to be linked to impaired liver function, and for them milk thistle extract can be helpful.

While I question the safety of many "cleansing programs" being touted by health gurus today, milk thistle extract can provide critical support for liver function during a detoxification program. It assists normal liver clearance of toxins as well as protects liver cells.

HOW TO USE MILK THISTLE EXTRACT

For persons with liver disease and impaired liver function, the daily dose of milk thistle extract, standardized to 70 or 80 percent silymarin content, should deliver 420 milligrams of silymarin in three divided doses. I recommend that this dose be used until clinical improvement is verified by laboratory tests (don't try to self-diagnose or treat liver disease!). According to research and clinical experience, improvement should be noted in about 8 weeks. Once that occurs, the daily dose may be reduced to 280 milligrams of silymarin. This lower dosage may also be used for preventive purposes.

Milk thistle extract is virtually devoid of any side effects and may be used by a wide range of people, including pregnant and lactating women. Since silymarin does stimulate liver and gallbladder activity, it may have a mild, transient laxative effect in some individuals. This will usually cease within 2 to 3 days.

RELATED CONDITIONS DISCUSSED IN PART 6

- Alcohol-related liver disease
- Depression
- HIV infection/AIDS
- Premenstrual syndrome
- Psoriasis

St. John's Wort

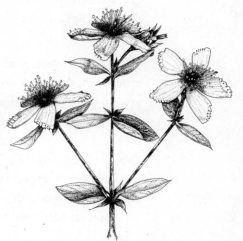

BOTANICAL NAME   *Hypericum perforatum*
PART USED   The flowering tops

COMMON USES
• Mild to moderate depression

ACTIVE CONSTITUENTS   Research has focused on the constituents hypericin and pseudohypericin. Although these substances have a clear antiviral effect, their contribution to the antidepressant properties of St. John's wort are unclear.

HOW IT WORKS   The antidepressant actions of St. John's wort are due to its ability to inhibit the action of the enzyme monoamine oxidase. Hypericin and related constituents also have antiviral activity.

RECOMMENDED USE   Dosage is typically based on hypericin concentration in the extract. The recommended daily hypericin dose is approximately 1 milligram. For example, an extract standardized to contain 0.2 percent hypericin would require a daily dose of 500 milligrams (usually given in two or three divided doses). Current treatment of mild to moderately depressed persons with St. John's wort extract (0.3% hypericin) consists of a daily dosage of 300 milligrams three times daily.

SIDE EFFECTS   St. John's wort makes the skin more light sensitive. People with fair skin should avoid exposure to strong sunlight and other sources of ultraviolet light (such as tanning lights) when taking St. John's wort. It is also advisable to avoid tyramine-containing foods such as red wine, cheese, yeast, and pickled herring.

SAFETY ISSUES St. John's wort should not be used at the same time as prescription antidepressants. In contrast to current European monographs, it is this author's opinion that St. John's wort should not be used during pregnancy or lactation.

ST. JOHN'S wort extracts are widely used in Europe for the treatment of mild to moderate depression. Like the use of valerian and kava for anxiety, St. John's wort offers a gentler and less toxic alternative to many prescription antidepressants. For persons with milder forms of depression, this herbal treatment offers a logical alternative to drugs, such as Prozac, that are being overprescribed in the United States. St. John's wort also offers a suitable option for people, in the recovery phase of a program for depression, who wish to work with their doctor on stopping stronger prescription antidepressants.

PLANT FACTS

St. John's wort, also known as *Hypericum perforatum,* is a shrubby perennial plant with numerous bright yellow flowers. Close examination of the flowers reveals small black dots. When rubbed between the fingers, these produce a red stain. This red pigment contains the constituent hypericin. Held up to the light, the leaves of the plant display a number of bright, translucent dots. This perforated look led to the Latin name *perforatum.*[1]

St. John's wort is found in dry, gravelly soil and grows best in sunny areas. It is native to many parts of the world, including Europe and the United States. It is especially abundant in northern California and southern Oregon. Modern herbal preparations are made from flowering tops of the plant.

HISTORY

St. John's wort has a long and colorful history. Dioscorides, the foremost physician of ancient Greece, as well as Pliny and Hippocrates, recommended the herb for a host of ailments, including sciatica, and for the treatment of poisonous reptile bites. The Latin name *Hypericum* derives from the Greek and means "over an apparition"—a reference to the belief that the herb was so obnoxious to evil spirits that a whiff of it would cause them to quickly depart the premises. Early English lore suggests that the flowers could protect one from the "evil eye," and would banish witches.

The name "St. John's wort" has its origins in Christian folk traditions. One belief held that the red spots appeared on the leaves during the anniversary of St. John's beheading and symbolized his blood. Another legend asserted that if you slept with a piece of the plant under your pillow the saint himself would appear in a dream, bless you, and prevent some loved one from dying the following year. Whether he gave any odds on the Battle of Hastings is open to speculation.

St. John's wort has a long history of medical use in Europe. It was, and continues to be, very popular for the topical treatment of wounds and burns. It has also been used as a folk remedy for kidney and lung ailments as well as depression.[2]

MEDICALLY ACTIVE CONSTITUENTS

St. John's wort has a complex and diverse chemical make-up. Hypericin and pseudohypericin have received the most attention, because of their contributions to both the antidepressive and antiviral properties of St. John's wort.[3] That's why in Europe, most modern St. John's wort extracts are standardized to contain measured amounts of hypericin. Recent research indicates that other constituents, such as xanthones and flavonoids, contribute to the medicinal actions of St. John's wort.[4]

HOW ST. JOHN'S WORT WORKS

Antidepressive Actions

St. John's wort inhibits the enzyme monoamine oxidase (MAO). Monoamine oxidase is responsible for the breakdown of two brain chemicals: serotonin and norepinephrine. Norepinephrine acts as a brain stimulant. By inhibiting MAO and increasing norepinephrine, St. John's wort exerts a mild antidepressive action.[5]

More powerful MAO inhibitors are available for the treatment of depression. One example is Nardil. These prescription MAO inhibitors are much stronger than St. John's wort and more likely to cause side effects.

The MAO-inhibiting actions of St. John's wort were originally thought to be due to hypericin.[6] We now know that hypericin does not act alone. Like many herbal medicines, St. John's wort relies on the complex interplay of many constituents for its antidepressant actions.[7]

Antiviral Activity

Hypericin and pseudohypericin are the undisputed champs when it comes to antiviral activity. Experimental studies have found that these constituents exhibit strong antiviral activity against herpes simplex virus types 1 and 2 (the viruses that cause herpes sores on the mouth and genitals) and two different flu viruses (influenza virus types A and B).[8] Hypericin has also shown strong antiviral activity against Epstein-Barr virus.[9] This is the virus that causes mononucleosis. It also has weak antiviral activity against a member of the hepatitis B virus family, duck hepatitis B virus (I think Donald Duck was the test case).[10]

In 1988, hypericin and pseudohypericin drew attention when a report by researchers at New York University Medical Center and the Weizmann Institute of Science (Rehovot, Israel) showed that these constituents could inhibit the activity of animal retroviruses.[11] Since human immunodeficiency virus (HIV) is also a retrovirus, focus quickly shifted to hypericin's effect on the viral cause of acquired immunodeficiency virus (AIDS).

The research team demonstrated that hypericin has the ability (in test tubes) to prevent uninfected T lymphocytes (the cells of the immune system targeted by HIV) from being infected by HIV.[12] In addition, the action of hypericin was found to be different from that of drugs currently popular for treating HIV—AZT and ddI.[13]

Human studies are currently underway with isolated hypericin as an antiviral treatment for HIV infection.

Wound Healing and Antibacterial Properties

Oil-based preparations of St. John's wort are recommended for the topical treatment of burns and wounds. Its antibacterial actions are one factor assisting with wound healing.[14,15]

HEALTH CARE APPLICATIONS

Depression

The diagnosis and treatment of depression can be a very complex process. If you choose to use a mild antidepressant such as St. John's wort, be sure it is part of a complete program that includes a sound nutritional program, exercise, and counseling.

A small, pilot study[16] with fifteen depressed women, ages 55 to 65 years, provided a starting point for further studies investigating the use of St. John's wort for depression. The study used a standardized extract supplying a daily dose of 1.0 milligram of hypericin. The patients showed improvements in mood, sleep, and feelings of self-worth. No side effects were reported.

Two recent studies have looked at larger numbers of patients. The first compared the effects of St. John's wort with those of a placebo in fifty depressed patients. The extract supplied 1.0 milligram of hypericin daily and was administered for 8 weeks. Patients receiving St. John's wort showed a remarkable improvement in mood and ability to carry out their daily routine. Again, no side effects were noted.[17]

The second study examined the effect of 900 milligrams of a St. John's wort extract (supplying 2.7 milligrams of hypericin daily) in 105 persons with mild to moderate depression. After only 2 weeks, the group taking St. John's wort showed notable improvement. Symptoms such as feelings of sadness, hopelessness, worthlessness, exhaustion, and poor sleep decreased throughout the 4-week study.[18]

St. John's wort extracts are effective over longer treatment periods. However, like any medication being used for depression, it should not be thought of as a cure or as a substitute for life-style modifications that will result in long-term change.

HIV Infection/AIDS

It is often the case that a plant constituent can look awfully darn good in the test tube and then fail miserably when people use it. This seems to be the story with St. John's wort for treatment of HIV infection.

The research at New York University Medical Center led to the widespread use by HIV-infected individuals of St. John's wort extracts with small, measured amounts of hypericin. Early reports in *AIDS Treatment News* indicated some success.[19,20]

However, more extensive studies[21,22] proved disappointing. A major frustration was the inability to pinpoint the suitable dose necessary for an anti-HIV effect. The major effect noted was a decrease in depression! One side effect noted with high doses of St. John's wort was an elevation in liver enzymes (an indication of liver toxicity) in some individuals.

Clinical studies have shifted from a standardized extract to a highly purified hypericin. Studies in Boston, Minneapolis, and New York are using an intravenous preparation of hypericin at very high doses. It remains to be seen how these studies will come out. In the meantime, it appears that standardized St. John's wort extracts do not possess an anti-HIV effect.

Other Viral Conditions

A similar dilemma exists with the use of St. John's wort as a prevention or treatment of other viral illnesses. Are we achieving an effect with an extract that provides relatively low amounts of hypericin? I have chosen to make the leap of faith (no, I haven't had a visit from St. John recently) in treating two conditions: herpes and mononucleosis.

The extract seems to be of particular value in persons with mononucleosis. I've noticed quicker recovery and a return of energy in mononucleosis patients using St. John's wort.

HOW TO USE ST. JOHN'S WORT

For treatment of depression, you should use an extract providing at least 1.0 milligram of hypericin daily. For children between 6 and 12 years old, I recommend half the adult dose. This means you're going to have to take your calculator to the store. St. John's wort extracts can vary in hypericin content from 0.14 to 0.5 percent hypericin. Please note that current research is pointing to a St. John's wort extract containing 0.3 percent hypericin for treatment of depression. The daily dose is 900 milligrams in three divided doses. As an antidepressant, St. John's wort should be monitored for 4 to 6 weeks to check effectiveness.

I prefer to err on the side of safety: my current dosage recommendation for persons using the extract for treatment of mononucleosis or as a prevention or treatment program for herpes is the same as that used for depression.

Hypericin makes the skin more sensitive to sunlight and other sources of ultraviolet light, such as sun lamps. In the 1970s, the U.S. Food and Drug Administration (FDA) put an "unsafe" label on St. John's wort. This proved to be overkill. Their warning was based on grazing animals who had consumed huge amounts of St. John's wort and developed a blistering skin disease.[23] The FDA failed to consider the fact that the hypericin content of most St. John's wort extracts is quite low and that most consumers are not "grazing." Skin reactions to St. John's wort have not been reported at the dosages recommended in this chapter. However, if you have fair skin, minimize your sunlight exposure while using St. John's wort.

Even though St. John's wort is a mild MAO inhibitor, we should pay attention to harmful interactions that stronger MAO inhibitors may have. This includes avoiding smoked or pickled foods and alcoholic beverages (especially red wine). I do not recommend the use of St. John's wort with other antidepressants.

The German Commission E monograph for St. John's wort lists no contraindications to its use during pregnancy and lactation.[24] However, I'd like to see a few more safety studies completed on this herb before agreeing. I also do not recommend administering St. John's wort to children under the age of 2 years.

RELATED CONDITIONS DISCUSSED IN PART 6

- Chronic fatigue syndrome
- Cold sores
- Depression
- Vitiligo

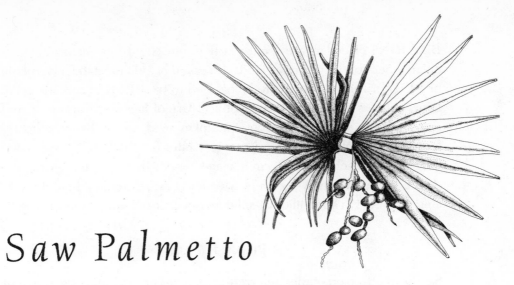

Saw Palmetto

BOTANICAL NAMES   *Serenoa repens, Sabal serrulata*
PART USED   The berries of the plant

COMMON USES
- Benign prostatic hyperplasia (BPH)
- Chronic nonbacterial prostatitis

ACTIVE CONSTITUENTS   Free fatty acids and esters in the berry

HOW IT WORKS   The lipophilic (fat-soluble) extract of saw palmetto berries reduces prostate size by reducing the amount of dihydrotestosterone and estrogen in the prostate. It also discourages the actions of inflammatory substances that contribute to BPH.

RECOMMENDED USE   Take 320 milligrams daily of a lipophilic extract rich in the fatty acids from the berry. This can be taken all at once, or in two separate doses.

SIDE EFFECTS   Side effects are rare with use of the lipophilic extract. Mild gastrointestinal disturbances have been reported on rare occasions.

SAFETY ISSUES   There are no known contraindications to long-term use of saw palmetto extract. There are no known interactions with commonly prescribed drugs. Use of any medication for BPH should begin only after accurate medical diagnosis and under the supervision of a health care professional.

BILLIONS of dollars are spent yearly in our country to manage benign enlargement of the prostate gland, also called benign prostatic hyperplasia or BPH. In Europe, herbs are being used to treat BPH, a condition that largely affects men over 50 years of age. Use of herbal extracts prepared from pygeum bark, nettle root, pumpkin seed oil, and saw palmetto berries has resulted in a drop in surgery rates for BPH and a more cost-efficient approach to long-term management of the condition. Without a doubt, the most widely recommended and best researched herbal medicine for BPH is a lipophilic (fat-soluble) extract from saw palmetto berries.

PLANT FACTS

Saw palmetto (sometimes referred to as *Sabal* in Europe) is a native of North America. Primarily found in Florida, Georgia, Louisiana, and South Carolina, it is a member of the fan palm family. Also known by the Latin names *Serenoa repens* and *Sabal serrulata*, it grows to approximately 10 feet with leaf clusters that grow to 2 feet or more. The plant produces a brownish-black berry. These berries are harvested and used in the preparation of modern lipophilic medicinal extracts.[1]

HISTORY

In the early part of this century, saw palmetto berry tea was commonly recommended for BPH by health care professionals. It was also used to treat chronic urinary tract infections. The berry was also thought to increase sperm production and increase sex drive in men, and became a popular tonic for males. The tea was listed in the National Formulary of the United States until the 1950s. As with many herbal medicines, it was deleted as a therapeutic option by the U.S. medical community.[2]

MODERN DEVELOPMENT OF SAW PALMETTO

On the basis of the above-mentioned use for BPH, French researchers in the 1960s began to examine the chemical composition of the saw palmetto berry. They found that the berry contained about 1.5 percent oil and that this fraction was high in free fatty acids. This led to work on isolation of the fatty acid portion of the berry and its ethyl ester and sterol content.[3]

The real breakthrough came with the development of a lipophilic extract of saw palmetto berries known as Permixon. *Lipophilic* means that the fat-soluble portion of the fruit is used medicinally. Lipophilic extracts of the berry are rich in fatty acids and sterols. Extracts using ethanol in the extraction process are also high in medicinally active esters. Lipophilic extracts of saw palmetto berries are currently approved by both the French and German governments for the treatment of BPH.

A BRIEF PRIMER ON BENIGN PROSTATIC HYPERPLASIA

Benign prostatic hyperplasia is a nonmalignant enlargement of the prostate. It can start in men as young as 40 years of age. However, symptoms usually do not develop until after the age of 50. According to U.S. estimates, the incidence of BPH in men 40 to 59 years of age is 50 to 60 percent. Treatment of BPH costs about $1 billion annually.[4]

Enlargement of the prostate leads to a narrowing of the outlet of the bladder, known as the urethra. This results in poor urine flow out of the bladder and a host of other signs and symptoms. Please see "Male Health Conditions" in Part 6 for a more detailed discussion of BPH.

It is believed that dihydrotestosterone (DHT), an extremely active form of testosterone, is the culprit behind prostate enlargement. High DHT levels have been found in the prostate tissue of men with BPH.[5] High levels are also associated with increased risk of prostate cancer.

A closer look reveals the real cause of high DHT levels. An enzyme known as 5-α-reductase (5-AR) converts testosterone to DHT. The activity of 5-AR increases as men age and appears to have a major influence in the development of the disease.[6]

Other hormones may also contribute to the development of BPH. These include estrogen, progesterone, and prolactin.

HOW SAW PALMETTO WORKS

Saw palmetto extract has been shown to reduce dihydrotestosterone (DHT) in prostate tissue by blocking the action of 5-α-reductase. It also blocks the binding of DHT to prostate cells.[7–9]

Recently, some herbal publications have compared the effects of saw palmetto extract and the drug Proscar. This recently approved drug for BPH also inhibits 5-α-reductase. Saw palmetto is clearly not as strong as 5-α-reductase inhibitor.[10] However, recent clinical studies in Europe have shown saw palmetto extract to be equally effective in the treatment of BPH and with fewer side effects. This is a classic example of how herbal medicines often differ from drugs. Drugs are often based on an aggressive model of manipulating one pathway or system in the body. Most herbal medicines act more gently and affect different pathways simultaneously.

The extract also reduces the effects of estrogen and progesterone on the prostate.[11] It also inhibits the effect of inflammatory substances.[12]

Collectively, these actions make the lipophilic extract of saw palmetto berry one of the most effective and comprehensive long-term medical interventions for BPH.

HEALTH CARE APPLICATIONS

The goal of any long-term therapy for BPH is to reduce the size of the prostate. This leads to relief from the common signs and symptoms of BPH such as increased frequency of urination, increased nighttime urination, dribbling after urination (that's urine, not basketballs!), decreased force and stream of urine flow, and painful urination. Numerous clinical trials have demonstrated that saw palmetto extract is effective in the management of these symptoms, with virtually no side effects. It's also a whole heck of a lot cheaper than the drugs commonly prescribed for BPH!

Optimally, men with BPH should be followed for at least 6 to 9 months to determine whether a medication is truly working on reducing BPH. While many of the early studies with saw palmetto were relatively brief, recently published studies have extended the period of observation to 6 to

12 months. Collectively, they have established saw palmetto as a safe and effective treatment for mild to moderate BPH.

The short-term studies, however, do indicate that there is a fairly quick response to saw palmetto. One 28-day study[13] with 110 BPH patients found 320 milligrams daily was effective in reducing painful urination (dysuria), nighttime urination (nocturia), and posturination residue in the bladder. There was also a significant improvement in urine flow rate. Forty-seven patients were then followed for 15 to 30 months and were found to have continued improvement.

Another study found a 43 percent increase in urine flow rate after only 60 days of treatment with 320 milligrams of saw palmetto extract daily.[14] In a 12-week study, saw palmetto compared favorably with the drug Prazosin, another commonly prescribed medication for BPH.[15] Finally, researchers followed 305 BPH patients taking 160 milligrams of saw palmetto extract twice daily.[16] At the end of 90 days, 88 percent of the patients rated the treatment a success. Their physician's evaluation was equally favorable. Urinary flow rate improved significantly and there was a notable decrease in prostate size.

A handful of studies, now completed, have monitored the effect of saw palmetto administered for 6 months or more. A 1-year study in Hungary[17] found that 320 milligrams of saw palmetto extract daily led to a reduction in residual urine (the urine left in the bladder after urination), and an increase in urinary flow rates. These results were clinically significant by the sixth month of treatment. A 6-month trial using the same daily dosage successfully reduced BPH symptoms in 24 patients.[18]

Two recent studies[19,20] have used a combination of saw palmetto extract and nettle root to treat BPH. These have been impressive because of the large number of patients followed in the first study and the head-to-head comparison with Proscar in the second.

The first study[19] followed 2,080 BPH patients for 12 weeks. Men in the study were treated with a combination of saw palmetto extract (160 milligrams) and urtica (stinging nettle) root extract (120 milligrams) twice daily. The saw palmetto/urtica combination produced a 26 percent increase in maximum urinary flow, 44.7 percent reduction in residual urine,

62.5 percent reduction in painful urination, 53.6 percent reduction in posturination dribbling, and 50 percent reduction in nighttime urination.

In early 1995, a 1-year study comparing the saw palmetto and nettle root combination with Proscar reached its halfway point.[20] Analysis of patients taking either saw palmetto/nettle root (at the dosage used above) or Proscar (5 milligrams daily) showed equal improvement in both groups after 6 months of treatment. This study, which is due to be completed in late 1995, is another step in establishing saw palmetto as a safe and cost-effective alternative to the drugs being used to treat BPH.

HOW TO USE SAW PALMETTO

The lipophilic extract of saw palmetto berries, rich in fatty acids and sterols, is recommended for BPH and chronic nonbacterial prostatitis. The recommended daily dose is 320 milligrams, taken either once daily or in two divided doses. I usually tell patients to use the extract for 4 to 6 weeks to determine its effectiveness. If it's working for you at that point, plan on it being a part of your ongoing, daily supplement regimen. Optimally, this decision should be made with the advice of a health care professional.

No significant side effects have been noted in clinical studies with saw palmetto extracts. It is important to understand that BPH can be diagnosed only by a physician. You should use saw palmetto extract only after a thorough work-up and diagnosis by your doctor.

RELATED CONDITION DISCUSSED IN PART 6

- Benign prostatic hyperplasia

Valerian

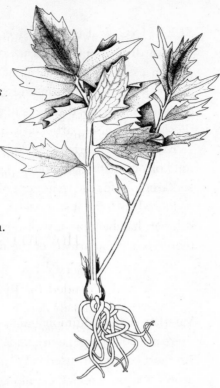

BOTANICAL NAME *Valeriana officinalis*

PART USED The root

COMMON USES
- Insomnia
- Mild anxiety and conditions of restlessness

ACTIVE CONSTITUENTS Not yet known. Constituents of the essential oil component portion of the root (e.g., valerenic acid) are commonly used as markers for quality control during extraction.

HOW IT WORKS Valerian root exerts a mild sedating effect on the central nervous system. It improves the ability of a person to get to sleep and sleep more soundly.

RECOMMENDED USE Concentrated root extract containing no less than 0.5 percent essential oils—300 to 400 milligrams once or twice daily

SIDE EFFECTS Research has indicated minimal side effects using valerian. A small percentage of persons using the extract may experience mild, transient stomach upset.

SAFETY ISSUES Persons currently taking sedative drugs or antidepressants should take valerian only under the supervision of a health care professional. European monographs list no contraindication to use of valerian root during pregnancy or lactation. Valerian does not lead to dependence or potential addiction. Valerian will not impair your ability to drive or operate machinery.

SLEEPING well is an elusive goal for millions of Americans. While a class of drugs known as benzodiazepines (e.g., Valium and Xanax) have proven useful in the treatment of severe cases of insomnia and anxiety, they can cause addiction and serious side effects, including withdrawal symptoms. Clearly, there is a need for gentler, nonaddictive medicines for these conditions—particularly in less severe forms of these conditions.

Extracts of valerian root, often in combination with one or two other mild plant sedatives, are often prescribed in Europe as a substitute for benzodiazepines for the treatment of insomnia and sometimes mild anxiety.

Paired with the historical use of the plant in our country for insomnia, valerian has become a well-researched herbal sedative that promises to increase in popularity over the next decade.

PLANT FACTS

Valerian is the common name given to the genus *Valeriana*, of which there are 200 species worldwide. In herbal medicine, the species of valerian most commonly used is *Valeriana officinalis*, an upright perennial that grows wild in woodlands, along river banks, and in damp meadows all over Europe. Most of the plants used for medicinal extracts are cultivated. As mentioned above, the root of the plant has the sedating properties and is used in herbal preparations.

HISTORY

Our old friend and Greek physician Dioscorides rears his herbal head again! He recommended valerian for a host of medical problems including digestive problems, nausea, liver problems, and even urinary tract disorders. Galen (131–201 A.D.) was the first to note the use of valerian as a treatment for insomnia.

Use of valerian for insomnia and nervous conditions gained momentum in the late sixteenth century. By the eighteenth century, it was an accepted sedative and was also used for nervous disorders associated with a restless digestive tract. It was also recommended for a nervous condition in women, referred to as "vapors." This label referred to a hysterical condition involving noises in the head, chills, impatience, and involuntary movements.[1] Use of the label faded away when they figured it was the sexist doctors who were really full of vapors—primarily hot air!

Valerian was listed in medical textbooks in both the United States and England until the 1940s. Currently, it is an approved over-the-counter medicine for insomnia in Germany, Belgium, France, Switzerland, and Italy.[2]

MODERN DEVELOPMENT

Research in Europe led to the discovery that the root of valerian contains oils that may contribute to the sedating properties of the plant. Even though research has pointed to the contribution of constituents known as valepotriates, most European medicinal preparations currently focus on essential oil content and constituents of the oil such as valerenic acid. This is partially because valepotriates are very unstable chemicals and are probably not very active in the body. Also, alcohol extracts of valerian contain minimal amounts of these compounds. According to the standards developed in herbal monographs, the current concentrated extracts contain a minimum essential oil content of 0.5 percent.[3]

Combining valerian root with other mildly sedating herbs is common both in Europe and the United States. Chamomile, hops, passion flower, and lemon balm are popular choices. Another popular development in Europe has been the creation of odor-controlled valerian root products. For those of you who have had the pleasure of smelling the typical valerian root product, the applause is deafening. For those of you who don't now what I'm talking about, let me just say three words: "old gym socks."

HOW VALERIAN WORKS

Even though studies in the early to mid-1980s found valerian to be an effective treatment for insomnia, no one really knew why it worked. This changed in 1989 when J. Holzl and P. Godau of the Institute of Pharmaceutical Biology (Marburg, Germany) demonstrated that valerian weakly binds the same receptors in the brain as benzodiazepines. In test tube studies, they found that valerian displaced benzodiazepines off these receptor sites.[4]

A follow-up study was able to show that constituents of valerian root actually bind GABA-A receptors (okay, we're going to stop the snooze-inducing scientific facts soon!).[5] Sedation in the central nervous system and brain is regulated by these receptors. Benzodiazepines and barbiturates act on these receptors.

Before you drag this book to the fireplace for recommending something that acts like benzodiazepines and barbiturates, let me finish! The active compounds in valerian *weakly* bind these receptors when compared to drugs like Valium and Xanax. While this activity helps us to at least partially understand valerian's action as a sedative, it still lets valerian off the hook as a potential addictive substance. This also makes it an intriguing therapeutic choice for those trying to withdraw from benzodiazepines.

HEALTH CARE APPLICATIONS

Insomnia

Population surveys have found that approximately one-third of the adult population suffers from initial sleep disorders.[6] While famous insomniacs like Philip Marlowe have turned the condition to their advantage, most people suffer in their personal and professional lives when sleep deprived.

Valerian root makes getting to sleep easier. It increases deep sleep as well as dreaming. Best of all, it doesn't cause any morning "hangover"—a side effect common to prescription sleep drugs.

In the early to mid-1980s, research completed at the Nestlé Research Laboratories in Switzerland proved the ability of valerian to help a person both get to sleep easier and have a deeper, more restful night's sleep. Bedtime valerian doses of 400 to 450 milligrams helped participants get to sleep quicker and reduced night awakenings. Dream recall was also increased the following day with no morning hangover.[7,8]

Unfortunately, chocolate won out and the jingle "N-E-S-T-L-E-S, Nestlé makes the very best valerian" was never heard.

Recent studies have shown similar results using valerian combined with other herbs. A Swedish study examined the effect of a valerian root combined with lemon balm and hops (in a capsule, not a beer bottle!). Twenty-seven people with sleep disorders were given either one tablet of the combination product (containing 400 milligrams of valerian root) or a weaker preparation containing only 4 milligrams of valerian. Eighty-nine percent of the people taking the full-strength combination reported better sleep; 44 percent reported "perfect" sleep.[9] Nightmares, frequent among many of the patients previously taking prescription sedatives, were nonexistent.

A German study[10] compared the effect of a combination product containing an extract of valerian root (320 milligrams at bedtime) and extract of lemon balm (*Melissa officinalis*) with the benzodiazepine Halcion. Sleep was monitored for 9 nights. The herbal duo matched Halcion in boosting the ability to get to sleep, as well as quality of sleep. However, the Halcion group reported the old hangover and loss of concentration the next day. People taking the valerian/lemon balm combination reported no negative effect on their daily routine.

On the basis of these reports and regular medical use, valerian has become the natural medicine treatment of choice for people suffering from insomnia both in Europe and the United States. Valerian's nonaddictive properties make it a logical alternative to the potentially addictive drugs commonly recommended for sleep in this country.

Anxiety

It's hard to avoid stress and the anxiety it breeds in our culture. Successfully dealing with anxiety includes stress reduction, proper diet, and support for the adrenal glands. In recent years valerian and kava have emerged as herbal alternatives for the treatment of less severe cases of anxiety.

Although anxiety reduction is not currently listed as a therapeutic use for valerian in the German Commission E monograph, it regularly wins recommendations from physicians and pharmacists. Valerian appears to be safe and effective in the early treatment of anxiety as well as in the long-term management of those unable to use or attempting to withdraw from benzodiazepines.[11] Kava is another primary herbal prescription in this area.

Valerian can be used during the day as well as night for anxiety. The daytime dosage is typically somewhat lower than the nighttime dosage used for sleep. Use of valerian during withdrawal from benzodiazepines should be done only under the supervision of a health care professional.

HOW TO USE VALERIAN

For insomnia, 300 to 500 milligrams of valerian root 1 hour before bedtime is recommended. Try to use extracts that contain at least 0.5 percent essential oils. Combination products with lemon balm, hops, and scullcap can also be used. Children ranging in age from 6 to 12 years will usually respond to one-half the adult dose. Consult a health care professional before administering valerian to young children.

For mild anxiety, a morning dose of 150 to 300 milligrams is recommended in addition to the bedtime dosage listed above. I like to use valerian combined with passion flower for daytime management of anxiety.

The current German Commission E monograph on valerian root lists no contraindications on its use during pregnancy or lactation.[12] Avoid taking it with alcohol. Recent research indicates that valerian does not impair your ability to drive or operate machinery.[13] Valerian root products do not lead to addiction or dependence.

RELATED CONDITIONS DISCUSSED IN PART 6

- Anxiety
- Insomnia

Vitex
agnus-castus

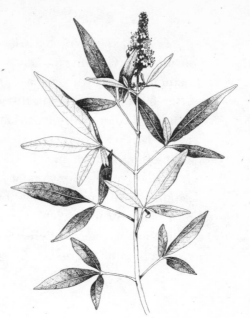

COMMON NAMES   Chaste tree, Monk's pepper

PART USED   The ripe, dried fruit

COMMON USES

- Premenstrual syndrome (PMS)
- Heavy or frequently occurring menses
- Amenorrhea (lack of menses)
- Infertility
- Hot flashes associated with peri-menopause

HOW IT WORKS   Vitex stimulates the pituitary gland to produce more luteinizing hormone. This leads to greater production of progesterone during the second half (luteal phase) of a woman's cycle. Vitex also reduces high levels of prolactin in the second half of the menstrual cycle.

RECOMMENDED USE   Forty drops of a liquid, standardized extract or one capsule of the equivalent powdered extract, once daily in the morning with some liquid. Use vitex over a period of several months continuously. Once improvement occurs, continue treatment for an additional 4 to 6 weeks.

SIDE EFFECTS   Side effects are rare using vitex. Minor gastrointestinal upset and a mild skin rash with itching has been reported in less than 2 percent of the women monitored while taking vitex.

SAFETY ISSUES   Vitex is not recommended for use during pregnancy. It should not be taken together with hormone therapy.

NATURAL therapies have made a dramatic contribution to women's health care. Growing numbers of women are opting for safe and effective natural medicines to manage gynecological conditions for which drugs offer short-term relief but threaten long-term health. This is particularly true for women with menstrual abnormalities stemming from hormonal imbalances. Nutritional and herbal interventions such as vitamin B_6, magnesium, and vitamin E, black cohosh, dong quai, and evening primrose oil offer relief for women with menstrual cycle abnormalities such as premenstrual syndrome and fibrocystic breast disease.

The unique ability of vitex to correct female hormonal imbalances in a gentle manner makes it effective against premenstrual syndrome, amenorrhea (lack of a period), and even infertility.

PLANT FACTS

Vitex agnus-castus, also known as chaste tree, is a shrub with finger-shaped leaves and slender violet flowers. The plant grows in creek beds and on river banks in valleys and lower foothills in the Mediterranean and central Asia. The plant blooms in high summer. After pollination, it develops dark-brown to black fruit the size of a pepper corn. The fruit possesses a pepper-like aroma and flavor. The ripe, dried fruit of *Vitex agnus-castus* is the part of the plant used in medicinal preparations today.

HISTORY

Vitex belongs to the official plants of antiquity (although I'm not sure whether it was ever featured on *American Bandstand*). Hippocrates, Dioscorides, and Theophrast mention the use of the plant in their writings. In the fourth century B.C., Hippocrates wrote that vitex was effective for a wide variety of conditions, including hemorrhaging following childbirth, and also assisted with the "passing of afterbirth." Decoctions of the fruit and plant were also used in sitz baths for diseases of the uterus.

Vitex was also believed to inspire chastity. This is the source of one of its common names, "chaste tree." This name partially developed from the ancient Greeks, who used it in festivals honoring the goddess Demeter. During the festival young women were expected to refrain from sexual activity and were adorned with blossoms of vitex to demonstrate their chastity.

The Christian church in Europe later developed a variation on this theme by placing the blossoms along the path leading to the monastery at the initiation of novice monks. The vitex blossoms supposedly suppressed libido and served as a deterrent to the temptation to run off to town and lose one's monkhood! This practice is said to continue in parts of Italy today.

Monks were also responsible for another common name for vitex—"monk's pepper." This name is derived from the fact that the fruits, which taste and smell like pepper, were commonly used as seasoning by the chef-in-residence at the monastery.[1]

MODERN DEVELOPMENT

Modern medical work with vitex began with the introduction of a concentrated extract of the dried vitex fruit in the 1950s. Produced by Madaus of Cologne, Germany, the extract was concentrated so that 100 ml of the solution contained 9 grams of the fruit. This is the form that has been employed in modern clinical research.

The German Commission E monograph (see Part 2 for an explanation of the German monograph system) lists the whole extract as "medicinally active."[2] This implies a cooperative effort among the different components of the fruit. Contrast this with an herbal extract such as milk thistle, which has one specific active compound.

A QUICK PRIMER ON LUTEAL PHASE DEFECT

If you are a woman with menstrual cycle irregularities or imbalances, there's a good chance you're not producing enough progesterone during the second phase of your cycle (also known as the *luteal phase*). This means that estrogen, the dominant female hormone during the first phase of the cycle (*follicular phase*), continues to dominate the second half. The result leads to a shortening (by as much as 50 percent) of the luteal phase, or "luteal phase defect."

The net effect of luteal phase defect and low progesterone production is a host of menstrual cycle abnormalities. These include heavy periods (hypermenorrhea), abnormally frequent periods (polymenorrhea), and also lack of menstruation (amenorrhea). Luteal phase defect may also contribute to premenstrual syndrome.[3]

Another problem frequently found with luteal phase defect is overproduction of the pituitary hormone prolactin. Prolactin, which assists with lactation in nursing mothers, has been shown to be abnormally elevated in 70 percent of women with luteal phase defect.[4] High levels of prolactin in the latter part of a woman's cycle can lead to breast tenderness and pain. More importantly, high levels are associated with infertility in some instances.

How Vitex Works

Vitex does not contain hormones. Its benefits stem from its actions on the pituitary gland—specifically on the production of estrogen and progesterone.[5] Vitex increases the pituitary's production of the regulating hormone luteinizing hormone (LH).[6] The LH boosts the secretion of progesterone during the luteal phase. The resulting increase in progesterone production leads to a normal balance between estrogen and progesterone and a normal two-phase cycle.

Vitex also keeps prolactin secretion in check.[7] The ability to decrease excessive prolactin levels has made it a treatment consideration for women with infertility.

Health Care Applications

Premenstrual Syndrome

Following more than 1,500 women for an average of 166 days, two surveys of gynecology practices in Germany[8,9] have shown vitex to be a valuable treatment for premenstrual syndrome (PMS).

Women were placed on a daily dose of 40 drops of a vitex liquid extract—taken once in the morning with some water. The success of treatment with vitex was determined through questionnaires given to both gynecologists and their patients. Physicians rated the treatment as very good or good 92 percent of the time. Fifty-seven percent of the patients reported improvement while another 33 percent had complete symptom relief. Mild side effects (mild upset stomach and short-term skin rash with itching) were reported in only 2 percent of the women.[8] These results have been verified in other studies with PMS sufferers.[9]

Another benefit for women taking vitex for PMS has been reduced cyclical breast pain, a result of the rise in progesterone levels.[10]

Other Menstrual Cycle Irregularities and Infertility

Research and clinical experience have also pointed to vitex as useful in a host of other menstrual cycle imbalances and irregularities. This has ranged from women with periods occurring too frequently (polymenorrhea) to women who aren't menstruating at all (amenorrhea). One study found that regular use of vitex over several periods normalized periods in women suffering from polymenorrhea. Vitex also reduces excessive bleeding during periods—a condition known as menorrhagia.[11]

At the other end of the spectrum, vitex may be used to treat women suffering from secondary amenorrhea (absence of a period after a history of normal menstruation). In one study, ten of fifteen women with secondary amenorrhea began having a normal period after 6 months of treatment with vitex. Hormone measures indicated a rise in progesterone and LH levels.[12]

Vitex has also made a significant impact in the treatment of infertility—particularly those cases with established luteal phase defect and high prolactin levels. Forty-eight women diagnosed with infertility, 23 to 39 years of age, were given vitex once daily for 3 months. Forty-five women completed the study.

Seven women became pregnant during the study. In twenty-five women progesterone levels were restored to normal—a factor that bodes well for potential pregnancy. Seven women had a rise in serum progesterone that did not reach normal levels during the 3 months of treatment. However, the upward trend in their progesterone levels probably means they'd achieve normal levels in another two to three cycles.[13,14]

High Prolactin Levels

As mentioned previously, vitex exerts a modulating effect on prolactin levels in the body. One study found that vitex was able to lower levels after 3 months of use.[15] It is interesting that the fifty-two women in this study also had luteal phase defect. A lengthening of the luteal phase and increased progesterone were also noted. No side effects were noted and two women actually became pregnant during the study.

Hot Flashes Associated with Pre- and Perimenopause

Even though there are no published clinical trials on the use of vitex for hot flashes (also known as *climacteric*) at the beginning of menopause, it is commonly recommended for this condition in Europe. The success of vitex in the treatment of this condition is believed to be due to elevated progesterone levels.

So, if you suffer from hot flashes (or "power surges" as they were called by one woman), include vitex as a potential natural therapy. After menopause, vitex should be discontinued, since there is no target organ for its actions.

HOW TO USE VITEX

With its emphasis on long-term balancing of a woman's hormonal system, vitex is not a fast-acting medication. If you have PMS or frequent or heavy periods, use vitex continuously for 4 to 6 months. Women with amenorrhea and infertility should remain on vitex for at least 12 to 18 months unless pregnancy occurs during treatment. Vitex should not be used once a woman becomes pregnant. Use of vitex with hormone therapy is not recommended.

The best news for women taking vitex is the one-a-day dosage. The recommended daily dose for the liquid extract is 40 drops in the morning with some liquid. A powdered equivalent of the liquid has been developed and is currently available in the United States. The recommended daily dose is one capsule in the morning.

RELATED CONDITIONS DISCUSSED IN PART 6

- Acne
- Fibrocystic breast disease
- Hot flashes associated with perimenopause
- Infertility
- Premenstrual syndrome

part 6

HERBAL PRESCRIPTIONS FOR COMMON HEALTH CONDITIONS

REMEMBER all that stuff I told you at the beginning of Part 5? Well, it's applicable here, too. Many of the conditions that we're about to discuss require accurate medical diagnosis and careful monitoring by your doctor. Many of them may also require a combination of standard medical treatment along with your complete natural health care plan.

This section is organized by body system. So, if you're having problems with angina look under "Cardiovascular System." If you have diabetes, refer to the appropriate section under "Endocrine System."

Each condition (with the exception of a few miscellaneous conditions) begins with a brief description and then offers herbal prescriptions to consider. The "Herbal Prescriptions" section is reserved for those herbs that I highly recommend. My recommendations are based on research and history of effective use for that particular ailment. Herbs under "Other Herbal Considerations" either support the primary herbal prescriptions or warrant some mention because of traditional use.

I've also added sections on nutritional supplements, diet, and lifestyle. The "Nutritional Supplement Considerations" section includes key vitamins, minerals, or other dietary supplements you should consider adding to your comprehensive natural health care program. I've tried to supply you with one or two key references for each recommendation. Please note that this is not intended to be a complete overview of the nutritional research literature. If you need a more complete overview, I suggest Melvyn Werbach's book, *Nutritional Influences on Illness* (Third Line Press, Tarzana, California, 1994).

A good diet and positive lifestyle changes (e.g., stress reduction and exercise) are the cornerstone of any wellness program. Although herbal treatments can play a critical part in your attempt to get well, how you eat and live your life should form the foundation of your wellness program.

Cardiovascular System

RELATED CHAPTERS IN PART 5

- Bilberry
- Evening Primrose
- Garlic
- Ginger
- *Ginkgo biloba*
- Ginseng
- Hawthorn

ATHEROSCLEROSIS (PREVENTION)

ATHEROSCLEROSIS, the primary villain in most major cardiovascular disease, contributes to angina, cerebrovascular insufficiency, congestive heart failure, and intermittent claudication. It also contributes to strokes. So, even though it's not first alphabetically, we need to talk about it first.

Let's start with arteriosclerosis. Arteriosclerosis is a hardening of the arteries. The hardening results when the arteries lose their elasticity and begin to thicken. This leads to narrowed arteries and less blood flow to many parts of the body.

When fatty plaques build up on the walls of these narrowed arteries, we call it *atherosclerosis*. If blood vessels that supply the heart (coronary arteries) become atherosclerotic, the condition is known as *coronary artery disease* (CAD). Coronary artery disease contributes to angina, congestive heart failure, and even heart attacks.

You've all been beaten over the head with some of the requirements for reducing your risk of atherosclerosis. Diet, exercise, and stress reduction all are important tools for reducing risk. Herbs, particularly those that are a common part of our normal diets, also play a key role in reducing your risk.

By altering your eating habits and lifestyle as described further on in this chapter, you'll:

- Reduce the levels of cholesterol and triglycerides in the bloodstream
- Reduce the "stickiness" of platelets in the blood
- Improve the strength of blood vessel walls
- Improve the flow of blood through the body
- Provide antioxidant protection to the cardiovascular system

The payoff: A reduced risk of atherosclerosis.

HERBS AND HERBAL CONSTITUENTS THAT REDUCE YOUR RISK OF ATHEROSCLEROSIS

Bilberry
Bioflavonoids
Evening primrose
Fenugreek
Garlic
Ginger
Ginkgo biloba
Ginseng
Gugulipid
Hawthorn
Psyllium

NUTRITIONAL SUPPLEMENTS THAT REDUCE YOUR RISK OF ATHEROSCLEROSIS

Vitamin C
Vitamin E
Vitamin B_6
Vitamin B_{12}
Folic acid

Note: Vitamins B_6, B_{12}, and folic acid reduce the level of homocysteine; a high homocysteine level is associated with increased risk of cardiovascular disease.

Niacin

Magnesium

Chromium

Selenium

Beta-carotene and other carotenoids

Coenzyme Q-10

Carnitine

Essential fatty acids (e.g., evening primrose oil and fish oil)

DIETARY RECOMMENDATIONS THAT REDUCE YOUR RISK OF ATHEROSCLEROSIS

- Increase your intake of complex carbohydrates from vegetables, grains, and fruit sources. This will provide you with more dietary fiber and valuable antioxidants.
- Reduce your dietary fat from animal sources. This includes red meat and milk. Some kinds of fats are healthier than others. Avoid heating polyunsaturated fats that may be transformed to saturated fats. A good bet is to cook with olive oil, which doesn't change when heated. The fat from fish and nuts is also preferable.
- Increase your dietary sources of the herbs listed above. These include garlic and ginger. Also, don't forget turmeric, onions, and green tea.

LIFESTYLE CONSIDERATIONS THAT WILL REDUCE YOUR RISK OF ATHEROSCLEROSIS

STRESS REDUCTION   Seek an outlet for your frustrations and anger so your cardiovascular system doesn't have to bear the brunt. Above all, try to avoid writing any lengthy herb books!

REGULAR EXERCISE   Regular exercise helps work off stress and also keeps weight down. Best of all, it strengthens and builds up the efficiency of your cardiovascular system.

ANGINA

Atherosclerosis can disrupt blood flow to many parts of the body. When it harms the arteries that supply the heart muscle (the coronary arteries), a lack of oxygen to the heart results. This leads to *angina*—a squeezing or pressure-like pain in the chest.

Angina attacks are most common during exercise, when the heart is forced to work harder. Stress can also bring on an attack. In addition to pressure in the chest, pain may radiate to the left shoulder and arm. Angina can sometimes be a warning sign of a heart attack.

Angina caused by atherosclerosis occurs most commonly; it is called *secondary angina*. Another, less common form of angina results from spasms of the coronary arteries. This is known as *primary* or *Prinzmetal's variant angina*. This form commonly occurs when a person is at rest.

When angina becomes more severe, drug therapy is usually needed. Examples are nitroglycerin, beta-blockers, and calcium channel blockers. These relieve symptoms but do not address the key problem, which is insufficient blood flow to the heart muscle.

Herbal and nutrient interventions work best in the early stages of angina. By increasing blood flow to the heart muscle and improving the work efficiency of the heart, they may actually slow the progression of angina.

HERBAL PRESCRIPTION
- Hawthorn extract (standardized to 18.75 percent oligomeric procyanidins)—160 milligrams daily in two divided doses. Individuals requiring more intensive treatment initially, should use 160 milligrams three times daily.
  Action: Increases blood flow and oxygen to the heart muscle

OTHER HERBAL CONSIDERATIONS
See the recommendations listed under "Atherosclerosis (Prevention)."

NUTRITIONAL SUPPLEMENT CONSIDERATIONS
- Coenzyme Q-10—90 to 120 milligrams daily in two to three divided doses[1]
- L-Carnitine—500 milligrams two to three times daily[2]
- Magnesium—300 milligrams twice daily[3]

DIETARY RECOMMENDATIONS

See the recommendations under "Atherosclerosis (Prevention)."

LIFESTYLE CONSIDERATIONS

Stress reduction is critical. Try yoga, meditation, or biofeedback. Settle on a method of relaxing that works for you and stick with it. I like listening to *Kind of Blue* by Miles Davis.

Regular exercise is important, but ease into it. Too much, too soon can worsen the problem. Try reducing caffeine consumption and stopping smoking.

BRUISING

If you're a perfectly healthy person who suddenly begins to develop bruises on the thighs, buttocks, or upper arms, it may be that your small blood vessels (primarily the capillaries) are fragile. It's not uncommon for people experiencing such bruising to seek the help of their doctor, only to be told that there's nothing wrong—just avoid bumping into things and take aspirin. Easy bruising does not mean you've got a terrible bleeding disorder.

Easy bruising is often more noticeable with aging. The capillaries become more fragile and pressure on the skin is more likely to create a bruise. In older individuals, these bruises may linger longer than in younger people. Again, this is not a serious medical condition.

HERBAL PRESCRIPTION

- Bilberry extract—80 to 160 milligrams three times daily
  Action: Strengthens and stabilizes the walls of the blood vessels

OTHER HERBAL CONSIDERATIONS

You can choose from a host of bioflavonoid products, including quercetin, hesperidin, and pycnogenol; these are all excellent options. Like bilberry, these compounds will assist in strengthening blood vessels.

NUTRITIONAL SUPPLEMENT CONSIDERATIONS

- Vitamin C (preferably with bioflavonoids)—1,000 milligrams twice daily

Increase your intake of blueberries and cherries. Also, increase your consumption of foods high in bioflavonoids, such as green tea, onions, and apples.

CEREBROVASCULAR INSUFFICIENCY

Cerebrovascular insufficiency means there's not enough blood flow getting to the brain. Reduced blood flow to the brain can lead to depression, memory loss, and disorientation.[1] Symptoms associated with cerebrovascular insufficiency[2] include:

Difficulty with concentration and memory
Absentmindedness
Confusion
Lack of energy and fatigue
Decreased physical performance
Depression
Anxiety
Dizziness
Tinnitus (ringing in the ears)
Headaches

Cerebrovascular insufficiency is commonly associated with arteriosclerosis. As noted in the chapter on ginkgo in Part 5, the condition is believed to play a role in Alzheimer's disease and senility associated with old age.

HERBAL PRESCRIPTION

- *Ginkgo biloba* extract—240 milligrams daily in two to three divided doses. Once improvement is noted, this can be reduced to 120 milligrams daily as a maintenance dose
  Actions: Improves blood flow to the brain. It also exerts a protective effect on the brain and central nervous system

NUTRITIONAL SUPPLEMENT CONSIDERATIONS[3]

- Vitamin B_6—50 milligrams daily
- Vitamin B_{12}—1,000 micrograms daily
- Folic acid—800 micrograms daily
- Vitamin E—800 international units (IU) daily

DIETARY RECOMMENDATIONS

See the recommendations listed under "Atherosclerosis (Prevention)."

CONGESTIVE HEART FAILURE

When a weakened heart fails to provide adequate blood flow to the extremities of the body, the condition is called *congestive heart failure* (CHF). A number of factors can lead to CHF, including a history of heart attack(s). As the condition progresses, fluid can accumulate in the lungs and around the ankles. Once the condition reaches this stage, the prognosis is poor.

The New York Heart Association has defined four stages of CHF. Medical treatment is usually reserved for stages III and IV. Digitalis is a common treatment in these later stages. Table 6.1 lists the four stages and their characteristics.

Table 6.1
STAGES OF CONGESTIVE HEART FAILURE AS DEFINED
BY THE NEW YORK HEART ASSOCIATION

Stage	Symptoms
Stage I	Patient is symptom free when at rest and on treatment
Stage II	Patient experiences impaired heart function with moderate physical effort. Shortness of breath with exertion is common. There are no symptoms at rest
Stage III	Even minor physical exertion results in shortness of breath and fatigue. There are no symptoms at rest
Stage IV	Symptoms such as shortness of breath and fluid around the ankles (edema) are present when the patient is at rest

How about stages I and II? Typically, treatment is not recommended during these stages, owing to the potential side effects of digitalis. This is where herbal and nutritional interventions play an important role. By improving the heart's efficiency in supplying blood to the body and by enhancing circulation to the extremities, natural medicines offer an opportunity to slow the progression of CHF and improve a person's quality of life.

HERBAL PRESCRIPTION

- Hawthorn extract (standardized to 18.75 percent oligomeric procyanidins)—160 milligrams daily in two divided doses. Individuals requiring more intensive treatment initially, should use 160 milligrams three times daily.

  Actions: Hawthorn improves the efficiency of the heart muscle. This means greater blood flow throughout the body. It also reduces the resistance to blood flow in the blood vessels of the extremities of the body.

NUTRITIONAL SUPPLEMENT CONSIDERATIONS

- Coenzyme Q-10—60 to 100 milligrams daily in two divided doses[1]
- L-Carnitine—500 milligrams two to three times daily[2]
- Taurine—2 grams three times daily[3]

DIETARY RECOMMENDATIONS

See the recommendations listed under "Atherosclerosis (Prevention)."

HYPERCHOLESTEROLEMIA (HIGH CHOLESTEROL)

A high cholesterol level usually triggers atherosclerosis. Usually, when we talk about a high cholesterol level, we're also talking about high levels of another set of fats in the blood known as *triglycerides*.

In western culture, the primary culprit causing high cholesterol is diet. The atherosclerosis prevention program outlined earlier is intended to prevent high cholesterol. Incorporate those recommendations into your cholesterol-lowering program.

A small percentage of people are genetically predetermined to have high cholesterol and triglycerides. Because their levels of blood fats can rise to dangerous heights, an aggressive cholesterol-lowering drug (e.g., Mevacor) is sometimes best at first. Following a drop in cholesterol and triglycerides, long-term treatment should focus on gentler medications, such as garlic, and the atherosclerosis prevention program outlined earlier.

HERBAL PRESCRIPTIONS
- Garlic—Tablets providing at least 5,000 micrograms of allicin daily in two divided doses
  Actions: Lowers cholesterol and triglycerides while raising high-density lipoprotein (HDL)-cholesterol levels. Garlic also reduces platelet stickiness and improves blood flow
- Gugulipid (*Commiphora mukul*)—Extract standardized to provide 25 milligrams of guggulsterones three times daily
  Action: Standardized extract of an ancient Ayurvedic herbal remedy (the name is easily pronounced by two-year-olds). It lowers cholesterol and triglycerides in a manner comparable to clofibrate. It also raises the HDL-cholesterol level and reduces platelet stickiness[1]

OTHER HERBAL CONSIDERATIONS
- Fenugreek seed—4 to 5 grams three times daily[2]

NUTRITIONAL SUPPLEMENT CONSIDERATIONS
- Niacin—1 to 3 grams daily in two to three divided doses[3]
  Note: Research indicates that the immediate-release form of niacin is the safest. Time-release forms are more likely to cause harm to the liver. However, immediate-release niacin can cause severe flushing in some individuals that can be quite uncomfortable.
      Even with use of immediate-release niacin you should have your liver enzymes checked by your doctor every few months. I will often recommend milk thistle extract with niacin therapy to add some liver protection

- Chromium—200 micrograms twice daily
- Vitamin E—400 to 800 IU daily

DIETARY RECOMMENDATIONS

See the recommendations listed under "Atherosclerosis (Prevention)."

INTERMITTENT CLAUDICATION

Atherosclerosis can also harm blood flow to the extremities, causing poor oxygen supply to the muscles. This often results in a condition known as *intermittent claudication,* characterized by pain or aching in the calf muscles on exertion. It is relieved by rest but returns as soon as exercise begins again. As the condition becomes more severe, the pain limits a person's walking distance.

Treatment of intermittent claudication in its early stages can prevent the condition from worsening. It will also allow greater freedom to exercise and help you maintain an active lifestyle.

HERBAL PRESCRIPTIONS

- *Ginkgo biloba* extract—120 to 160 milligrams daily in two to three divided doses
  Action: Improves blood flow to the extremities
- Garlic (standardized to allicin potential)—Tablets providing at least 5,000 micrograms of allicin daily in two divided doses
  Action: Makes platelets less sticky, which results in more efficient blood flow

OTHER HERBAL CONSIDERATIONS

- Padma 28—560 milligrams twice daily[1] (Padma 28 is a combination of 28 herbs and is based on an ancient Tibetan formula)

NUTRITIONAL SUPPLEMENT CONSIDERATIONS

- Vitamin E—400 to 800 IU daily[2]
- Inositol nicotinate—2 grams twice daily[3]

Note: This form of niacin will not cause flushing. However, your doctor should monitor your liver enzymes while you are taking the high dose recommended

- L-Carnitine—2 grams twice daily[4]

DIETARY RECOMMENDATIONS
See the recommendations listed under "Atherosclerosis (Prevention)."

LIFESTYLE CONSIDERATIONS
Don't stop exercising! You should try to walk at least an hour daily. When the pain starts, stop walking, allow it to disappear, and then resume walking. The distance you are able to walk pain-free tells you how successfully your treatment program is progressing.

RAYNAUD'S DISEASE

Raynaud's disease is characterized by a spasm of the midsized blood vessels, known as *arterioles*, in the hands. This interrupts blood flow to the fingers and causes a loss of color in the hands. Raynaud's disease is not usually painful but leads to a lack of sensation in the hands. It's triggered by exposure to cold or by emotional upsets. Color and sensation will return to the hands after they are warmed up. It usually affects both hands and is most common in younger women.

A related condition, Raynaud's phenomenon, is often due to connective tissue diseases such as scleroderma, lupus, and rheumatoid arthritis. Other conditions associated with the nervous and cardiovascular system can also contribute to Raynaud's phenomenon. This condition frequently involves only one hand. The herbal approach to treatment is similar with both forms.

HERBAL PRESCRIPTION
- *Ginkgo biloba* extract—120 to 160 milligrams daily in two to three divided doses[1]
  Actions: Improves circulation to the extremities and has a mild dilating effect on the blood vessels

- Evening primrose oil—4 to 6 grams daily with meals in two divided doses[2]

  Action: Reduces prostaglandins, which may contribute to vasospasm and inflammation

NUTRITIONAL SUPPLEMENT CONSIDERATIONS
- Vitamin E—400 to 800 IU daily
- Inositol nicotinate—2 grams twice daily[3]

VARICOSE VEINS

Healthy veins return blood from the extremities to the heart, where it is reoxygenated and recycled to the body. When the elastic walls of the veins break down, the veins become dilated. Dilated veins lose the ability to block backflow of blood. When this occurs, blood pools in the extremities and leads to complications such as thrombophlebitis (inflammation of veins associated with a blood clot).

Varicose veins usually occur in the veins closest to the surface of the skin. This causes a rather unsightly bulging in the back of the legs. Varicose veins can also cause aching and a feeling of heaviness in the legs.

Varicose veins most commonly affect women past 50 years of age. However, they can also occur during pregnancy. This is most likely to happen during the third trimester, when gravity and baby pull blood flow toward terra firma. Obesity also increases your chances of developing varicose veins.

Treatment for varicose veins includes:

- Improving the tone of the walls of the veins
- Reducing the pooling of blood that contributes to swelling
- Improving circulation through the veins

HERBAL PRESCRIPTIONS
- Horse chestnut extract—Standardized extract delivering 150 milligrams of aescin (the active constituent of horse chestnut) daily in three divided doses. This should be used in conjunction with a topical

aescin gel preparation. Apply the gel to the affected area three to four times daily[1]

Action: Reduces the breakdown of the walls of the veins and adds tone for more efficient blood flow. The topical gel adds an astringent action (see "Astringents" in Part 4)

Note: Internal use of horse chestnut is not recommended during pregnancy. The topical gel is safe to use

- Bilberry extract—80 to 160 milligrams three times daily

Action: Anthocyanosides (active bioflavonoids) strengthen the walls of the veins by improving proper collagen formation

Note: Highly recommended for varicose veins associated with pregnancy

OTHER HERBAL CONSIDERATIONS

- Butcher's broom—1,000 milligrams two to three times daily, or a standardized extract supplying 50 to 100 milligrams of ruscogenins daily[2]
- Gotu Kola—1,000 milligrams twice daily
- Bioflavonoids—A host of excellent bioflavonoid products are on the market. These include quercetin, hesperidin, and pycnogenol. As is the case with bilberry, these will strengthen blood vessels

NUTRITIONAL SUPPLEMENT CONSIDERATIONS

- Vitamin C (with bioflavonoids)—1,000 milligrams twice daily

LIFESTYLE CONSIDERATIONS

Regular exercise is a great way to prevent varicose veins. Along with diet, this will not only make blood flow more efficient, it will also keep weight down. If you have varicose veins, try to avoid standing still for long periods of time. You may also benefit from the use of support stockings while on your feet.

Digestive System

RELATED CHAPTERS IN PART 5

- Chamomile
- Eleuthero (Siberian ginseng)
- Ginger
- Milk Thistle

ALCOHOL-RELATED LIVER DISEASE

Alcohol abuse can lead to gastritis (inflammation of the stomach), pancreatitis (inflammation of the pancreas), malabsorption of important nutrients, nerve disorders, heart disease, and liver disease.

The area of the body most directly affected by alcohol abuse is the liver. The liver is the major detoxifying organ of the body and is responsible for clearing alcohol and some other drugs from the body. Overconsumption of alcohol wears down the liver, lessening its ability to clear toxins, and eventually leads to destruction of liver cells.

Alcohol disrupts the membrane surrounding liver cells. Inflammation of the liver cells (i.e., *hepatitis*) follows and this leads to infiltration of fat into the liver cells. The final stage in liver destruction is known as cirrhosis. Once this stage is reached, alcohol-related liver disease becomes irreversible. Cirrhosis is topped only by cardiovascular disease and cancer as a cause of death in the 45-to-65 age group in the United States.

Treatment of alcohol-related liver disease needs to begin with abstinence from alcohol. Get into a good alcohol rehabilitation center and stick with the initial withdrawal program and follow-up. Remember, alcoholism involves addiction: long-term treatment is necessary.

Treatment should then aim to reestablish normal liver function. The chapter on milk thistle in Part 5 covers the functions of the liver and offers a glimpse at the importance of reestablishing optimal liver function.

HERBAL PRESCRIPTION

- Milk thistle extract (standardized to 70 or 80 percent silymarin)—420 milligrams of silymarin in three divided doses. Once improvement occurs a maintenance dosage of 280 milligrams of silymarin daily may be used for long-term treatment

  Note: It's easy to figure out silymarin content. If it's a milk thistle extract that contains 70 percent silymarin, take 200 milligrams of the extract three times daily. An 80 percent extract would require 175 milligrams of the extract three times daily

  Actions: Milk thistle regenerates injured liver cells and helps them reestablish normal function. It also strengthens the liver cells' antioxidant defense system, which is impaired by alcohol abuse

OTHER HERBAL CONSIDERATIONS

- Eleuthero (Siberian ginseng)—Standardized dry extract of the root and rhizomes—300 to 400 milligrams daily; dried, powdered root and rhizomes, 2 to 3 grams daily in two or three divided doses[1]

  Note: Eleuthero is recommended for use during an alcohol-withdrawal program. It is noted for decreasing the recurrence of alcoholism

- Schizandra—2 grams three times daily[2]

NUTRITIONAL SUPPLEMENT CONSIDERATIONS

Alcoholism can lead to a number of nutritional deficiencies. It is important that you work closely with a health care professional trained in nutrition to establish and treat any nutritional deficiencies. Then use supplements to help maintain normal liver function. Some considerations are the following:

- Multiple vitamin/mineral supplement
- Vitamin E—400 to 800 IU daily
- Chromium—200 micrograms daily

DIETARY RECOMMENDATIONS

Liver disease hinders the digestion of fats. It's wise, therefore, to reduce fats in your diet and increase sources of complex carbohydrates (leafy green vegetables, legumes, and fruit). Get your protein from low-fat and easy-to-digest sources such as soy. Use the "hypoglycemic" diet outlined in the discussion on stress and fatigue under "Endocrine System" to help with proper blood sugar balance.

COLIC

A distressing experience for new parents is their first encounter with a colicky baby. Infant colic is characterized by bouts of crying, abdominal pain, and irritability. Infants will often draw their legs up and have excessive gas and a tight abdomen. A gentle stomach massage will often relieve some of the abdominal distress.

Even though a colicky infant can turn your otherwise tranquil world upside down, the condition usually doesn't cause long-term difficulty for a child. Most colicky infants eat and gain weight normally.

HERBAL PRESCRIPTION

- Chamomile—2 to 3 ml of a liquid extract in warm water three to four times daily
  Actions: Eases intestinal cramping and exerts a mild sedating effect, aiding sleep

DIETARY RECOMMENDATIONS

A few general considerations:

- If your colicky baby has a strong sucking urge when eating and then fusses after stopping, he or she may need to feed longer.
- If they're bottle feeding, make sure that the hole in the nipple is not too big. Also, some infants swallow air with bottle feeding if allowed to suck on an empty bottle after feeding.
- If your infant has started on formula and becomes colicky, the problem may be an intolerance to lactose in the cow's milk formula or an allergy to the milk proteins. Try substituting a soy formula for the cow's milk formula. However, about 40 percent of infants with cow's

milk allergies also react to soy. If this occurs, then a nonallergenic formula such as Nutramigen should be tried.

CONSTIPATION

The urge to be "regular" has resulted in a multimillion-dollar industry. Laxatives have become one of the biggest selling over-the-counter medications in our society.

Constipation implies a difficulty in having bowel movements or a decreased frequency of bowel movements. Right off the bat, you should notice that this is very subjective. What's normal for one person may be totally unacceptable to another. See the father in the novel *Portnoy's Complaint*.

Here are some of the possible causes of constipation:

Diet high in refined foods and low in fiber
Inadequate fluid intake
Physical inactivity
Pregnancy
Drugs such as anesthetics, antacids, antidepressants,
    and muscle relaxants
Iron supplements
Low thyroid function
Irritable bowel syndrome
Nerve disorders of the bowel
Overuse of enemas and laxatives

It's interesting that the first two items listed are diet and physical activity. We'd probably cure a lot of constipation by focusing on more fiber in the diet and a regular exercise program!

Chronic constipation is a major concern among the elderly. This is particularly true in rest homes and among people who are bedridden. Loss of intestinal tone results from inactivity and also from impaired nerve control of the bowels.

Bowel health ranks high in an overall wellness program. Sluggish movement of food through the digestive tract can lead to irritation and cause a harmful buildup of bacteria in the intestines.

HERBAL PRESCRIPTIONS

Stimulant Laxatives

For people with severe constipation, stimulant laxatives are a good short-term consideration. Long-term use of stimulant laxatives can lead to sluggish bowel function and dependence on the laxatives for a normal bowel movement (see discussion of laxatives in Part 4).

- Senna or *Cascara sagrada*—These are the most commonly used stimulant laxatives (cascara being somewhat more gentle). These herbs are approved over-the-counter medicines, so the dosage is fairly consistent. Carefully follow the instructions on the product you decide to buy. *Action:* These herbal laxatives produce anthraquinones that increase bowel motility

Bulk-forming Laxatives

Bulk-forming laxatives, when consumed with sufficient liquid, expand in volume and stimulate the bowels to move. They are considered safer for long-term use than the stimulant laxatives.

- Psyllium seeds—7.5 grams of the seeds (2 teaspoonfuls) or 1 teaspoon of the husks one to two times daily. Mix it up with some water or juice and down the hatch! Be sure your intake of fluids remains regular throughout the day.

Combination Products

Over the past few years, research has indicated that a combination of senna and psyllium is the best choice for treatment of chronic constipation in the elderly. Please see the discussion at the end of "Laxatives" in Part 4.

NUTRITIONAL SUPPLEMENT CONSIDERATIONS

- Magnesium—300 milligrams twice daily[1]

DIETARY RECOMMENDATIONS

Increase your consumption of vegetables, grains, and fruit. These are all sources of dietary fiber. Decrease red meat, cow's milk, and fried foods. Work with a health care professional trained in nutrition to rule out food allergies. Be sure to drink plenty of liquids during the day. Reduce coffee intake.

DIARRHEA

Diarrhea is the result of irritation or inflammation of the intestinal tract. This is often due to an infection in the intestinal tract. In these cases, the diarrhea can be frequent and explosive. During serious bouts, make sure you have close medical monitoring. Proper amounts of fluid and electrolytes must be administered or life-threatening dehydration can occur.

Diarrhea can be a symptom of inflammatory bowel conditions such as ulcerative colitis or Crohn's disease. It can also result from the foods that we eat—particularly if we are allergic to them. A classic example is mild diarrhea and loose stools in infants who are allergic to cow's milk.

Note: The following recommendations are for self-treating milder forms of diarrhea. They should be used for more serious cases only after proper medical monitoring takes place.

HERBAL PRESCRIPTIONS

The following substances are all rich in tannins, which have an astringent action in the intestines. Please see the discussion on astringents in Part 4.

- Carob powder—One to 2 tablespoons mixed with applesauce three to four times daily (particularly useful for diarrhea in young children and infants)[1]
- Other common astringents used for diarrhea—Blackberry leaves, blackberry root bark, blueberry leaves, and raspberry leaves[2]

OTHER HERBAL CONSIDERATIONS

- Chamomile—Reduces cramping and helps ease irritation of intestinal tissue (see the instructions for use provided in "Irritable Bowel Syndrome")
- Marshmallow root—1,000 milligrams two to three times daily
  Action: Soothing effect on irritated intestinal tissue

NUTRITIONAL SUPPLEMENT CONSIDERATIONS

Acute and chronic diarrhea can lead to a host of nutritional deficiencies—particularly the fat-soluble vitamins, vitamins A and D. Work closely with a health care professional trained in nutrition to avoid loss of nutrients. This is particularly important for infants recovering from diarrhea.

- Acidophilus/bifidus supplements—Excellent for use during diarrhea and also for long-term use afterward. An excellent preventive of traveler's diarrhea[3,4]

HEARTBURN

Heartburn involves a backflow of stomach contents and acid into the esophagus. It often results in a burning pain in the chest that may radiate to the neck, throat, and face. It frequently occurs following meals or when a person is lying down.

Heartburn is a symptom and not an actual disease. It is most commonly a sign of gastroesophageal reflux, a condition caused by an inability of the lower esophageal sphincter (a valve between the lower esophagus and the stomach) to properly block the reflux of stomach contents into the esophagus. Repeated reflux of stomach contents into the esophagus leads to inflammation and often ulceration. If you're experiencing repeated heartburn, seek the attention of a physician for proper diagnosis and treatment.

HERBAL PRESCRIPTIONS

- Deglycyrrhizinated licorice (chewable tablets)—Chew one to two tablets 5 to 10 minutes before major meals during the day and before bed at night

Action: Soothes irritation of the tissue on the inside of the esophagus. Please see note on deglycyrrhizinated licorice in the section "Peptic Ulcer Disease"

- Chamomile—Follow the instructions for preparing a tea as outlined in the chapter on chamomile in Part 5
  Action: Antiinflammatory and soothes irritation of tissue inside the esophagus

NUTRITIONAL SUPPLEMENT CONSIDERATIONS
- Vitamin B complex—50 milligrams daily[1]
  Note: A deficiency of vitamin B_3 (niacin) should be ruled out by your health care practitioner
- Calcium carbonate (either liquid or chewable tablet)—600 milligrams every 2 to 3 hours during an acute attack of heartburn

DIETARY RECOMMENDATIONS
Eliminate caffeine, alcohol, and chocolate. Reduce saturated fats in your diet from meat and dairy products. A diet high in fiber and complex carbohydrates from vegetables, fruits, and grains will stimulate normal emptying of stomach contents, reducing reflux into the esophagus.

IRRITABLE BOWEL SYNDROME

Irritable bowel syndrome (IBS) affects one in seven people and accounts for half of all referrals to outpatient gastroenterology clinics. It is characterized by pain in the abdomen, accompanied by a change in bowel habits. This change can be either diarrhea or constipation. Increased flatulence is also common.

Since IBS affects more women than men, our sexist medical community has presumed that the condition is 90 percent psychological. However, research in Great Britain has indicated that IBS patients have no higher levels of anxiety than persons suffering from intestinal conditions with similar symptoms.

Herbal Prescriptions

- Peppermint oil (enteric-coated)—One to two capsules (0.2 ml of oil per capsule) three times daily between meals[1,2]

  Action: Carminative action eases intestinal cramping and soothes irritation.

  Note: Be sure to use the enteric-coated form. It is released in the intestines and not the stomach, where it would cause irritation. Some people may experience a burning sensation in their rectum with regular use of the enteric-coated form (affectionately known as "irritable buns syndrome"). They may be better off opting for chamomile.

- Chamomile—Chamomile is typically taken in a tea form. Pour boiling water over a heaped tablespoon of dried flowers, cover it, and after 5 to 10 minutes pass it through a tea strainer. Drink a cup of freshly brewed tea three to four times daily between meals. An alternative is to take a dried, encapsulated product or alcohol-based tincture and mix it with hot water. The dosage should be 2 to 3 grams of the encapsulated product or $1/2$ to 1 teaspoon of the tincture three times daily between meals.

  Action: Carminative action eases intestinal cramping and soothes irritation.

- Psyllium (or another high-fiber, bulk-forming laxative)—See previous instructions for use of psyllium seeds under "Bulk-forming Laxatives"

  Action: Helps regulate normal bowel activity and reduce the alternating constipation/diarrhea noted with IBS patients.

Nutritional Supplement Considerations

- Acidophilus/bifidus supplements

Dietary Recommendations

Please refer to the dietary recommendations under "Constipation." Rule out food allergies and lactose intolerance by consulting a health care professional trained in nutrition.

LIFESTYLE AND MEDICAL CONSIDERATIONS

Hypnotherapy and relaxation techniques have proven successful in the treatment of IBS.[3,4] Stress reduction should also be a part of your long-term approach to IBS.[5] Be sure to ask your doctor to check your thyroid function to see if it is low.

NAUSEA ASSOCIATED WITH MOTION SICKNESS

Please refer to the chapter on ginger in Part 5 for a discussion of nausea associated with motion sickness.

HERBAL PRESCRIPTION

- Ginger—1 gram of the dried rhizome powder daily. For prevention of motion sickness, begin taking 2 days before the planned trip

PEPTIC ULCER DISEASE

Peptic ulcer disease describes ulceration of either the stomach or duodenum (the first part of the small intestine). Duodenal ulcers are the most common, occurring about five times more frequently than gastric ulcers. Duodenal ulcers are about four times more common in men than in women. Gastric ulcers can occur with overconsumption of alcohol, aspirin, and nonsteroidal antiinflammatory drugs (NSAIDs).

People with duodenal ulcers have a fairly consistent pain pattern. The pain is usually absent first thing in the morning. By midmorning it begins to rear its ugly head and can sometimes be relieved by food. This is only temporary, as pain returns 2 to 3 hours later. Pain will often wake a person afflicted with a duodenal ulcer at 1 or 2 A.M. Pain may occur daily for one to several weeks and then resolve without treatment. Recurrence, however, is normal.

Gastric ulcers do not follow the same pattern. Eating will often make symptoms worse, producing heartburn, bloating, or nausea. Gastric ulcers are often preceded or accompanied by a condition known as gastritis, or inflammation of the stomach lining. The treatment for gastritis is virtually the same as that for ulcers.

Recently, high levels of a bacterial species known as *Helicobacter pylori* have been linked to gastritis and ulcers. This has led to the use of bismuth and antibiotics in the treatment of these conditions.

Note: Peptic ulcer disease can be a dangerous condition, especially if it's causing bleeding. The following herbal and nutritional recommendations should be used only following proper medical diagnosis.

HERBAL PRESCRIPTIONS

- Deglycyrrhizinated licorice (chewable tablets)—250 to 500 milligrams 15 minutes before meals and 1 to 2 hours before bedtime[1,2]

  Actions: Heals the tissue lining of the duodenum and stomach and promotes protection against stomach acid and other irritants

  Note: Deglycyrrhizinated licorice is an extract of licorice root that has had the constituent glycyrrhizic acid removed. This is the portion of licorice that has been blamed for increasing blood pressure in some individuals who consumed large amounts of licorice root supplements or licorice tea. By removing the glycyrrhizic acid, the healing portion of the licorice root remains and the risk of side effects is erased. Deglycyrrhizinated licorice is an approved treatment for ulcers in Great Britain and is widely used in this country by alternative practitioners as a substitute for cimetidine (Tagamet)

- Catechin—1,000 milligrams five times daily[3]

  Action: As is true with other bioflavonoids, catechin reduces the formation of histamine, a proinflammatory substance in the body

  Note: Other bioflavonoids or bioflavonoid-containing extracts can be substituted for catechin. Examples are quercetin and bilberry

OTHER HERBAL CONSIDERATIONS

- Chamomile—See instructions for use under "Irritable Bowel Syndrome"
- Marshmallow root—1,000 milligrams two to three times daily

NUTRITIONAL SUPPLEMENT CONSIDERATIONS

- Zinc (monomethionine or citrate)—25 to 30 milligrams daily[4,5]
- Vitamin C—1,000 milligrams daily[6]

- Manuka honey[7]

   Note: Recent research indicates that this New Zealand honey inhibits the growth of *Helicobacter pylori,* the bacterial species associated with ulcers and gastritis. It's premature to suggest this can replace treatment of *H. pylori* with bismuth, antibiotics, and antiparasitic medications. However, adding a few tablespoons daily to your diet can't hurt.

DIETARY RECOMMENDATIONS

Increase your consumption of foods high in fiber and complex carbohydrates (leafy green vegetables, fruits, and legumes). These foods will also be higher in antioxidant nutrients such as beta-carotene, vitamin A, and vitamin C. Reduce your intake of sugar, saturated fats (primarily from meat, milk, and cheese), coffee (including decaffeinated) and black tea (green tea is fine), and alcohol. With the help of a health care professional, identify and eliminate potential food allergens. Don't use milk to treat your ulcer!

LIFESTYLE CONSIDERATIONS

Reduce risk factors including smoking, aspirin, and nonsteroidal anti-inflammatory drugs such as ibuprofen. Stress reduction through meditation, relaxation training, and so on, is essential.

Ears, Nose, and Throat

EAR INFECTIONS (RECURRENT)

Chronic ear infection, also known as otitis media with effusion, is a chronic inflammation of the middle ear. Loss of hearing can result from the prolonged buildup of fluid behind the tympanic membrane (the membrane separating the middle ear and external ear). Otitis media with effusion (OME) is a major cause of hearing loss in young children, especially those 3 years of age and under.

Fluid buildup results from obstruction in the eustachian tube, the canal draining the middle ear. The eustachian tube of young children sits in a somewhat horizontal position, which hinders drainage of fluid. Obstruction occurs as a result of inflammation caused by repeated acute ear infections, frequent colds, and allergic reactions starting in the nose. When the eustachian tube does not drain and fluid builds up, the eardrum does not move properly in response to sounds. It is then that hearing is damaged.

The following are important questions if your child has OME:

- Does your child have allergies? Environmental allergies to animal dander, dust, and pollen can cause inflammation in the nose and impair proper draining. Also, food allergies are very important. Early weaning and introduction of cow's milk are linked to an increased risk of OME.
- Does your child get frequent colds or upper respiratory tract infections? A sluggish immune system can make your child more susceptible to these infections—particularly if they attend day care. Also, chronic use of antibiotics can contribute to a sluggish immune response.[1]
- Does either parent smoke? Secondhand smoke increases the risk of OME.[2]

HERBAL PRESCRIPTION

- *Echinacea purpurea* (expressed juice of the herb)—40 drops of the juice two to three times daily for 6 to 8 weeks continuously. A 2-week break should be taken before resuming use of echinacea
  Actions: Strengthens the immune response and decreases the risk of colds and upper respiratory tract infections. This serves to lower the risk of ear infections recurring

NUTRITIONAL SUPPLEMENT CONSIDERATIONS

- Vitamin C
  In children less than 1 year of age—100 to 200 milligrams daily
  In children 1 to 3 years of age—250 milligrams daily
  In children 3 years of age and older—250 milligrams twice daily
- N-Acetyl-L-cysteine (NAC)—400 to 600 milligrams daily[3]
  Note: N-Acetyl-L-cysteine is a mucolytic. This means it thins the mucus and helps with drainage from the middle ear. (It's also useful for chronic sinus congestion. N-Acetyl-L-cysteine tastes horrible! Try to hide it in sweet potatoes or applesauce.) N-Acetyl-L-cysteine can cause loose stools or diarrhea in some children

DIETARY RECOMMENDATIONS

Breast-feeding is the best preventive medicine. Children breast-fed for at least 9 to 12 months have a greatly reduced risk of OME.[4,5] Children with OME should be evaluated for food allergies as part of an entire treatment program involving environmental allergens.[6] Once specific food allergens are identified, a systematic elimination should be carried out under the supervision of a health care practitioner. Major allergens to consider include cow's milk, eggs, wheat, soy, citrus, and peanut butter. Make an attempt to decrease sugar and simple carbohydrates in your child's diet. These can contribute to a "sluggish" immune system.

TINNITUS AND HEARING LOSS

Tinnitus is simply a ringing or buzzing noise in the ear. However, the complexity of managing the condition can be overwhelming. Part of the frustration is the fact that an underlying disease is identified only about 5 percent of the time.

One person out of ten has some form of hearing impairment or ear problem; 85 percent of these sufferers have tinnitus. Tinnitus affects more than 37 million Americans. It's most common in elderly persons, but can occur at any age. The most common causes are noise-induced damage to the inner ear and age-related hearing loss. Contributing factors to tinnitus include smoking, caffeine, aspirin, some prescription drugs (examples include indomethacin, Elavil, and Gantrisin), and stress.

Tinnitus may be a sign of conditions such as Meniere's disease and sensorineural hearing loss (hearing loss originating in the inner ear). In addition, tinnitus may be a sign of circulation problems to the inner ear, high blood pressure, hyperthyroidism, or high cholesterol.[1]

You should consider the following suggestions for possible treatment of tinnitus, sensorineural hearing loss, and Meniere's disease.

HERBAL PRESCRIPTION
- *Ginkgo biloba* extract—120 to 240 milligrams daily in two or three divided doses[2]

  Action: Improves blood flow to the inner ear. Ginkgo seems to be effective in a subset of persons with tinnitus (most likely those with tinnitus caused by noise damage or atherosclerosis).

NUTRITIONAL SUPPLEMENT CONSIDERATIONS
- Vitamin B_{12}—1,000 micrograms daily (sublingual lozenges are best if used orally). Be sure to take with at least 400 micrograms of folic acid. If you have a health care professional willing to help out, the better option is to have an intramuscular injection of 1,000 micrograms (1 milliliter) of B_{12} weekly for 4 to 5 months.[3]
- Zinc (monomethionine or citrate)—50 milligrams three times daily between meals. Use for 12 to 24 weeks. Additional supplementation of copper should take place during this time (2 to 3 milligrams daily).[4]

DIETARY RECOMMENDATIONS
Reduce your dietary sources of saturated fats, such as beef and dairy products. Also lower your dietary intake of sodium (salt is usually the

culprit) as well as sugar and other simple carbohydrates. Eating more frequent, smaller meals that are higher in protein and complex carbohydrates helps regulate sugar metabolism.[5]

LIFESTYLE CONSIDERATIONS

There appears to be some correlation between stress and tinnitus.
Stress reduction through meditation, biofeedback, or yoga should be part
of your long-term strategy to combat tinnitus.[6]

OTHER EARS, NOSE, AND THROAT CONDITIONS

HAY FEVER
- Nettle herb—450 milligrams two to three times daily[1]
- Quercetin—500 milligrams two to three times daily[2]
- Vitamin C—2 to 3 grams daily[3]

SINUS INFECTIONS (RECURRENT)

See the recommendations listed under "Ear Infections (Recurrent)."
For adults, the doses should be adjusted as follows:
- *Echinacea pupurea* (expressed juice of the herb)—40 drops of the
  juice three times daily or one capsule of the dried juice three or four
  times daily for 6 to 8 weeks
- *N*-Acetyl-L-cysteine (NAC)—500 milligrams three times daily[1]
- Vitamin C—2 to 3 grams daily

Additional Considerations
- Tea tree oil—place 1/4 teaspoon in boiling water and breathe in the
  steam for 15 minutes
- Goldenseal root—500 milligrams two to three times daily for 14 to 21
  days

SORE THROAT

Note: The following recommendations are for symptom relief. A sore
throat can indicate a more serious infection (e.g., strep throat). Please
seek medical attention if you have a sore throat accompanied by swollen

lymph glands in the neck or if you've been exposed to someone with strep throat.

- Slippery elm—take one or two lozenges every couple of hours for symptomatic relief
- Goldenseal root (liquid extract or tincture)—2 ml every 2 to 3 hours for 7 to 10 days. Gargle with the preparation before swallowing

Other Herbal Considerations
- Cayenne, garlic, and echinacea

Nutrient Considerations
- Zinc lozenges, vitamin C

Endocrine System

Related Chapters in Part 5

- Eleuthero (Siberian Ginseng)
- Evening Primrose
- *Ginkgo biloba*
- Asian Ginseng

Diabetes

Diabetes mellitus is a chronic disease that is caused by insufficient production of insulin by the pancreas. This causes blood sugar to rise. Chronically high blood sugar leads to a host of complications in other parts of the body. Examples include retinopathy (see the following chapter on eye conditions), neuropathy (see the chapter on nervous system conditions), cardiovascular disease, and kidney disease. Diabetes is one of the leading causes of blindness and kidney disease in our country.

More than 11 million people have diabetes in the United States. Each year, 500,000 new cases are reported. Treatment of diabetes and its eye, nerve, cardiovascular, and kidney complications leads to a yearly medical cost of approximately 20.4 billion dollars!

Diabetes mellitus comes in two forms. Type I, also known as *juvenile-onset diabetes*, begins in childhood or adolescence. It is the most serious form and requires a lifetime of daily injections of insulin to maintain normal blood sugar levels. In type I diabetes, the immune system attacks the cells in the pancreas that produce insulin—hence the need for an external source of insulin. Another term for this type of diabetes is *insulin-dependent diabetes mellitus*. Type I diabetics represent less than 10 percent of the cases of diabetes in the United States.

Type II diabetes is called *adult-onset* and affects older people. The most common characteristic of the adult-onset diabetic is obesity. Type II diabetics have a lower rate of complications and their condition can sometimes be controlled with diet and noninsulin medications that lower blood sugar (also known as hypoglycemic drugs). In medical circles, this form of diabetes is referred to as non-insulin-dependent. It represents more than 90 percent of diabetes cases nationwide.

So, where does herbal medicine fit into the picture? Type I diabetics require insulin. It should not be assumed that they'll ever be able to do without it. However, diet, nutritional supplements, and herbal medicines play an important supporting role. Research is showing that these may prevent complications and even lower the requirement for insulin.

Dietary and herbal prescriptions also directly benefit type II diabetics. In many cases, healthy changes in a diet and sticking to a good exercise plan can work wonders in lowering blood sugar. Nutritional and herbal supplements can sometimes serve as primary therapies with type II diabetes. *Gymnema sylvestre* leaves and fenugreek seed can reduce the need for antidiabetic (hypoglycemic) medicines, which have well-known side effects.

As we'll see in the discussion of HIV (human immunodeficiency virus) infection under "Immune System," diabetics need to become the captain of their health care ship. Create a team of health care providers that addresses the condition from different and yet complementary perspectives. The complex and chronic nature of diabetes requires an eclectic approach.

Note: Remember that chronically high blood sugar is dangerous! Every optimal health care plan for diabetes needs to start with regular monitoring of blood sugar and include other important laboratory measures. Regular visits to your doctor will not only keep an eye on these measures but will also give you direct feedback about the effectiveness of your dietary and supplement program.

HERBAL PRESCRIPTIONS

Herbal Medicines That Help Lower and Control Blood Sugar

- Fenugreek seeds (defatted)—10 to 15 grams with each meal[1,2]
  Action: Effectively lowers blood sugar following meals
  Note: Defatted fenugreek seeds are available in capsules. At the recommended doses, you may simply want to add it in with your food

- *Gymnema sylvestre* leaf extract—400 milligrams daily[3,4]
  Actions: Enhances the ability of the pancreas to produce insulin in type II diabetics. Also, helps insulin work more effectively in lowering blood sugar in both type I and type II diabetes. This is an excellent substitute for oral blood sugar-lowering drugs in type II diabetics
- Asian ginseng—See dosage recommendations under "Stress and Fatigue"
  or
- Eleuthero (Siberian ginseng)—See dosage recommendations under "Stress and Fatigue"
  Actions: These adaptogenic herbs have been used historically in the long-term management of diabetes. Both promote normal blood sugar balance. Their antioxidant actions are also useful for lowering the risk of some diabetic complications

Herbal Medicines That Lower the Risk or Can Be Used to Treat Diabetic Complications

Diabetic Cataracts
- Quercetin—500 milligrams two to three times daily[5]
  Note: Since bilberry is also high in bioflavonoids and useful for prevention of retinopathy, I usually recommend bilberry so that prevention of both conditions is covered

Diabetic Retinopathy
See the section on herbal prescriptions in the treatment of diabetic retinopathy in the following chapter ("Eyes").

- Bilberry extract
- *Ginkgo biloba* extract

Diabetic Neuropathy
Please turn to the chapter on nervous system conditions and review the herbal recommendations for the treatment of diabetic neuropathy (they're near the end of the chapter).

- Evening primrose oil
- *Ginkgo biloba* extract

NUTRITIONAL SUPPLEMENT CONSIDERATIONS

Note: Start with a good multiple vitamin and mineral supplement. The following recommendations are total daily doses, so don't forget to include the amount in your multiple vitamin/mineral supplement.

- Vitamin C—1 to 2 grams daily[6]
- Chromium (polynicotinate)—200 micrograms twice daily[7]
- Magnesium—200 to 400 milligrams daily[8]
- Zinc (monomethionine or citrate)—25 milligrams daily[9] (be sure copper is also supplemented)
- Vitamin E—800 international units (IU) daily[10]
- Niacinamide—500 to 1,000 milligrams daily (for type I diabetics)[11]

DIETARY RECOMMENDATIONS

Research suggests an ideal diet is a cross between a whole-foods, high complex carbohydrate diet and a Mediterranean diet high in monounsaturated fats such as olive oil. To tell you the truth, I'd rather have my complex carbohydrates with some olive oil and garlic than without!

It's critical to increase your dietary fiber. High complex carbohydrate foods (vegetables and fruits) are high in dietary fiber. Fiber from beans, peas, and oats have all been shown to reduce blood sugar and prevent diabetic complications such as retinopathy and neuropathy.

Avoid processed grains and white bread. Drink fruit juice in moderation and definitely avoid soda pop, candy, and other sugary junk foods.

Get your protein from cold-water fish (e.g., salmon), soy, and other healthy sources. Avoid red meat and other animal sources of protein and fat. Eliminate fried foods and other sources of saturated fats.

LIFESTYLE CONSIDERATIONS

If you have type II diabetes, get on an exercise program immediately! Exercise increases the body's response to insulin and also reduces your risk for heart disease. Type I diabetics also benefit from exercise, but should be careful about overdoing it and disrupting blood sugar control.

Todd Bell—A Friend and Hero

Storytellers are always indebted to the characters who shape their stories. Many of my stories are richer because of people who've woven their experiences with mine. Todd Bell, my friend and brother-in-law, enriched my life greatly during the short time I knew him.

Todd was diagnosed with diabetes at the age of 11. After battling with retinopathy and other complications, Todd had kidney failure in December 1985. After a successful kidney transplant in June 1986, we all breathed a sigh of relief and assumed Todd would get back to his life in the restaurant business.

One of the most determined and stubborn people I've ever met, Todd decided only one year after his transplant to ride a bicycle across the country to increase public awareness of organ donation. He set about raising money through connections in Florida, as well as New York.

His route took him from Los Angeles to Miami. Todd completed the trip with flying colors. Newscasts along the way carried the story of his trip and his message, "Don't take your organs to heaven; heaven knows we need them here."

He became the president of the Southwest Florida Branch of the National Kidney Foundation in 1990 and continued to increase awareness about organ donation. He also participated in the National Transplant Olympics in the same year. He won a bronze medal for swimming.

After the transplanted kidney failed in early 1993 and chronic hepatitis dealt another blow to his health, Todd began his final journey with the courage and stubborn determination that were his trademarks. He died December 27, 1993.

The National Kidney Foundation created a research grant in Todd's name in June 1994.

OK, Todd, I'll join the battle cry, "BE AN ORGAN DONOR!!"

Stress can affect your ability to monitor blood sugar. Try yoga, meditation, or any other favorite method—listening to *Impressions* by John Coltrane is a favorite of mine—to keep stress in check.

Stress and Fatigue (Adrenal Exhaustion)

Stress is usually defined in terms of impaired balance. It can be triggered by both mental and physical stimuli. When stress occurs, it shifts your body's equilibrium or balance. How efficient you are at rebalancing often determines how little or how much effect stress will have on your body.

In the 1930s, Hans Selye developed a model for the way we react and adapt to stress. His model, referred to as the general adaptation syndrome (affectionately abbreviated "GAS"), is divided into three stages.[1]

The first stage is called the *state of alarm*. During this phase, a person is ready to react ("fight or flight"). The hypothalamus–pituitary–adrenal gland axis in the endocrine system kicks into high gear. The adrenal glands begin producing hormones, including epinephrine and cortisone-like substances. This explains the "keyed up" feeling a person gets when reacting to stress. Fat stores are also mobilized to offer extra energy. All of these factors contribute to a nonspecific resistance to stress.

The second stage is the *state of resistance*. After either trying to make the stress go away or avoid it during stage one, our body begins to adapt to the stress and the adrenals and other glands begin to return to a normal, balanced state. The resistance thus becomes specific to the stress and not a generalized reaction.

The third stage, termed *exhaustion*, represents the body finally breaking down under the pressure of stress. Selye observed in animal studies that damage to organs in the body occurred during this phase.

The organs most directly affected by constant stress are the adrenal glands. When your body is bombarded with stress on a regular basis, your adrenal glands can become run down. What happens then?

In the late 1940s, John Tintera, a medical doctor living in New York, picked up where Selye left off. Tintera began to look at patients in his practice who complained of chronic fatigue and unexplained aches and pains. He observed that many of these people had been experiencing recurring stress and had poorly functioning adrenal glands. The term *hypoadrenocorticism* was created to describe their condition.[2]

Tintera then assembled a list of specific symptoms common to people with sluggish adrenal function:

Excessive fatigue
Nervousness and irritability
Depression
Anxiety
Excessive weakness
Inability to recover from exercise
Insomnia
Headaches
Inability to concentrate
Increased allergies
Enlarged lymph nodes on the neck

What's fascinating is the remarkable similarity of these signs and symptoms to those associated with what is now called chronic fatigue syndrome (please see "Immune System" for a discussion of chronic fatigue syndrome). Anxiety and depression are also components of this condition. Tintera also noticed that people with low adrenal function were likely to have problems with hypoglycemia (low blood sugar).

Tintera's solution for reestablishing normal adrenal function was to give his patients regular injections of an extract made from animal adrenal glands. He found that this allowed the adrenal glands some rest and recuperation time, which allowed them to build up some reserves. He also placed these patients on a diet similar to the one I outline here, and used nutritional supplements such as vitamin C and pantothenic acid, which help support normal adrenal function.

Unfortunately, Tintera didn't know about adaptogenic herbs such as eleuthero (Siberian ginseng) and Asian ginseng (see "Adaptogens" in Part 4). These herbs are the perfect fit for both treating and preventing adrenal exhaustion. It's interesting to note that the term *adaptogen* implies an ability to help the body adapt to stress in its various forms. So, when you've got Selye's "GAS" try a little herbal tonic!

HERBAL PRESCRIPTIONS

Choose One of the Following Adaptogens:

- Eleuthero (Siberian ginseng)—Standardized, concentrated extract of the root and rhizomes, 300 to 400 milligrams daily; dry, powdered root and rhizomes, 2 to 3 grams daily in two or three divided dosages; alcohol-based extract, 8 to 10 milliliters in two to three divided doses. Use continuously for 4 to 6 weeks with a 1- to 2-week break before resuming. *Action:* Promotes and supports normal adrenal function. Eleuthero is my personal favorite for long-term support of adrenal function.
- Asian ginseng—100 milligrams twice daily of an extract standardized to contain 4 to 7 percent ginsenosides. Use for 4 weeks continuously with a 1- to 2-week break before resuming. *Action:* Promotes and supports normal adrenal function

OTHER HERBAL RECOMMENDATIONS

See the chapter "Nervous System" for recommendations for management of anxiety and mild depression.

NUTRITIONAL SUPPLEMENT CONSIDERATIONS

- Vitamin B complex—50 to 100 milligrams daily
- Pantothenic acid—250 milligrams daily
- Vitamin C—2 to 3 grams daily
- Chromium (polynicotinate form)—200 micrograms twice daily

DIETARY RECOMMENDATIONS

Low adrenal function often leads to low blood sugar (hypoglycemia). A good way to counter low blood sugar is to eat smaller, more frequent meals. In addition to your three major meals, try a midmorning and midafternoon snack. Snacks don't mean a candy bar or diet soda! Try fruit, a salad, or a bag of mixed nuts. Breakfast is an important meal. Don't skip it! Move your dietary focus away from simple carbohydrates (primarily sweets) toward complex carbohydrates and dietary fiber found in vegetables and fruits. Keep your protein intake at a normal level by consuming soy, fish, and nuts.

Eyes

CATARACTS

Cataracts result when the normal transparency of the eye degenerates. As the eye (usually the lens or capsule) becomes less transparent, it turns cloudy or opaque. The cardinal symptom of cataracts is a progressive and painless loss of vision. Cataracts may occur because of injury or surgery, diseases such as diabetes, overexposure to X-ray and ultraviolet light, and even some medications.

Cataracts afflict 50 million people worldwide. In the United States, it is a leading cause of blindness. Conservative estimates indicate that 18 percent of people from 65 to 75 years of age have cataracts. This figure jumps to 46 percent for people more than 75 years old.[1] In the United States, more than 541,000 surgeries for cataracts are performed annually at a cost of over 3.8 billion dollars. It has been estimated that if cataract formation could be delayed by only 10 years, the need for lens surgery could be cut in half.[2]

As will be noted in the following discussion of macular degeneration, free radical damage to the lens of the eye is a major factor. Thus, prevention centers on using antioxidant supplements to block free radical buildup.

Note: These recommendations are made with the understanding that herbal and nutritional interventions are preventive in nature. Those of you with documented cataract formation should be under the close care of an ophthalmologist.

HERBAL PRESCRIPTION

- Bilberry extract (25 percent anthocyanosides)—80 to 160 milligrams three times daily[3]
  Action: Potent antioxidant for the eyes

NUTRITIONAL SUPPLEMENT CONSIDERATIONS

- Vitamin C—1 to 2 grams daily[4]
- Vitamin E—800 international units (IU) daily with meals
- Beta-carotene (preferably a mixed carotene supplement)—25,000 IU daily with meals[5]

DIETARY RECOMMENDATIONS

To keep free radicals from forming, avoid fried foods and animal products such as red meat and milk. Add leafy, green vegetables and also yellow and orange veggies to your diet. Increase your consumption of fruits—particularly berries and others high in bioflavonoids.

LIFESTYLE CONSIDERATIONS

I'm probably going to cause rioting in Scottsdale and Boca Raton, but I've got to say it anyway: Reduce sun exposure to avoid ultraviolet radiation. This is one of the major sources of eye-related free radical damage. Get some good sunglasses or start thinking of places like Seattle and London as new retirement havens.

DIABETIC RETINOPATHY

The leading cause of blindness among diabetics is retinopathy. This condition causes the capillaries in the eye to become fragile and begin leaking. This in turn causes swelling in the retina and eventual loss of normal vision. Advanced complications include scarring and retinal detachment.

The onset of diabetic retinopathy appears to be linked to how long a person has had diabetes. It most commonly appears around the tenth year following diagnosis of diabetes. Two factors that are important in delaying onset are control of blood sugar level and keeping blood pressure down. Yearly retinal exams should begin 5 years after diabetes has been first diagnosed.

Note: With the exception of bilberry, the recommendations given are for prevention. Please review the general nutritional and dietary recommendations given in the section on diabetes in "Endocrine System," as well as the nutritional supplement recommendations just cited for cataracts in the preceding section.

HERBAL PRESCRIPTIONS

- Bilberry extract (25 percent anthocyanosides)—80 to 160 milligrams three times daily
  Actions: Strengthens capillaries and reduces hemorrhaging in the retina
- *Ginkgo biloba* extract—120 to 240 milligrams daily in two to three divided doses
  Action: Protects the retina of the eye, primarily by antioxidant properties[1]

MACULAR DEGENERATION

Also known as age-related macular degeneration (AMD), this condition is the leading cause of irreversible blindness in adults over 50 years of age. The incidence of AMD in persons over 65 years of age is 10 percent and increases to more than 28 percent in those over 75 years old. Cases in the United States are predicted to rise from 2.7 million in 1970 to more than 7.5 million by the year 2030. Approximately 20 percent of new cases of blindness in the United States are due to AMD.

Age-related macular degeneration refers to a degeneration of the macular disk—the portion of the retina of the eye responsible for precise vision. Age-related macular degeneration destroys central vision and affects the ability to read or do close work, to drive, and to differentiate colors and faces. A classic early symptom of AMD is a person complaining that door frames appear bent or wavy. The condition can often be aggravated by high blood pressure, diabetes, and high cholesterol.[1]

A major focus of research on AMD over the last few years has been the role of free radical damage in the macula caused by high sun exposure and ultraviolet B light. As with cataracts, AMD occurs more frequently in areas of year-round sunlight.

HERBAL PRESCRIPTIONS

Treatment of Early-Stage Macular Degeneration and Prevention

- *Ginkgo biloba* extract—120 to 240 milligrams daily in two to three divided doses[2]
  Actions: Protects the retina of the eye and slows the progression of macular degeneration in the early stages

Prevention

- Bilberry extract—See the instructions for use under "Cataracts"

NUTRITIONAL SUPPLEMENT CONSIDERATIONS

In addition to the recommendations listed previously for the prevention/treatment of cataracts, consider the following:

- Lutein and zeaxanthin—Oral supplement providing 6 to 10 milligrams of each carotenoid[3]
- Zinc (monomethionine or citrate)—30 milligrams daily[4]
  Note: The research study cited used 80 milligrams of zinc daily. I think this is too high for long-term use

DIETARY RECOMMENDATIONS

Please review the dietary recommendations in the "Cataracts" section. For prevention of macular degeneration, it's best to get plenty of vegetables high in carotenes—especially lutein and zeaxanthin. Examples include kale, spinach, and collard greens.[5]

EYE GEAR RECOMMENDATION

If you have AMD or are at risk for AMD, you should consult an ophthalmologist to obtain protective eye wear for use in bright sunlight.

OTHER EYE CONDITIONS

BLOCKED TEAR DUCT

Note: A common condition in young infants is a temporary blockage of the tear duct in one or both eyes. This can lead to an infection and often requires antibiotic treatment and dilation of the tear duct. The recommendations made here are early measures, meant for use before infection sets in.

- Chamomile—Place a warm chamomile tea bag over the eye for 5 to 10 minutes. Repeat every 2 to 3 hours. Be sure the tea bags are not too hot!
- Breast milk—Many mothers and midwives tell me that the best cure for a blocked tear duct is simply to squirt breast milk into the child's eye. I hear this is a good cure for the ol' Oedipus complex in boys!

POOR NIGHT VISION
- Bilberry extract—See dosage instructions under "Cataracts"
- Vitamin A—5,000 IU daily
- Zinc—30 milligrams daily

DRY EYES ASSOCIATED WITH SJÖGREN'S SYNDROME
- Evening primrose oil—3 grams daily with meals[1]
- Vitamin C—1 gram three times daily
- Vitamin B_6—50 milligrams twice daily

UVEITIS (CHRONIC)
- *Ginkgo biloba* extract—Follow the instructions under "Macular Degeneration"
  Action: Ginkgo counters a proinflammatory substance known as platelet-activating factor. This factor is elevated in the eyes of people with chronic uveitis[1]

Female Health Conditions

RELATED CHAPTERS IN PART 5

- Echinacea
- Evening Primrose
- Garlic
- Ginger
- Milk Thistle
- *Vitex agnus-castus*

FIBROCYSTIC BREAST DISEASE

Fibrocystic breast disease (FBD) is a benign (noncancerous) condition that affects approximately 40 percent of premenopausal women. This makes FBD the most common breast disease.

It is characterized by the formation of cysts within the breasts and usually involves both breasts. There are often multiple cysts and, if located near the surface of the breast, can be freely moved and are usually tender to touch. Symptoms of pain often accompany cyst formation and can range from mild to severe. Some women with FBD have no pain and discover cyst formation only by breast self-examination.

Fibrocystic breast disease is usually cyclic and often precedes a woman's period. Commonly, it accompanies premenstrual syndrome and usually becomes worse during the later part of the luteal phase. This may be explained by the increase in estrogen levels during this phase of the cycle (see the section "A Quick Primer on Luteal Phase Defect" in the chapter on vitex in Part 5).

Women with FBD who have a family history of breast cancer should be under the close supervision of a physician and have regularly scheduled breast examinations and mammography.

Note: For a more comprehensive look at prevention and treatment of breast cancer, I highly recommend *Breast Cancer: What You Should Know (But May Not Be Told) about Prevention, Diagnosis, and Treatment* by Steve Austin and Cathy Hitchcock (Prima Publishing, Rocklin, California, 1994).

HERBAL PRESCRIPTIONS
See the recommendations for vitex and evening primrose oil in the section on premenstrual syndrome (PMS) below.

NUTRITIONAL SUPPLEMENT CONSIDERATIONS
The recommendations for PMS apply here also.[1]

DIETARY RECOMMENDATIONS
For FBD, the first step is to eliminate methylxanthines (caffeine), common in coffee, tea, colas, and chocolate.[2,3] Reduce dietary fats, especially red meat and dairy products, and follow the rest of the dietary instructions for PMS.

HOT FLASHES (ASSOCIATED WITH PERIMENOPAUSE)

I found myself in the midst of a near-riot 2 years ago during a lecture in Fort Lauderdale, Florida. Speaking to a group of senior citizens in a large health food store, I was asked to recommend treatment for hot flashes during perimenopause. Before I had a chance to answer, a loud voice from the other side of the room boomed, "They're not flashes, darling, they're flushes." Within seconds, the flashes and flushes had squared off in a battle reminiscent of the Yooks (butter side up) and Zooks (butter side down) in the *Butter Battle Book* by Dr. Seuss.

Two weeks later I finally discovered the truth. While I was relating the story of the flashes versus the flushes, a woman calmly raised her hand and set us all straight. "Dr. Brown, they're simply power surges."

So, I'll save you from medical ramblings about your power surges. I highly recommend reading *Perimenopause: Preparing for the Change* by Nancy Lee Teaff and Kim Wright Wiley (Prima Publishing, Rocklin,

California, 1995). It provides a thorough overview of the symptoms associated with perimenopause and also evaluates issues such as hormone-replacement therapy.

HERBAL PRESCRIPTION

- Black cohosh root—In Europe, 8 milligrams daily of a highly concentrated extract is used. If you can't find an equivalent extract, try 100 milligrams of the powdered root twice daily.[1]
  Actions: Black cohosh has weak estrogen-like activity. Its ability to reduce hot flashes was thought to be due to a reduction in luteinizing hormone (LH) levels. This has been challenged in the past few years.

OTHER HERBAL CONSIDERATIONS

- *Vitex agnus-castus*—Forty drops of a liquid, standardized extract or one capsule of the equivalent powdered extract taken with some liquid, once daily in the morning.
- Dong quai (*Angelica sinensis*)—2 to 3 grams daily in two to three divided doses

NUTRITIONAL SUPPLEMENT CONSIDERATIONS[2]

- Calcium—1200 milligrams daily
- Magnesium—600 milligrams daily
- Vitamin C—2 to 3 grams daily
- Vitamin E—800 IU daily with meals

DIETARY RECOMMENDATIONS

Increase your consumption of foods high in phytoestrogens (see the following discussion on phytoestrogens). The all-purpose one here is soy. One cup of soy beans daily delivers close to the equivalent amount of conjugated estrogens as one tablet of Premarin.[3]

Reduce your intake of saturated fats from animal sources and eat plenty of complex carbohydrates and fiber from vegetables, fruits, and legumes.

A Note on Phytoestrogens: The term *phytoestrogen* implies a plant or food that has estrogen-like constituents and actions. The most popular example is soy, which contains a substance known as genistein. Currently, the most we can say about phytoestrogens is that eating foods or taking herbs high in these compounds offers promise against breast cancer, osteoporosis, and many of the maladies that women suffer from in the United States.

Herbs that qualify as phytoestrogens include black cohosh, red clover, licorice root, and Asian ginseng. Dong quai is often mistakenly listed as a phytoestrogen.[4]

We don't know whether these plant estrogen sources can replace Premarin for the prevention of osteoporosis and heart disease in menopausal women. The safest bet is to use them for the treatment of conditions such as hot flashes. Including soy in the diet and perhaps black cohosh in your regular supplement regimen makes sense as part of a complete prevention program before you reach menopause.

Research on phytoestrogens as a substitute for estrogen-replacement therapy in menopausal women will, it is hoped, become a priority in medical circles over the next few years.

INFERTILITY

Please see the related discussion in the chapter on vitex in Part 5. I'm limiting the focus here to infertility caused by high production of prolactin by the pituitary and an abnormal estrogen-to-progesterone balance during the second phase of the menstrual cycle.

HERBAL PRESCRIPTION

- *Vitex agnus-castus* (liquid, concentrated extract or dried, powdered extract equivalent)—40 drops of the liquid or one capsule of the dried extract once daily in the morning with some liquid
  Actions: Restores normal balance of progesterone and estrogen. Also reduces excess prolactin production in the latter part of the luteal phase

NUTRITIONAL SUPPLEMENT RECOMMENDATIONS

- Zinc (monomethionine or citrate)—50 to 75 milligrams daily[1]
- Vitamin B_6—100 milligrams twice daily[2]

Morning Sickness during Pregnancy

Please refer to the discussion in the chapter on ginger in Part 5.

Herbal Prescriptions

- Ginger root powder—1 gram daily as needed for nausea
  Actions: Decreases nausea and improves digestion. Ginger can also be used in the treatment of hyperemesis gravidarum, a more severe condition characterized by severe vomiting and nausea. This should be considered only after proper medical consultation

Nutritional Supplement Considerations

- Vitamin B_6—50 to 100 milligrams daily[1]
  Note: I find that an intramuscular injection of vitamin B_6 works wonders. The dosage is $1^1/_2$ milliliters and should be performed by a trained health care professional

Dietary Recommendations

Smaller, more frequent meals will sometimes help. My midwife friends also recommend some dry toast upon rising in the morning (yummy!).

Premenstrual Syndrome

If you're a woman 30 to 40 years of age, there's a better than even chance you've suffered premenstrual syndrome (PMS). Premenstrual syndrome is a condition marked by nervousness, irritability, mood swings, depression, and often headaches, water retention, and breast tenderness. Other symptoms that appear include nausea, constipation, backache, and abdominal bloating. Symptoms usually start 7 to 10 days before the onset of your period and will often resolve with the onset of menstrual flow. Symptoms can vary in severity from month to month.

The exact cause of PMS is unknown and probably involves a number of different factors. These factors also vary from woman to woman. One area of focus has been the production of high estrogen and low progesterone during the luteal or second phase of a woman's cycle. See the chapter on vitex in Part 5 for further discussion.

HERBAL PRESCRIPTIONS

- *Vitex agnus-castus* (liquid, concentrated extract or dried, powdered extract equivalent)—40 drops of the liquid extract or one capsule of the dried extract once daily in the morning with some liquid
  Actions: Restores normal balance of progesterone and estrogen. Also reduces excess prolactin production in the latter part of the luteal phase
- Evening primrose oil—3 to 4 grams daily with meals
  Actions: Corrects abnormal essential fatty acid metabolism. Gamma-linolenic acid (GLA) increases the production of hormones known as prostaglandins, which reduce uterine cramping and breast tenderness

OTHER HERBAL CONSIDERATIONS

- Dong quai (*Angelica sinensis*)—2 to 3 grams daily in two to three divided doses
  Note: Dong quai is especially useful if you're having a lot of premenstrual uterine cramping and pain. Also consider using it for dysmenorrhea (painful periods)[1]
- Milk thistle extract (standardized to 70 or 80 percent silymarin)—420 milligrams of silymarin daily in three divided doses
  Note: The liver is a forgotten organ in the management of PMS. Many women with PMS have excess estrogen. Since estrogen is metabolized by the liver, use milk thistle to support normal liver function

NUTRITIONAL SUPPLEMENT CONSIDERATIONS

Note: Dosage recommendations for single nutrients are based on a daily total. These should be adjusted in light of nutrient levels contained in the multiple vitamin/mineral formulation.

- Multiple vitamin/mineral supplement—Formulation should be free of allergens and contain adequate amounts of B vitamins (especially vitamin B_6), magnesium, vitamin E, and iron[2]
- Vitamin B_6—100 milligrams twice daily[3]
- Magnesium—400 to 600 milligrams daily[4]
- Vitamin E—400 IU daily with meals[5]

DIETARY RECOMMENDATIONS

Dietary modifications are at the heart of any strategy against PMS. The following guidelines should be helpful:

- Reduce or eliminate sugar, salt, and saturated fats from animal sources such as red meat and dairy products. Cut down on simple carbohydrates such as white flour and concentrated carbohydrates, including fruit juices and dried fruits. Avoid junk foods, diet sodas, and caffeine, which is present in coffee, tea, chocolate, and even some over-the-counter drugs. Limiting alcoholic beverages is also recommended.
- Increase your intake of complex carbohydrates and fiber from vegetables, fruits, and grains. Get your protein from sources such as soy and fish.
- Eat small, more frequent meals. This will keep weight down while stabilizing blood sugar.

LIFESTYLE CONSIDERATIONS

An aerobic exercise program is highly recommended. The goal should be four times weekly for 20 to 30 minutes for each session. Relaxation exercises such as yoga or meditation are also recommended.

VAGINAL YEAST INFECTIONS (RECURRENT)

HERBAL PRESCRIPTIONS

To Reduce Recurrence:
- *Echinacea purpurea*—40 drops of the expressed juice three times daily or one capsule of the dried juice three or four times daily for 6 to 8 weeks
  Action: Strengthens the immune response to resist reinfection
- Garlic—Tablets providing at least 5,000 micrograms of allicin daily in two divided doses
  Action: Antimicrobial activity includes *Candida albicans* and other yeast organisms

Topical Treatments:

- Tea tree oil suppository—200 milligrams of oil in a vegetable oil (e.g., coconut oil) base. Insert one suppository in the vagina once daily on alternating days for 7 to 10 days[1]

  Action: Powerful antiyeast activity

  Warning: Some women may experience a burning sensation with use of tea tree oil intravaginally. Use with caution and do not exceed the dilution recommended here

  Note: This is also an excellent treatment for bacterial vaginosis[2]

OTHER HERBAL CONSIDERATIONS

- Pau d'Arco—500 to 1,000 milligrams twice daily for 2 to 3 weeks
- Grapefruit seed extract—130 milligrams twice daily with plenty of water

  Note: Both of these herbal options are short-term and should not be taken for more than 2 to 3 weeks

NUTRITIONAL SUPPLEMENT CONSIDERATIONS

- Acidophilus/bifidus probiotic supplement—Use internally one or two times daily. Also effective when used topically either by inserting a gelatin capsule directly into the vagina (don't worry, it will dissolve!) or in a douche[3]

DIETARY RECOMMENDATIONS

Increase your intake of garlic and yogurt. Try to cut down on sugar in your diet. Consume more complex carbohydrates and fiber from vegetables, fruits, and legumes.

Immune System

Related Chapters in Part 5

- Echinacea
- Eleuthero (Siberian Ginseng)
- Evening Primrose
- Garlic
- Milk Thistle
- St. John's Wort

Chronic Fatigue Syndrome

It has taken the medical world some time to accept chronic fatigue syndrome (CFS). Initially thought to be all in the mind, CFS was targeted as the "yuppie flu," and was also believed to be caused by *Epstein–Barr virus* (the virus causing mononucleosis). It's now an official diagnosis known as chronic fatigue immunodeficiency syndrome. While we still don't know for sure what causes the condition, new evidence may help unlock the key to successful treatment of CFS.

Table 6.2 lists the signs and symptoms for CFS. To be diagnosed with CFS, a person must meet both the major criteria and eight of the minor symptom criteria, which sounds a bit like trying to figure out who's going to be in the wild card playoffs in football!

I try to address these three major areas with all of my CFS patients:

- Adrenal function
- Immune function
- Psychological issues

Let's consider these individually.

Adrenal Function: Evidence is mounting that CFS is a condition caused by sluggish or exhausted adrenal glands.[1,2] Turn to the chapter "Endocrine System" and review the section on stress and fatigue. Compare the criteria for hypoadrenocorticism (low adrenal function)

Table 6.2
DIAGNOSTIC CRITERIA FOR CHRONIC FATIGUE SYNDROME[3]

Major criteria

1. New onset of persistent or relapsing, debilitating fatigue with no previous history of similar symptoms. Average daily activity reduced or impaired below 50 percent for 6 months
2. Exclusion of other conditions that may produce similar symptoms

Minor symptom criteria:

1. Minor fever or chills
2. Sore throat
3. Painful lymph nodes in the neck and underarms
4. Unexplained generalized muscle weakness
5. Muscle tenderness or pain (myalgia)
6. Twenty-four hours of fatigue after exercise that is usually tolerated
7. Generalized headaches, unlike previous headaches
8. Joint pain that moves to different parts of the body
9. Depression and/or anxiety
10. Sleep disturbance (insomnia)
11. Symptoms developing over a few hours to a few days

established by John Tintera back in the late 1940s. They include excessive fatigue and weakness, depression, headaches, insomnia, swollen lymph nodes, and increased allergies; these criteria are remarkably similar to those currently used to describe CFS.[4]

A telltale sign of adrenal exhaustion is excessive fatigue following exercise. This means that the usual rush you get from exercise never comes and your recovery from a workout is slow and drawn out. In other words, exercise makes you feel worse. This shows up in both hypoadrenocorticism and CFS.

Low adrenal function also upsets blood sugar metabolism, causing hypoglycemia (low blood sugar). It also hampers the body's ability to fight inflammation and pain. This is because of the drop-off in production of natural, cortisone-like substances by the adrenals. It's interesting to note that a common condition associated with CFS is fibromyalgia. The generalized aches and pains associated with this condition could very well be linked to sluggish adrenal function.

It's my opinion that CFS is the current embodiment of hypoadrenocorticism. By supporting adrenal function through herbs, nutrients, diet, and stress reduction, you may be 90 percent of the way toward solving the puzzle of CFS.

Immune Function: The immune system of people with CFS is also out of balance. Some CFS patients show a depressed immune system that resembles the profile seen with HIV (human immunodeficiency virus)-infected patients. Other patients actually have overactive immune systems resembling those of people with autoimmune conditions such as lupus.[5,6]

Restoring balance to the immune function is critical. The herbs that work best on the adrenal glands (i.e., eleuthero and ginseng) also promote a balanced immune system. Adaptogens are the perfect starting point for an herbal offensive against CFS (see "Adaptogens" in Part 4).

Psychological Issues: While I don't support the premise that most of CFS resides in the mind, I do find that many of my CFS patients are depressed when they first visit my office. Of course, who wouldn't be with the uncertain nature of CFS?

I often use a mild herbal antidepressant such as St. John's wort to counter depression. This is usually short-term because once adrenal function begins to make a comeback, depression will often be one of the first things to go.

HERBAL PRESCRIPTIONS

Choose One of the Following Adaptogens:
- Eleuthero (Siberian ginseng)—Standardized, concentrated extract of the root and rhizomes, 300 to 400 milligrams daily; dry, powdered root and rhizomes, 2 to 3 grams daily in two or three divided dosages; alcohol-based extract, 8 to 10 milliliters in two to three divided dosages. Use continuously for 4 to 6 weeks with a 1- to 2-week break before resuming

Actions: Promotes and supports normal adrenal function and immune system activity. Eleuthero is my personal favorite for long-term treatment of CFS

- Asian ginseng—100 milligrams twice daily of an extract standardized to contain 4 to 7 percent ginsenosides
  Actions: Promotes and supports normal adrenal function and immune system activity
- Astragalus—3 to 6 grams daily
  Action: Promotes healthy, balanced immune function

OTHER HERBAL CONSIDERATIONS

- St. John's wort extract—A daily dose that delivers approximately 1 milligram of hypericin is recommended. For example, an extract standardized to contain 0.2 percent hypericin would require a daily dose of 500 milligrams (usually given in two or three divided doses)
  Note: Excellent for the initial treatment of depression
- Evening primrose oil—4 to 6 grams daily with meals[7]

NUTRITIONAL SUPPLEMENT CONSIDERATIONS

- Magnesium—200 to 300 milligrams twice daily[8]
- Vitamin B complex—50 to 100 milligrams daily
- Pantothenic acid—250 milligrams daily
- Vitamin C—2 to 3 grams daily

DIETARY RECOMMENDATIONS

Low adrenal function often leads to low blood sugar (hypoglycemia). A good way to counter low blood sugar is to eat small, frequent meals. In addition to your three major meals, try a midmorning and midafternoon snack. Snacks don't mean a candy bar or diet soda! Try fruit, a salad, or a bag of mixed nuts. Breakfast is an important meal. Don't skip it!

Move your diet away from simple carbohydrates (primarily sweets) and toward the complex carbohydrates and dietary fiber found in vegetables, fruits, and legumes. Keep your protein intake at a normal level by consuming soy, fish, and nuts.

Recent reports have also indicated that food allergies may play a part in CFS.[9] Work with a qualified health care professional to identify and eliminate food allergens.

OTHER CONSIDERATIONS

Be sure your doctor rules out low thyroid function.[10] Follow a good relaxation program. If you also have fibromyalgia (generalized aches and pains originating in the soft tissues of the body), add acupuncture or massage to your treatment plan.

COLD AND FLU

The common cold is the bane of mainstream medicine. Everybody gets colds but modern medicine doesn't know how to cure them. A good case of the flu and you're in the same boat. The best we're offered is decongestants, cough medicines, and acetaminophen to chase away our symptoms. Problem is, none of that stuff makes a difference.

In fact, the aches and fever associated with the flu and the nasal congestion, sore throat, and headache that accompany a cold are really signs that the body is doing its best to end the infection. It's not pleasant while it's occurring, but our immune systems should be applauded for their efforts and not be interfered with.

Herbal medicines also relieve symptoms (see the discussions on coughs, sinus infections, and sore throats in "Ears, Nose, and Throat" and diarrhea in "Digestive System"). Where they really shine, however, is in their ability to support the immune system. First, they support the immune system in its fight to keep the system infection free. This means that around cold and flu season, the herbal prescriptions listed below are perfect defenses to prevent a cold or flu.

Second, they speed the healing process once you've become sick. Your best friend here is echinacea. You may ache and feel lousy but echinacea will usually shorten your time of suffering.

Last, but not least, don't use flu vaccines if you're basically a healthy individual. Flu vaccines may be necessary for the very young and very old as well as those with impaired immune systems, but the rest of us don't need them! Follow the recommendations below—you'll be healthier and your immune system will thank you.

HERBAL PRESCRIPTIONS

Prevention

- *Echinacea purpurea* (expressed juice of the herb)—40 drops of the juice three times daily or one capsule of the encapsulated dried juice three or four times daily for 6 to 8 weeks continuously. A 2-week break should be taken before resuming use of echinacea. Great to use right before cold and flu season begins
  Action: Strengthens the immune response and decreases the risk of colds, flu, and upper respiratory tract infections
- Eleuthero (Siberian ginseng)—Standardized, concentrated extract of the root and rhizomes, 300 to 400 milligrams daily; dry, powdered root and rhizomes, 2 to 3 grams daily in two or three divided doses; alcohol-based extract, 8 to 10 milliliters in two to three divided doses. Use continuously for 4 to 6 weeks with a 1- to 2-week break before resuming
  Actions: Promotes a healthy immune response and supports normal adrenal function. Offers particularly good support for a person under a lot of stress
- Garlic—Tablets providing at least 5,000 micrograms of allicin daily
  Actions: Garlic has proven antiviral properties

Treatment

- *Echinacea purpurea* (expressed juice of the herb)—At the onset of a cold or flu use an initial dose of 40 drops or two capsules of the dried encapsulated juice. Two hours later begin taking 40 drops of the liquid or one capsule of the dried juice every 2 hours throughout the day for 48 hours or until symptom relief is noted. After symptom relief is noted, use 40 drops of the juice three times daily or one capsule three or four times daily for an additional 7 to 10 days

- Vitamin C—1 gram every 3 to 4 hours
- Zinc—one chewable lozenge two to three times daily is good for sore throats

And from the "because it's good for you, bubeleh" department:

- Rest
- Lots of water
- Chicken soup

HIV INFECTION/AIDS

Excuse me while I vent.

I was reading in the newspaper last week that Senator Jesse Helms thinks we're spending too much money on research for anti-HIV drugs and treatments for acquired immunodeficiency syndrome (AIDS). Carrying the homophobic banner forward, Senator Helms suggested that those who had AIDS essentially deserved it.

I'd like to suggest that Senator Helms be reminded of the fact that a large part of his financial base comes from the tobacco industry. Ironic that a self-proclaimed health expert like Senator Helms has been responsible for shielding an industry that is directly responsible for thousands of deaths yearly.

Thanks, I feel better.

Numerous resources offer a wide range of information about HIV infection. Here are two organizations and a publication I highly recommend:

Seattle Treatment Exchange Project (STEP)
127 Broadway E., #200
Seattle, Washington 98102
(800) 869-STEP

The STEP produces a publication, three times yearly, known as the *STEP Perspective*. The articles cover treatment issues ranging from antiviral drugs, supportive therapies for prevention of secondary infections, and alternative therapies. The STEP has also produced a set of "Fact Sheets" on HIV testing, general treatment strategies, nutrition, and alternative therapies, including some herbal treatments.

Gay Men's Health Crisis (GMHC)
129 West 20th Street
New York, New York 10011
(212) 807-6664

The GHMC produces the publication *Treatment Issues*. It is a monthly newsletter that provides reliable information on experimental AIDS therapies.

AIDS Treatment News
P.O. Box 411256
San Francisco, California 94141
(415) 255-0588

AIDS Treatment News is one of the most popular and well-written guides to experimental and complementary AIDS treatments. Edited and published by John James, the publication attempts to increase awareness of different treatments and their combinations that may serve to make HIV infection a manageable condition.

OK, let's talk about herbal medicines and where they fit into your treatment choices for HIV infection. First, let me say that this is my spin on the whole picture. How herbs fit into long-term treatment of HIV infection is not totally clear. As is true with most therapies for HIV, we need more research and clinical feedback. Bastyr University (Seattle, Washington) was given a grant by the National Institutes of Health's Office of Alternative Medicine in 1994 to gather information on alternative treatments for HIV infection and AIDS. Let's hope their work begins to uncover which therapies are actually working.

Second, it's my opinion that herbs, vitamins and minerals, and other alternative medicines are best viewed as complementary at this point. In other words, use them to increase your chances of long-term survival. I don't know of any natural therapies that will replace AZT or ddI in the antiviral arena.

Last, make educated choices. Read as many articles, books, and case studies as you can. Talk to long-term survivors and find out what they do. Use the resources listed here. Don't get caught up in the latest "miracle cure." The so-called miracle workers are usually trying to take short cuts based on commercial greed.

The cornerstone of my herbal prescriptions for HIV infection begins with support of the immune system (see the discussion on immunomodulators in Part 4). Herbs can steer the immune system toward a state of healthy balance and complement more aggressive antiviral drugs such as AZT and ddI. The following is a partial list of herbal medicines with known immunomodulating properties:

Astragalus
Eleuthero (Siberian ginseng)
Asian ginseng
Reishi
Schizandra
Shiitake

Note: I've included reishi and shiitake, which technically qualify as mushrooms; but you'll probably find them in the herb section of your health food store.

Immune-enhancing herbs offer the greatest benefit when started as early as possible in the course of HIV infection. If you start with a helper T lymphocyte (CD4 cell) count over 200, you'll have better odds of a successful response (i.e., an increase in your count). If you're below 200 in your CD4 count, don't expect a significant increase, but don't give up on using adaptogens. Other benefits, including adrenal support and antioxidant activity, are useful at all stages of HIV infection. These herbs can be used safely with standard antiviral drugs.

Herbal prescriptions may also play a role in decreasing your chance of getting certain secondary infections or complications. I regularly recommend garlic as a preventive tool to help the body combat yeast, cytomegalovirus, and *Mycobacterium avium* (the bacterium that causes tuberculosis in AIDS patients) infections.

Herbs can also protect you against the negative consequences of AIDS drugs. I've found that milk thistle extract reduces the side effects caused by AZT and helps keep the liver functioning optimally.

Finally, a comment on using herbal medicines for their anti-HIV activity: Since 1989, the National Cancer Institute (NCI) has been screening thousands of plants yearly for anti-HIV actions. This screening has uncovered numerous plants and plant constituents that show anti-HIV activity in a test tube. For various reasons, most of them have not advanced to clinical uses. Many of these plants are toxic when consumed at dosages that would cause an antiviral effect (examples include St. John's wort and trichosanthin).

Plants or plant constituents with antiviral activity that have made their way into the treatment programs of HIV-infected persons or community-based research trials include the following:

- Hypericin—A component of St. John's wort (please see the discussion in the chapter "St. John's wort" in Part 5)
- Bitter melon (*Momardica charantia*)—A protein named "MAP-30" has shown anti-HIV activity[1]
- Curcumin (from the spice turmeric)[2]
- Glycyrrhizin sulfate—A constituent of licorice root. Widely used in Japan for treatment of chronic hepatitis. It is administered intravenously.[3]

To date, we can only say that more research needs to be completed. I cannot recommend any of these herbal antivirals as substitutes for established antivirals such as AZT and ddI.

HERBAL PRESCRIPTIONS

Immunomodulators
Each of the following is high in complex polysaccharides—pick one and take the recommended dosage.

- Eleuthero (Siberian ginseng)—Standardized, concentrated extract of the root and rhizomes, 600 to 800 milligrams daily in two divided doses; dried powder of the root and rhizomes, 4 to 6 grams daily in

two or three divided dosages, alcohol-based extract (33 percent alcohol), 16 to 20 milliliters in two to three divided doses. Use continuously for 4 to 6 weeks with a 1- to 2-week break before resuming[4]
- Astragalus—6 to 12 grams daily[5]

  Note: Immunomodulating herbs provide excellent support if you're receiving chemotherapy for Kaposi's sarcoma. They will help the bone marrow bounce back and produce white blood cells following chemotherapy.[6]

Antimicrobial
- Garlic—Tablets providing at least 5,000 micrograms of allicin daily or one clove of raw garlic daily[7-9]

Liver Support
- Milk thistle extract (standardized to 70 or 80 percent silymarin)— 420 milligrams of silymarin daily in three divided doses

NUTRITIONAL SUPPLEMENT CONSIDERATIONS
Note: Recent research promotes antioxidant nutrients for people with HIV infection. Don't forget bioflavonoids from herbal and dietary sources!

Multiple Vitamin and Mineral Supplement
- Selenium—200 micrograms daily[10]
- Vitamin E—400 IU daily[11]
- Vitamin C—1 gram three to five times daily[12]
- Vitamin B_{12}—1,000 micrograms daily[13]

  Note: I prefer to use an intramuscular injection of 1,000 micrograms (1 milliliter) twice monthly. This should be done by a qualified health care professional.
- Folic acid—800 micrograms daily[14]

DIETARY RECOMMENDATIONS
A key consideration if you have HIV infection is your weight—not if you have too much, but if you have too little. Unexplained weight loss is a warning sign that should be shared with your doctor. Also, if you're having diarrhea, see your doctor.

The easy way out would be to recommend a vegetarian diet with a whole-foods focus. Unfortunately, it's not that simple if your immune system is working poorly. Be very cautious of raw produce. Be sure it's washed well before using. Also, avoid consuming raw eggs (found in Caesar salad dressing) and raw milk. Use plastic cutting boards—wood harbors bacteria—for preparing meat and fish, and wash them thoroughly with hot soapy water after use. That goes for your hands also. The Food and Drug Administration has a good summary on food safety issues for persons with HIV.

OK, now you can think about the healthy, whole-foods diet. Remember, raw garlic, turmeric, and other recommended spices win favor with your immune system as well as your taste buds.

OTHER CONSIDERATIONS

Research continues to show that a large and loving personal support group helps people with HIV infection and AIDS to survive longer. Develop a moderate exercise program and try yoga, meditation, or any other discipline that encourages a healthy mind–body connection.

I recommend acupuncture for most of my HIV-infected patients. Acupressure or massage are other options.

Male Health Conditions

RELATED CHAPTERS IN PART 5

- *Ginkgo biloba*
- Asian Ginseng
- Saw Palmetto

BALDNESS

I don't have a clue! My glowing pate has defied attempts to save the follicles naturally. If you have any suggestions that warrant sharing with our bald brethren, please drop me a line and I'll put it in the next edition.

BENIGN PROSTATE ENLARGEMENT

If you are a male between 40 and 59 years of age, there is a 50 to 60 percent chance that you have benign enlargement of the prostate gland. This condition, known as benign prostatic hyperplasia (BPH), begins in many men in their fourth decade. Distressing symptoms usually begin after age 50 years.[1] The cause, which has yet to be discovered, may be related to hormonal changes in middle-aged and elderly men.

Problems with urine flow are the major symptoms of BPH. The symptoms occur when the enlarged prostate gland impinges on the outlet of the bladder and the urethra (the tube carrying urine from the bladder). Listed here are common signs and symptoms of BPH:

- Dysuria—painful urination
- Hesitancy to urinate
- Straining to urinate
- Decreased force and caliber of urinary stream
- Prolonged dribbling after urination

- Sensation of incomplete bladder emptying
- Increased frequency of urination
- Nocturia—frequent urination at night

In addition to these symptoms, complications may arise, including bladder infections, involuntary urination, and bleeding in the urinary tract.

Accurate medical diagnosis is critical in order to rule out prostate cancer.

HERBAL PRESCRIPTIONS

- Saw palmetto (lipophilic extract of saw palmetto berries)—320 milligrams daily, taken all at once or in two separate doses
  Actions: Reduces the size of the prostate by inhibiting 5-α-reductase formation of dihydrotestosterone. Also has antiinflammatory properties. This should be your first choice for long-term treatment of BPH

Get to Know Your Prostate!

Problems related to the prostate account for billions of health care dollars annually. Yet many of you males out there don't know much about the location or workings of the prostate! The March 26, 1995 *London Times* reports the results of a survey that asked men about their prostate glands. The survey found that 89 percent of men did not know where the prostate gland is located. Sixty-two percent of respondents mistook it for the bladder. Only one-half of the men responding knew that only men could suffer from prostate problems. Finally, women were slightly better informed—only 41 percent failed to identify the prostate correctly!

The prostate, which is the size of a walnut or chestnut (they actually say that in medical texts!), lies below the bladder and is wrapped around the urethra—the tube that carries urine away from the bladder. In conjunction with the Cowper's glands, the prostate produces seminal fluid, which is needed for sperm to survive.

- Nettle root extract—120 milligrams twice daily
  Actions: Antiinflammatory and decongestant (antiedema) properties.[2]
  European extracts are often used in combination with saw palmetto.
- Pygeum (lipophilic extract of the bark)—50 to 100 milligrams
  twice daily
  Actions: Antiinflammatory and decongestant (antiedema) properties[3]
  Note: These herbal prescriptions can also be considered for the treatment of chronic, nonbacterial inflammation of the prostate (also known as chronic prostatitis).

NUTRITIONAL SUPPLEMENT CONSIDERATIONS
These are primarily for prevention of both BPH and prostate cancer:

- Zinc (monomethionine or citrate)—30 milligrams daily
- Selenium—100 to 200 micrograms daily

DIETARY RECOMMENDATIONS
Again, the intent here is prevention of both BPH and prostate cancer.

Keep your intake of saturated fats low. This includes red meat, milk, and fried oils. Include more polyunsaturated fats by eating vegetables and fish, and use olive oil for cooking. A vegetarian diet has been shown to reduce the amount of circulating hormones in the body—this also reduces the risk of BPH as well as prostate cancer.[4,5] A vegetarian diet also adds dietary fiber and antioxidant nutrients. Soy products should be a staple of your vegetarian strategy against BPH and prostate cancer.[6]

IMPOTENCE

It's not uncommon after I give a public lecture for some middle-aged man to linger in the wings until the crowd has thinned out. The usual topic of conversation is impotence.

Male impotence affects about one-fourth of men over 50 years of age and is estimated to affect some 15 million men in our country.

Male impotence is the inability either to attain or sustain an erection sufficient for intercourse. It can sometimes be due to psychological or emotional problems, as opposed to physiological ones. Seeking counseling either alone or with your partner may be the first step toward solving the problem.

If the problem is not psychological, a thorough medical work-up by a urologist should take place. Diseases such as diabetes, hypothyroidism, and multiple sclerosis can cause impotence. Drugs used to lower blood pressure, tranquilizers, and sedatives (be sure to read the fine print on the drug insert) also can be at fault. Chronic alcohol abuse also is a common cause of impotence.

Contrary to popular belief, your age should have nothing to do with your ability to have a normal erection. In other words, impotence is a preventable condition in many men past 50! The most common cause of impotence in men over 50 is atherosclerosis. Poor blood flow to the erectile tissue of the penis results in an impaired ability to have an erection.

Another common cause of impotence in men over 50 is partial or complete surgical removal of the prostate as part of treatment for prostate cancer. See the dietary recommendations for prevention of prostate cancer in the earlier section "Benign Prostate Enlargement."

HERBAL PRESCRIPTIONS
- *Ginkgo biloba* extract—240 milligrams daily in two to three divided doses[1,2]

  Action: Improves blood flow to the erectile tissue of the penis
- Asian ginseng (standardized extract containing 4 to 7 percent ginsenosides)—100 to 200 milligrams twice daily. Use continuously for 3 to 4 weeks with a 1- to 2-week break between.

  Action: An adaptogenic herb, it has been used for centuries in traditional Chinese medicine as a tonic for impotence.

OTHER HERBAL CONSIDERATIONS
- Yohimbine—15 to 20 milligrams daily[3]

  Note: This is an approved treatment for male impotence in the United States. Derived from the bark of the West African yohimbe tree, this alkaloid also increases blood flow to erectile tissue. However, unlike ginkgo, it commonly causes side effects such as anxiety, high blood pressure, and headaches. Taking the risk-to-benefit ratio into consideration, you're better off starting with ginkgo and ginseng.

- Muria puama (*Ptychopetalum olacoides*)—1 to 1.5 grams daily[4]
  Note: This Brazilian herb has one study to its credit. Its mechanism of action is unknown; neither is its safety with long-term use.

NUTRITIONAL SUPPLEMENT AND DIETARY RECOMMENDATIONS

Please see the recommendations listed under "Atherosclerosis (Prevention)" in the chapter "Cardiovascular System."

Mouth and Gums

RELATED CHAPTERS IN PART 5

- Chamomile
- Echinacea
- St. John's Wort

CANKER SORES

Canker sores are small ulcers that occur inside the mouth. They are usually harmless but can be painful. Canker sores occur singly or in groups and last from 7 to 21 days, depending on the type.

The most common form of canker sore is the "minor" form, defined as being less than 1 centimeter in diameter. These usually last 10 to 14 days and heal without scarring. These occur chiefly in young adults. The less common, "major" form features sores greater than 1 centimeter in diameter. They last weeks to months, and usually heal with scarring. These are most common in younger children. Canker sores are usually recurrent.

HERBAL PRESCRIPTIONS

- Deglycyrrhizinated licorice (DGL)—Gargle with mouthwash (200 milligrams of powdered DGL mixed with 200 ml of warm water) and swish in mouth for 2 to 3 minutes and then spit out. This should be done morning and evening for 1 week.[1]
  Note: For a discussion on DGL, please see the section on peptic ulcer disease under "Digestive System."
- *Echinacea purpurea* (expressed juice)—Take 40 drops of the juice three times daily. Swish in mouth before swallowing

OTHER HERBAL CONSIDERATIONS

- Myrrh—Place powder or liquid extract in warm water and use as a mouthwash three to four times daily
- Chamomile—Same instructions as for myrrh

NUTRITIONAL SUPPLEMENT CONSIDERATIONS
- Vitamin B complex—50 milligrams daily[2,3]
- Zinc (chewable tablets)—One or two tablets daily (do not exceed 50 milligrams)[4]

DIETARY RECOMMENDATIONS
Under the supervision of a health care professional, eliminate potential food allergens. Wheat and other gluten-containing grains should be at the top of your list.[5]

LIFESTYLE CONSIDERATIONS
Stress is a major factor contributing to recurrent canker sores. Stress reduction should be a therapeutic goal. Relaxation training, guided imagery, and meditation are among some helpful techniques.[6]

COLD SORES

Cold sores, also known as fever blisters, are caused by the herpes simplex virus (HSV). Herpes can also cause outbreaks on the genitals and sometimes other areas of the body, including the buttocks, thighs, and abdomen. Highly contagious, herpes is often transmitted by physical contact.

A herpes outbreak is usually heralded by tingling and itching. The actual sore is a cluster of blisters that initially contain a honey-colored fluid. Later, they crust over and then disappear.

Herpes is a recurrent disease, and once it establishes residence in your body, it is with you for life. Recurrent HSV outbreaks on the lips or around the mouth (also known as herpes labialis) occur in 20 to 40 percent of the population.

If your doctor decides to treat you for herpes, it will usually be for the genital form. The treatment of choice is acyclovir. Herpes on the lips or mouth is usually treated with a host of topical preparations that reduce swelling and itching. Neither of these treatments reduces recurrence.

Note: The recommendations given here are primarily for self-treatment of HSV-related cold sores. Genital herpes may respond to these topical preparations, but often requires acyclovir treatment as well.

HERBAL PRESCRIPTIONS

Topical Options

- Glycyrrhizic acid ointment (5 percent concentration)—At the onset of the prodromal symptoms (itching and tingling before outbreak), begin applying the ointment to the affected area four times daily. Use for the duration of the outbreak.
  Actions: Glycyrrhizic acid, which is a component of licorice root, is antiviral and reduces the recurrence of HSV infections. It reduces swelling and discomfort and speeds healing time.
- Lemon balm cream (1 percent concentration)—At the onset of prodromal symptoms, apply the cream to the affected area five times daily. Use for the duration of the outbreak.[1]
  Actions: Same as those for glycyrrhizic acid

OTHER HERBAL CONSIDERATIONS

- *Echinacea purpurea*—40 drops of the expressed juice three times daily or one capsule of dried juice extract three or four times daily
- St. John's wort extract (standardized for hypericin content)— The daily dose of hypericin should be at least 1.0 milligram.

NUTRITIONAL SUPPLEMENT CONSIDERATIONS

- L-Lysine—2 to 3 grams daily in two to three divided doses. Begin at the onset of the prodromal period and take for the duration of the outbreak. A preventive dose of 500 milligrams is recommended after the infection has resolved (this is not recommended for those with high cholesterol levels).[2]
- Vitamin C with bioflavonoids—2 to 3 grams daily[3]

DIETARY RECOMMENDATIONS

Increase your consumption of foods high in the amino acid lysine and avoid foods high in the amino acid arginine. Lysine-containing foods include legumes, fish, and chicken. Peanuts, almonds, and other nuts, as well as chocolate, have high levels of arginine.

LIFESTYLE CONSIDERATIONS

Recurrence of herpes is often associated with stress. Reduce stress through the use of a relaxation program of yoga, meditation, or listening to *Monk's Dream* by Thelonius Monk.

PERIODONTAL DISEASE

Periodontal disease is a common disorder of the gums and teeth. It is normally broken into two categories: gingivitis and periodontitis. Gingivitis represents a swelling of the gums characterized by redness, change of normal contours, recession, and often bleeding. Gingivitis is often the precursor of the more serious condition, periodontitis. Periodontitis represents a progression of gingivitis to the point at which pockets form between the teeth and gums and the gums lose their attachment to the teeth. The end result is bone loss in the jaw.

The leading cause of periodontal disease is poor dental hygiene. This leads to the build-up of bacterial plaque. This can often be prevented by proper brushing and daily use of dental floss. Periodontal disease, however, may sometimes be part of a more serious condition such as diabetes, an allergic reaction, or vitamin deficiencies involving vitamin C and niacin. Gingivitis traced to hormonal changes is common during puberty and pregnancy. If you have gingivitis, work closely with your dentist to identify the underlying cause and halt the progression.

Goals in treating periodontal disease include (1) control of plaque and bacterial buildup, (2) assisting with gum healing, (3) decreasing inflammation and free radical (reactive substances in the body that may cause damage to healthy cells) damage, (5) improving collagen (connective tissue) integrity and strength in the gums, and (6) improving immune function to assist with resistance to infection.

Note: The recommendations listed here are intended to support a regular dental hygiene program that includes conscientious brushing and flossing.

HERBAL PRESCRIPTIONS

Use the Following Herbs in Mouthwash and Toothpaste for the Prevention and Treatment of Periodontal Disease:

- Bloodroot (*Sanguinaria canidensis*)[1]
- Licorice root[2]

Mouthwash Combination

- Sage oil, peppermint oil, mint oil, menthol, chamomile tincture, expressed juice from *Echinacea purpurea* herb, myrrh tincture, clove oil, and caraway oil—In cases of acute gum inflammation, take 0.5 ml of the herbal mixture in half a glass of water three times daily. Rinse slowly in the mouth before spitting out. For daily hygiene, use slightly less of the mixture in half a glass of water and repeat only one or two times daily.[3]

Actions: See Table 6.3 for a listing of each herb's action

Table 6.3
ACTION OF HERBS IN MOUTHWASH FOR PERIODONTAL DISEASE

Herb	Action
Sage oil, peppermint oil, caraway oil, and menthol	Inhibit the growth of microorganisms (e.g., bacteria) that may cause inflammation Prevent bad breath Caraway oil increases blood flow to affected tissue
Myrrh	Astringent effect on the gums, helping to tighten them. This helps stop bleeding
Clove oil	Alleviates pain
Echinacea	Increases the body's resistance to infections
Chamomile	Antiinflammatory actions

Toothpaste

- Sage oil, peppermint oil, chamomile tincture, expressed juice from *Echinacea purpurea* herb, myrrh tincture, and rhatany tincture[4]
Action: In addition to the actions listed in Table 6.3, rhatany tincture tightens the gums through its astringent properties

NUTRITIONAL SUPPLEMENT CONSIDERATIONS

- Vitamin C with bioflavonoids—250 milligrams twice daily[5]
- Zinc citrate—Use a chewable tablet or liquid so it can make contact with the gums[6]
- Coenzyme Q-10—50 milligrams daily[7]

DIETARY RECOMMENDATIONS

Reduce your simple carbohydrate (including sugar) intake. Eat healthy foods that are high in fiber and complex carbohydrates (vegetables, fruits, and grains). Consumption of foods high in bioflavonoids such as grapes and blueberries is also encouraged.

Musculoskeletal System

RELATED CHAPTERS IN PART 5

- Eleuthero
- Evening Primrose
- Ginger

RHEUMATOID ARTHRITIS

The term *arthritis* refers to a condition that causes inflammation and tissue damage in the joints of the body. Arthritic conditions include rheumatoid arthritis, osteoarthritis, psoriatic arthritis, juvenile arthritis, and ankylosing spondylitis.

Rheumatoid arthritis (RA) is the most common type of arthritis. Estimates are that 1 to 3 percent of the U.S. population suffers from RA. As opposed to osteoarthritis, which primarily affects an older population, RA most commonly begins around 20 to 40 years of age. Women seem to be more susceptible and have a three times greater incidence of RA than men.

The first appearance of RA is often preceded by a low-grade fever, fatigue, and generalized joint stiffness and pain. Within several weeks, the condition may affect several joints (in some people only one or two joints may be affected), causing swelling and pain. The joints of the hands, feet, wrists, ankles, and knees are most commonly affected. Rheumatoid arthritic joints are often referred to as "hot" because they are red, swollen, and warm to the touch.

Rheumatoid arthritis is usually relapsing. Bouts come and go. After time, however, chronic inflammation causes the joints to become deformed. The goal of any treatment plan should be early intervention to slow progression of joint destruction.

Rheumatoid arthritis is largely believed to be an autoimmune illness. *Autoimmune* refers to the fact that a person's own immune system is attacking a particular part of the body. In the case of RA, the site of action is the joints, specifically the synovial lining that acts to lubricate the joints and keep them working normally.

What causes RA? Like other autoimmune illnesses, we don't know for sure. Family history of RA may be one predictor. Evidence suggests an infection may trigger the onset of RA.

There's also compelling evidence that diet and the health of our intestinal tract may play a role in RA. As we'll note in the section on dietary recommendations, food allergies and also saturated fats can make RA worse. Without a healthy intestinal tract, allergens from food may pass into the bloodstream and spark an allergic response in the joints. A good diet and the addition of supplements high in healthy bacterial microorganisms (such as members of the *Lactobacillus* and *Bifidobacterium* groups) promote intestinal tract health.

HERBAL PRESCRIPTIONS

Long-Term Treatment

- Evening primrose oil (combined with fish oil)—The combination should equal approximately 80 percent evening primrose oil and 20 percent fish oil. Take twelve capsules daily with meals in two or three divided doses.[1]

  Action: Evening primrose oil and fish oil provide a balanced supply of essential fatty acids to help the body produce hormones known as prostaglandins. These substances help steer the body away from inflammation.

- Bromelain—125 to 450 milligrams three times daily on an empty stomach[2]

  Action: Bromelain is an enzyme contained in pineapple. It reduces inflammation and helps strengthen the connective tissue in the joints.

- Eleuthero (Siberian ginseng)—Standardized, concentrated extract of the root and rhizomes, 300 to 400 milligrams daily; dry, powdered root and rhizomes, 2 to 3 grams daily in two or three divided doses. Alcohol-based extract, 8 to 10 ml in two to three divided doses. Use continuously for 4 to 6 weeks with a 1- to 2-week break before resuming.

Actions: This one probably comes as a bit of a surprise. However, the immune system balance and adrenal support offered by eleuthero are important factors in any autoimmune disease.

Short-Term Relief
- Capsaicin ointment (0.025 percent concentration)—Apply to affected area four times daily. Be sure to avoid contact with eyes or mouth as this stuff is hot![3]
  Action: Capsaicin is the component of cayenne pepper responsible for its hot taste. It reduces pain by blocking the action of pain fibers and a transmitter chemical known as substance P.

OTHER HERBAL CONSIDERATIONS
- Ginger rhizome powder—2 to 3 grams daily
- Devil's claw root (*Harpagophytum procumbens*)—3 to 4 grams three times daily
- Yucca stalk (*Yucca schidigera*)—1 to 2 grams three times daily

NUTRITIONAL SUPPLEMENT CONSIDERATIONS
Note: Research suggests that people with RA may benefit from the use of antioxidant nutrients.[4] Remember that herbs high in bioflavonoids are powerful antioxidants (see "Antioxidants" in Part 4).

DIETARY RECOMMENDATIONS[5]
- Vitamin E—800 international units (IU) daily
- Selenium—200 micrograms daily
- Vitamin C (with bioflavonoids)—1 to 2 grams daily
- Zinc (monomethionine or citrate)—30 milligrams daily
- Manganese—15 milligrams daily
- Acidophilus/bifidus supplement

With the guidance of a health care professional trained in nutrition, eliminate potential food allergens from your diet. Recent research promotes a 7- to 10-day therapeutic fast as a powerful tool in the treatment of RA.[6]

Fasting not only clears allergens from your system, it also gives your intestinal tract a chance to recover and reestablish a normal balance of healthy microorganisms. Remember that fasting should be done only under the guidance of a qualified health care professional. Fasting is not recommended for persons with diabetes, HIV infection, or for young children.

Shift your diet in the vegetarian direction.[7] Increase your intake of onions, garlic, and turmeric. Reducing fats from animal sources such as red meat and dairy products is essential. Also, avoid fried foods and reduce your intake of sweets.

LIFESTYLE CONSIDERATIONS

Don't stop exercising! Try swimming or another exercise that places less pressure on the joints. Yoga is also an excellent form of exercise for people with RA. I also highly recommend acupuncture or some form of massage as part of your regular treatment program.

SPRAINS AND STRAINS

WHAT MY TRAINER TOLD ME

Immediately after the injury or sprain, apply RICE (rest, ice, compression, and elevation). This decreases circulation to the injured area and lessens swelling.

Also, don't forget to see your doctor. Ligament and tendon injuries may need to be stabilized for proper healing.

WHAT MY WIFE TOLD ME

"Oy vey, not another ankle injury!"

TOPICAL CONSIDERATIONS

• Horse chestnut extract gel (standardized to contain 2 percent escin)—
Apply a thin layer of the gel over the injured area once or twice daily and then gently rub it into the skin. Avoid contact with your eyes.[1]
Action: Widely used in Europe for sports injuries, horse chestnut extract gel contains escin, which has been proven to reduce inflammation and swelling at the site of the injury.[2]

SUPPLEMENTS FOR INTERNAL USE

- Bromelain—450 milligrams three times daily between meals[3]
- Curcumin—600 milligrams three times daily[4]
- Manganese—15 milligrams daily
- Vitamin C (with bioflavonoids)—2 to 3 grams daily
  Note: Bromelain and curcumin are excellent for both short-term and long-term recovery. Manganese and vitamin C with bioflavonoids are long-term therapies that will help strengthen injured ligaments or tendons.

PHYSICAL THERAPY CONSIDERATIONS

- Ultrasound
- TENS (transcutaneous electrical nerve stimulation)

Nervous System

Related Chapters in Part 5

- Chamomile
- Eleuthero (Siberian Ginseng)
- Evening Primrose
- Feverfew
- *Ginkgo biloba*
- Asian Ginseng
- Kava-Kava
- Milk Thistle
- St. John's Wort
- Valerian

Alzheimer's Disease (Prevention and Early Stage)

Except for cardiovascular disease and cancer, the major health care concern among elderly people in our society is dementia. *Dementia* refers to mental deterioration. The most common form of dementia is Alzheimer's disease. Close to 2 million Americans have Alzheimer's and the incidence is on the rise.

Alzheimer's disease that starts before age 65 is referred to as "presenile" dementia. After 65, you've got "senile" dementia (I believe people over 65 ought to resist the label "senile"). The condition starts with memory loss and signs of depression, including apathy and social withdrawal. As the brain degenerates, these symptoms progress to problems with speaking, impaired ability to make proper judgments, and personality changes including paranoid thoughts. In the advanced stages of the illness, people usually require full-time supervision to counter confusion and also aggressive behavior.

Although medicine really knows very little about the condition and how to prevent or treat it, there are a few findings of interest. Medical research has looked at the brains of people with Alzheimer's after they've died and found key areas destroyed and infiltrated with abnormal protein. Also, the neurotransmitters serotonin and acetylcholine—chemical substances that carry messages in the brain—are either low or don't have proper binding sites in Alzheimer's patients. Lastly, Alzheimer's patients show a 30 percent reduction in normal blood flow to the brain.

All of this makes for wonderful discussion among doctors. What *you* really want to know is how to prevent the condition. Although we're a long way from a clear answer, there is new information emerging that indicates prevention may involve reducing free radicals in the brain through the use of antioxidant herbs and nutrients.

Also, with the proven effectiveness of *Ginkgo biloba* extract in the early stages of Alzheimer's, we may be able to slow the progression of the disease and improve quality of life.

Note: The recommendations made here address prevention. In the case of ginkgo, new research indicates that it is effective in the early stages of Alzheimer's disease. Although I'm not opposed to using these recommendations for patients with moderate to advanced Alzheimer's, it is unrealistic to expect very significant results.

HERBAL PRESCRIPTIONS

- *Ginkgo biloba* extract—240 milligrams daily in two to three divided doses

  Actions: Improves blood flow to the brain. Protects the cells of the brain from free radical damage. Increases the number of and normalizes serotonin receptors in the brain. Very effective for treatment of patients with depression and memory loss in the early stages of Alzheimer's disease

- Asian ginseng—100 milligrams twice daily of an extract standardized to contain 4 to 7 percent ginsenosides[1]

  Actions: Protects cells of the brain and increases serotonin activity. Increases mental alertness

NUTRITIONAL SUPPLEMENT CONSIDERATIONS

- Folic acid—400 micrograms daily[2]
- Vitamin B_{12}—Intramuscular injection of 1,000 micrograms once monthly

Note: This treatment should be performed only by a skilled health care practitioner[3,4]

- Vitamin B$_6$—100 milligrams daily
  Note: A combination of vitamin B$_6$, B$_{12}$, and folic acid helps to counter the formation of homocysteine. This substance is believed to contribute to atherosclerosis, as well as depression and dementia, in the elderly.[5] These three nutrients should be paired with ginkgo.
- Vitamin E—800 international units (IU) daily[6]
- Selenium—200 micrograms daily[7]
- Acetyl-L-carnitine—1 gram twice daily[8]

ANXIETY

Anxiety is the most common psychiatric diagnosis in our society today. Five percent of the population is diagnosed with anxiety. It commonly afflicts younger adults.

Stress, feelings of isolation, and internal conflicts can all contribute to anxiety. The most obvious trigger is stress. People push themselves daily, forgetting their body's need to relax and recover. Anxiety is often a sign that body reserves (i.e., adrenal glands) have been exhausted.

Less obvious triggers can also lead to the same point. Repressed internal feelings are another source of anxiety. Modern society has also isolated many people, with the resulting feelings of detachment both physically and emotionally producing anxiety.

Acute anxiety attacks are known as panic attacks. Usually lasting a few minutes to 1 or 2 hours, these attacks can be frightening. Shortness of breath, rapid heart beat, and chest pain sometimes accompany these attacks. Although rarely a medical emergency, acute panic attacks can cause hyperventilation. This is dangerous and needs to be monitored by a medical professional.

Persons with chronic anxiety may go unnoticed. If they experience attacks of anxiety, they are usually less severe and of longer duration. These individuals are often uneasy in public and have uncertainty about the future. They commonly complain about chronic fatigue, insomnia, and a variety of physical problems.

As noted in the chapters on kava and valerian in Part 5, antianxiety drugs are among the most common prescriptions in our society today. The herbal recommendations made here are alternatives for the treatment of mild to moderate anxiety. I also recommend reviewing the discussion on stress and fatigue in the chapter "Endocrine System." A complete program for treating anxiety should include combating adrenal exhaustion.

HERBAL PRESCRIPTIONS

- Kava root extract (70 percent kava lactones)—100 milligrams three times daily
  Action: Relaxing effect on the body without a narcotic-like effect on the mind
- Valerian root extract—300 to 400 milligrams two times daily
  Action: Mild sedative effect on the body and mind. It is the treatment of choice if insomnia is a component of your anxiety.

Note: Valerian is commonly combined with passion flower or lemon balm in European herbal products used to treat anxiety. I do not recommend using valerian with kava.

For other herbal, nutritional, and lifestyle recommendations, please see the section on stress and fatigue in the chapter "Endocrine System."

ATTENTION-DEFICIT HYPERACTIVITY DISORDER

One need venture no further than the last few volumes of the American Psychiatric Association's *Diagnostic and Statistical Manual of Mental Disorders* to realize the uncertainty surrounding the diagnosis of attention-deficit hyperactivity disorder (ADHD). The last two to three decades have seen this condition labeled minimal brain damage, minimal brain dysfunction, behavior and learning disorder, hyperkinetic–impulsive disorder, hyperkinetic syndrome, developmental hyperactivity, and finally attention-deficit hyperactivity disorder. What is apparent is that ADHD is a collection of symptoms or criteria. The decision to label a child with the diagnosis of ADHD is fraught with the potential for error.

Nowhere is this more evident than in attempts to estimate the number of children with ADHD. Recent estimates place the numbers at 10 percent of boys and 3 percent of girls ranging in age from 4 to 11 years old. The central feature of ADHD is trouble getting things done, both at home and at school, and trouble getting along with adults and other children. The increased activity and short attention span of the child with ADHD have led to the use of stimulant drugs such as Ritalin to control behavior. Paradoxically, these medications work to "slow down" the ADHD child. Unfortunately, these medications are potentially harmful and act merely to mask symptoms without getting to the core of the problem.

Early intervention and successful treatment of ADHD have become even more important in light of recent studies that predict these children face greater problems as adults. Evidence is mounting that children with ADHD are at higher risk for depression, restlessness, alcoholism, and antisocial behavior as adults.[1]

HERBAL PRESCRIPTIONS
- Eleuthero (Siberian ginseng)—Please use one-half the recommended dose for adults listed under "Other Herbal Considerations" in the following section on depression.
  Actions: Helps correct blood sugar metabolism and adrenal function
- Evening primrose oil—2 to 3 grams daily[2]
  Action: Recommended by the Hyperactive Children's Support Group of Great Britain. It corrects the essential fatty acid deficiency noted in some ADHD children.

NUTRITIONAL SUPPLEMENT CONSIDERATIONS
- Vitamin B_6—50 to 100 milligrams daily[3]
- Zinc—5 to 10 milligrams daily[4]
- Copper—0.5 to 1 milligram daily
- Chromium—200 micrograms daily[5]

DIETARY RECOMMENDATIONS
A whole-foods diet, high in protein and complex carbohydrates. Cut down on sugar and simple carbohydrates.[6] Cut back on processed junk

foods high in additives and food colorings. The Hyperactive Children's Support Group of Great Britain recommends that the following food additives be avoided:

Tartrazine	Quinoline Yellow	Caramel
Sunset Yellow	FCF	Cochineal
Benzoic acid	Carmoiic acid	Sodium benzoate
Amaranth	Sulfur dioxide	Sodium nitrate
Red 2G	Potassium nitrate	BHA
Brilliant Blue FCF	BHT	Indigo
Carmine		

Try to avoid foods, such as the following, with high salicylate content:[7]

Plums (canned)	Prunes (canned)
Raspberries (fresh)	Strawberries (fresh)
Peppers	Tomatoes
Almonds	Peanuts
Peppermint tea	Honey

Many spices: cardamom, cinnamon, cloves, curry, oregano, paprika, pepper, rosemary, sage, turmeric

Lowering the intake of cow's milk, soy, eggs, wheat, citrus, and other potential allergenic foods may be helpful until your child's behavior improves.[8] Identification and elimination of food allergens should be done under the supervision of a trained health care practitioner.

LIFESTYLE CONSIDERATIONS
- Limit TV watching and video games.
- Work with a counselor to discover if there are any family relationship problems that may be triggering ADHD behaviors.
- Children with ADHD living in urban areas should be tested for possible lead poisoning.

DEPRESSION

The diagnosis of depression includes the presence, for at least 2 weeks, of at least four of the following signs and symptoms:

Poor appetite or significant weight loss

Either lack of sleep or abnormally long periods of sleep

Mental agitation or slowing of mental functioning

Loss of interest in usual activities, including decreased sex drive

Loss of energy and fatigue

Low self-esteem and feelings of worthlessness or self-reproach

Complaints or evidence of decreased ability to concentrate
or think clearly

Recurrent thoughts of death or talk of suicide or actual suicide attempts

Depression is a broad definition and can range from mild, situational depression to more serious states requiring medication and possible hospitalization. The depressed individual should be under the supervision of a health care professional. Treatment of depression is usually complicated and requires the input of many different medical specialties.

Older people with impaired blood flow to the brain (known as cerebrovascular insufficiency) are particularly susceptible to depression. Depression often occurs with memory loss and, sometimes, irritability. It's ironic that this form of depression is often described as "resistant" because it does not respond well to many prescription antidepressants. As noted in the chapter on ginkgo in Part 5, reestablishing healthy blood flow often leads to a dramatic reversal of these symptoms.

HERBAL PRESCRIPTIONS

Mild to Moderate Depression

- St. John's wort extract—A daily dose that delivers at least 1 milligram of hypericin is recommended. For example, an extract standardized to contain 0.2 percent hypericin would require a daily dose of 500 milligrams (usually given in two or three divided doses).
  Action: Mild monoamine oxidase-inhibiting action leads to increased levels of norepinephrine in the brain. This has an antidepressive effect

Older Individuals with "Resistant" Depression

- *Ginkgo biloba* extract—240 milligrams daily in two to three divided doses
  Action: Increases blood flow to the brain

OTHER HERBAL CONSIDERATIONS

- Eleuthero (Siberian ginseng)—Standardized, concentrated extract of the root and rhizomes, 300 to 400 milligrams daily; dry, powdered root and rhizomes, 2 to 3 grams daily in two or three divided doses; alcohol-based extract, 8 to 10 ml in two to three divided doses. Use continuously for 4 to 6 weeks with a 1- to 2-week break before resuming.
- Milk thistle extract (standardized to 70 or 80 percent silymarin)—420 milligrams of silymarin in three divided doses
  Note: Milk thistle extract protects the liver if you are taking prescription antidepressants.

NUTRITIONAL SUPPLEMENT RECOMMENDATION

- Vitamin B complex—50 milligrams twice daily[1]
- Folic acid—400 micrograms daily[2]
- Vitamin B_{12}—Intramuscular injection of 1,000 micrograms (1 milliliter) once monthly
  Note: The vitamin B_{12} treatment should be performed only by a skilled health care practitioner[3,4]
- Vitamin B_6—100 milligrams daily
  Note: A combination of vitamin B_6, B_{12}, and folic acid helps to counter the formation of homocysteine. This substance has been linked to atherosclerosis, as well as depression and dementia, in the elderly.[5] These three nutrients should be paired with ginkgo in elderly depressed individuals

DIETARY RECOMMENDATIONS

Identify and eliminate food allergens under the supervision of a trained health care practitioner. A trial elimination of wheat and cow's milk may prove beneficial. Small, frequent meals high in protein and complex carbohydrates help regulate blood sugar. Avoid excessive consumption of sugar and other simple carbohydrates.

OTHER MEDICAL CONSIDERATIONS

Be sure your doctor checks for anemia and low thyroid function.

INSOMNIA

More than one-third of the adult population has trouble sleeping. Stress is a major culprit. However, if stress is affecting your sleep and loss of sleep is making you a wreck the next day, the last thing you want to hear is a lecture on stress reduction. So, let's look at some approaches to help you sleep and when you're rested, you can read the section on fatigue and stress in the chapter "Endocrine System."

HERBAL PRESCRIPTIONS

- Valerian root extract (minimum of 0.5 percent essential oils)—300 to 500 milligrams 1 hour before bedtime. Valerian root extracts combined with passion flower, lemon balm, and scullcap can also be used. Children 6 to 12 years old will usually respond to one-half the adult dose.
  Action: Mild central nervous system sedative. Helps you get to sleep quicker and enjoy a deeper sleep. Valerian is not addictive and doesn't cause the "morning hangover" common to many sleep aids
- Passion flower (concentrated extract)—200 to 300 milligrams 1 hour before bedtime. Liquid preparations should be taken at a dose of 4 to 6 milliliters.[1]
  Action: Mild central nervous system sedative

OTHER HERBAL CONSIDERATIONS

- Chamomile—2 to 3 milliliters of a liquid extract in warm water before bed. Chamomile is a mild sedative and best reserved for infants or young children with restlessness caused by colic or teething.
- Other mild herbal sedatives—Scullcap and hops (herbal capsules or tinctures, not a six-pack!)

MIGRAINE HEADACHE

Migraine headaches are characterized by throbbing pain on one or both sides of the head, occasionally accompanied by nausea, vomiting, and sensitivity to light. Approximately 80 percent of migraine headaches are classified as "common" migraines. These migraines last from 1 to 3 days and seldom have any warning signals prior to the headache.

Other migraine sufferers report symptoms that precede their headaches, including "auras"—blurring or bright spots around certain objects. This may be accompanied by disturbed thinking, anxiety, fatigue, and numbness or tingling on one side of the body. These are referred to as "classic" migraines and may last from 2 to 6 hours. This type of migraine is usually localized to one side of the head and accounts for approximately 10 percent of migraines. The remaining 10 percent come from a migraine-like headache known as *cluster headaches*.

HERBAL PRESCRIPTIONS
- Feverfew—125 milligrams or more of a dried leaf preparation standardized to contain at least 0.2 percent parthenolide. The daily parthenolide dose should be at least 250 micrograms.
  Actions: Inhibits serotonin and inflammatory mediator release from platelets. Improves blood vessel tone in affected area.

OTHER HERBAL CONSIDERATIONS
- Ginger—1 to 2 grams daily of rhizome powder
- *Ginkgo biloba* extract—120 milligrams daily in two to three divided doses[1]

NUTRITIONAL SUPPLEMENT CONSIDERATIONS
- Magnesium—200 to 300 milligrams twice daily[2]
- MaxEPA (fish oil)—3 to 4 grams daily with meals[3]

DIETARY RECOMMENDATIONS
Ban foods high in vasoactive amines from your diet. Key among these are aged cheeses, red wine, chocolate, and pickled herring. Identify and eliminate food allergens under the supervision of a health care practitioner.[4] Use ginger in liberal amounts with your cooking. Drop aspartame-containing beverages and foods from your diet.

MISCELLANEOUS CONSIDERATIONS
Relaxation and stress reduction are critical to the long-term success of any program for migraines. Biofeedback, acupuncture, massage, and meditation are methods you can use to reduce stress.

Neuropathy (Diabetic)

Diabetic neuropathy is a common complication of diabetes. It affects approximately 28.5 percent of all diabetics. It's a progressive disorder of the nerves that leads to an initial sensation of "pins and needles" in the soles of the feet and palms of the hands.

Neuropathy can advance to a point at which sufferers have difficulty differentiating temperature and pressure changes in their extremities. This can lead to an inability to know when a burn or cut on the foot, for example, has occurred.

HERBAL PRESCRIPTIONS

- Evening primrose oil—4 to 6 grams daily with meals
  Action: Supplies essential fatty acids, such as gamma-linolenic acid (GLA), that are improperly metabolized by diabetics. GLA and other essential fatty acid metabolites increase the levels of protective hormone-like substances known as prostaglandins.

OTHER HERBAL CONSIDERATIONS

- *Ginkgo biloba* extract—120 to 160 milligrams daily in two to three divided doses

NUTRITIONAL SUPPLEMENT CONSIDERATIONS

- Vitamin B_6—50 milligrams twice daily
- Vitamin B_{12}—1,000 micrograms daily

DIETARY RECOMMENDATIONS

Please see the recommendations listed for diabetes in the chapter "Endocrine System."

Respiratory Tract

ASTHMA

Asthma is a tightening of the bronchial tubes that leads to wheezing and difficulty in breathing. While the precise cause of asthma is unclear at this point, we do know that many stimuli or stresses can induce an asthma attack. These include viral infections, exposure to allergens such as pollen or food, inhalation of cold air, airborne irritants (pollution, cigarette smoke), emotional distress, and exercise.

Standard drug treatment of asthma focuses on combating acute asthma attacks and reducing bronchial tightness between attacks. Unfortunately, these medications often must be taken for many years. While they're potentially life-saving in some situations, recent research has found that regular use of bronchodilating medications such as Alupent and albuterol may harm cardiovascular health.[1,2]

Research in the United States, England, and Australia has shown that medicine is failing miserably in the long-term treatment of asthma. The rate of death among asthmatics actually rose during the decade of the 1980s![3] Again, the finger points directly at the choice of medications for long-term treatment of asthma, although the rise in air pollution is probably another contributing factor.

While natural medicine has little to offer for the treatment of a serious asthma attack, it does possess tools to improve the long-term outlook. This is another example of the complementary way that medical doctors and alternative medical practitioners can work together to optimize patient care.

HERBAL PRESCRIPTIONS

- *Ginkgo biloba* extract—120 milligrams daily in two to three divided doses. For children 6 to 12 years old, reduce the dosage to 80 milligrams daily. Children under 6 years, use 40 milligrams daily[4,5]
  Actions: Inhibits the substance platelet-activating factor. Platelet-activating factor increases the tightness (hyperresponsiveness) of bronchioles. Ginkgo is also a scavenger of free radicals (i.e., it is an antioxidant).

- Quercetin—500 milligrams two to three times daily
  Action: Like other bioflavonoids, quercetin is a natural antihistamine. It is ideal if your asthma is linked to an airborne or food allergy.[6]

OTHER HERBAL CONSIDERATIONS

- Ma Huang (*Ephedra sinica*)—1 to 2 grams of the dried herb in two to three divided doses (this represents about 15 to 30 milligrams of ephedrine)[7]
  Note: This Chinese herb provides two constituents commonly used in over-the-counter medications for hay fever and asthma. The first, pseudoephedrine, is used as a nasal decongestant.

  The second, ephedrine, is included in products assisting with bronchodilation and providing relief from asthma attacks. The dosage of ephedrine should not exceed 150 milligrams in a 24-hour period for adults and children over 12 years old. While it provides excellent results, ephedrine can also strain the heart and adrenal glands. I do not favor prescribing it for children less than 12 years old. I will occasionally use Ma Huang in cough formulations to add a mild bronchodilating and decongestant effect. However, I am a strong opponent of its long-term use and do not think it is a suitable substitute for the treatment of acute asthma attacks.

  Another new herbal bronchodilator being touted is the Ayurvedic herb *Tylophora asthmatica*.[8] Like Ma Huang, it is high in alkaloids and is probably not suitable for long-term use.

- Marshmallow root—2 grams three to four times daily
  Note: Mucilage-containing herbs are excellent for irritated airways.

NUTRITIONAL SUPPLEMENT CONSIDERATIONS

Note: The recommended dosages listed here are for adults. Appropriate reductions should be made for children, under the supervision of a health care practitioner. All supplements should be free of additives and potential allergens.

- Vitamin B$_6$—50 milligrams twice daily[9]
- Vitamin C—500 to 1,000 milligrams twice daily[10]
  Note: If your asthma gets worse when you exercise, try taking 1,000 milligrams of vitamin C about 15 minutes before you start exercising.
- Magnesium—300 milligrams daily
- Selenium—200 micrograms daily[11]

DIETARY RECOMMENDATIONS

Identify and eliminate food allergens under the supervision of a health care practitioner. Omitting cow's milk from the diets of children with asthma makes sense, but be sure to make up for the loss of calcium and vitamin D. Avoiding food additives, particularly sulfites, and food colorings is essential. The following list includes commonly used food additives and colorings:

Benzoic acid	EDTA derivatives
Formic acid	Sulfites
Sodium benzoate	Tartrazine
Food Red 14	Sunset Yellow
Propionic acid	4-Hydroxybenzoic acid
Malic acid	Acetic acid
Nitrate compounds	Benzaldehyde
Carminic acid	Cyclamate

And here are some foods high in sulfites:

Commercially baked products	Beer
Canned seafood	Canned soups
Corn sweeteners	Dried fruits
Food starches	Gelatin
Maraschino cherries	Mushrooms
Salads (in restaurants)	Sausage meats
Shrimp (uncooked; outside the United States)	Wine
	Vinegar

Keeping down saturated fats, primarily from animal products, will also assist in lowering the amount of proinflammatory mediators being produced. Hate to sound like a broken record, but we're talking a whole-foods, low processed food diet here, folks!

Eat lots of onions and garlic unless you're allergic to them. Onions have been shown to be an excellent antiasthma food![12]

Last, but not least, asthma is another of those childhood diseases that goes down dramatically when breast-feeding is a part of a child's first 9 to 12 months of life.[13]

LIFESTYLE CONSIDERATIONS

There's a lot of stigma attached to childhood asthma! Work with your child on relaxation and breathing exercises. I like to use visualization that encourages the asthmatic child to "open up," both physically and men-

---

**Vegetarian Diet and Natural Medicines
Combine to Improve Asthma[16]**

A 1985 Swedish study looked at the effect of a vegetarian diet and lifestyle changes on thirty-five adult asthmatics. The treatment regimen included

- Vegetarian diet: mainly raw foods and soups with no meat, fish, eggs, or dairy products
- Fresh, spring water
- No chocolate, coffee, caffeinated tea, sugar, or salt
- Initial 7-day juice fast
- Herbal teas from licorice and marshmallow
- Vitamin C, garlic, nettles were added as supplements
- Fresh, unpolluted air
- Regular physical activity

Twenty-four patients completed the study. The results indicated a 71 percent improvement after 4 months and a 92 percent improvement after 12 months.

---

tally. Breathing exercises are fabulous and can be a lot of fun. Try huffing and puffing and blowing your house down.

For adults, research has shown that yoga breathing exercises and relaxation are great for reducing asthma attacks.[14]

Children exposed to second-hand cigarette smoke have a greatly increased chance of asthma. Stop smoking around your kids![15]

Also, remember that some asthma medications can deplete adrenal reserves. Use eleuthero (Siberian ginseng) or Asian ginseng to support adrenal function if you're taking steroids or bronchodilators long-term.

COUGHS

Instead of trying to give you the medical details on different kinds of coughs, let me just say to be careful with coughs. A tight cough that makes breathing difficult should always be monitored by your doctor—particularly if it's a child who is having problems. If a large amount of phlegm and mucus are being produced, it may be a sign of bronchitis or pneumonia. Chronic coughs that aren't resolving should also be brought to the attention of your doctor.

The categories of coughs listed here have a lot of overlap. So don't be afraid to mix and match from different categories. These remedies are my personal favorites.

Mild, Irritating Cough

- Loquat syrup—1 to 2 tablespoons every 2 to 3 hours for short-term relief of cough. This is excellent for young children.
- Marshmallow root, mullein flowers, and slippery elm—Equal parts of each, either from liquid extracts or prepared in a tea from the dried product. In the liquid extract, take 2 tablespoons every 2 to 3 hours. As a tea, combine 2 to 3 teaspoonfuls of each herb and brew for 10 to 15 minutes. Strain the preparation and drink 8 to 10 ounces every couple of hours.[1]

Dry, Spasmodic Cough

- Drosera (sundew) and thyme—Equal parts of both herbs either as liquid extracts or as the dried herbs prepared in a tea. One tablespoon of the liquid extract preparation every 3 to 4 hours. With the tea, brew 1 to 2 grams of each herb and then strain. Drink 8 to 10 ounces three to four times daily.[2,3]

Note: Drosera and thyme are grossly underused in this country. Call your favorite herb company and tell them you want cough syrups with these ingredients!

Cough with Congestion

- Ma Huang, thyme, licorice root—This combination includes a bronchodilating herb (Ma Huang), an antispasmodic and expectorant herb (thyme), and a soothing and expectorant herb (licorice root). It also tastes bad, so combine it with some honey or glycerin to sweeten it. Follow the instructions given for the preceding drosera and thyme combination. Remember that Ma Huang should be administered only to older children and is intended for short-term use.

  Note: I'll usually recommend a steam with either tea tree oil or eucalyptus oil as another means to loosen mucus and help clear the airways. Place ¼ teaspoon of either oil in a pot of boiling water and steam for 10 to 15 minutes. For younger children, use a hot-air vaporizer at night.

Skin Conditions

RELATED CHAPTERS IN PART 5

- Chamomile
- Evening Primrose
- Milk Thistle
- St. John's Wort
- *Vitex agnus-castus*

ACNE

Acne is a complex skin problem that involves interactions among hormones, hair, sebaceous (oil-secreting) glands (collectively known as pilosebaceous glands), and bacteria. Teenagers, both male and female, are more susceptible to acne around the onset of puberty. This is attributed to an outburst in production of the hormone testosterone. Boys produce more testosterone than girls, which probably accounts for the increased incidence of acne in teenage males (one of the "testosterone curses"—male pattern baldness is another).

Acne vulgaris is characterized by open *comedones* (blackheads) or closed comedones (whiteheads). Blocked pilosebaceous glands may also lead to the growth of the bacteria *Propionibacterium acnes*. This can lead to deeper lesions, known as *acne conglobata*. This will often result in scarring.

Some women will experience acne right before their menstrual period. This is sometimes referred to as *premenstrual acne*.

Acne rosacea is a form of acne most common in middle-aged to older adults with a history of alcohol abuse. We will not cover it here, but remember to read about milk thistle extract (in Part 5) and digestive bitters (in Part 4).

HERBAL PRESCRIPTIONS

- Tea tree oil (15 percent solution)—Apply topically to acne lesion three to four times daily[1]

Actions: Antiinflammatory, antibacterial, and cleansing actions. Tea tree oil is a proven alternative to benzoyl peroxide

Note: Use at the recommended dilution. Stronger concentrations may irritate the skin. Avoid contact with the eyes

- *Vitex agnus-castus*—Liquid, concentrated extract or dried, powdered extract equivalent—40 drops of the liquid or one capsule of the dried extract once daily in the morning with some liquid
  Action: Vitex is useful for women experiencing premenstrual acne

OTHER HERBAL CONSIDERATIONS

- Burdock root—2 to 3 grams daily in two to three divided doses

NUTRITIONAL SUPPLEMENT CONSIDERATIONS

- Vitamin A—25,000 to 50,000 international units (IU) daily with meals[2]
  Note: Daily doses of vitamin A above 5,000 IU should be used by women of child-bearing age only under the supervision of a health care practitioner. Severe cases of acne may require higher doses than those listed here. This should also be supervised by a health care practitioner
- Zinc (citrate or monomethionine forms)—50 to 75 milligrams daily[3,4]
  Note: Be sure your copper intake is sufficient (5 to 7 milligrams at the dosages of zinc recommended here)
- Vitamin E—400 IU daily with meals
- Selenium—200 micrograms daily[5]
- Vitamin B_6—50 to 100 milligrams daily (useful for premenstrual acne flare-ups)[6]

DIETARY RECOMMENDATIONS

Cut down on simple carbohydrates, meat, dairy products, fried foods, and soda pop (sorry, McDonald's). Adopt a whole-foods diet high in complex carbohydrates and fiber from vegetables, grains, and fruits. Consumption of cold-water fish such as salmon is also recommended.

ECZEMA

Also known as atopic dermatitis, eczema is a chronic, itching, inflammatory condition of the skin. Eczema that begins in infancy is characterized by red, weeping, crusted lesions on the face, scalp, and extremities. Older children and adults are more likely to suffer dry, thick, localized patches. The incidence of eczema is estimated at 2 to 7 percent of the population.

Atopic dermatitis involves an allergic reaction. Two-thirds of children with eczema have a positive history of allergic disease in their family. Children whose mothers have allergies have an even greater chance of developing eczema (see "Evening Primrose" in Part 5). Eczema often occurs with other allergy-associated diseases such as asthma and hay fever.

HERBAL PRESCRIPTIONS

Internal Use
- Evening primrose oil
  Adults: 4 to 6 grams daily with meals (this includes breast-feeding mothers with a history of allergic disease)
  Children 1 to 12 years old: 2 to 4 grams daily with meals
- Chinese herbal combination (Zemaphyte)—One or two packets of the combination in hot water daily[1,2]
  Note: This product was created in England and currently bears a patent for use with eczema. I don't think it's available in this country. Among the herbal ingredients are licorice root. I recommend that you consult a specialist well versed in traditional Chinese medicine before you try to put this herbal combination together.

External Use
Apply each of the following topically to the affected area three to four times daily.

- Witch hazel extract cream (with phosphatidylcholine)[3]—This is an approved treatment for eczema in Europe. It has been shown to be as effective as 1 percent hydrocortisone.
- Glycyrrhetinic acid (from licorice root)[4]

Note: I highly recommend the use of glycyrrhetinic acid-containing topical creams or ointments if you are using topical cortisone. Glycyrrhetinic acid has been shown to focus the topical antiinflammatory action of cortisone and reduce its potential systemic side effects (topical *Aloe vera* gel has a similar effect)[5]

- Chamomile cream or ointment[6]

OTHER CONSIDERATIONS
- Chickweed ointment, calendula ointment

NUTRITIONAL SUPPLEMENT CONSIDERATIONS
- Zinc (monomethionine or citrate)
  Adults—30 milligrams daily
  Children 3 to 12 years old—15 milligrams daily
       1 to 3 years old—5 to 10 milligrams daily
       Less than 1 year old—2.5 to 5 milligrams daily
  Note: Be sure copper is included at a dose one-tenth that of the zinc dosage

DIETARY RECOMMENDATIONS
For children with eczema, the best dietary move is to eliminate food allergens. This is most easily done under the supervision of a health care practitioner well versed in nutrition. Cow's milk, eggs, wheat, and tomatoes are among the leading food triggers of eczema. Food additives and colorings should be reduced also.[7] Mothers with a history of allergies who decide to breast-feed should reduce allergenic foods in their diet. Dietary planning should also include the reduction of saturated fats—particularly those from animal sources. Consume more cold-water fish unless you have an identified allergy to them.

PSORIASIS

Psoriasis is a chronic and recurrent skin disease affecting 2 to 4 percent of the population in the United States. Characterized by well-defined, dry, silvery, and scaling lesions, it can appear on the scalp, the elbows and knees, the back, and the buttocks. Psoriasis may cause pitting in the nails and sometimes is associated with arthritis.

The root problem in psoriasis appears to be accelerated growth of skin cells. The skin cells of psoriasis patients divide approximately 1,000 times faster than normal skin cells!

Other factors contributing to psoriasis are abnormal bowel function, poor protein digestion, and sluggish liver function. All of these boost the levels of toxins in the body. Psoriasis sufferers may have a problem with increased permeability of the bowel, allowing endotoxins to cross more freely across the bowel walls and into the circulation. Certainly, maintaining normal bowel health is important in managing psoriasis.

HERBAL PRESCRIPTIONS

- Capsaicin ointment (0.025 percent concentration)—Apply to the affected area four times daily. Be sure to avoid contact with your eyes or mouth, as this stuff is hot![1,2]
  Action: Capsaicin is the component that gives cayenne pepper its hot taste. Topically, it relieves pain and itching that occurs in cases of moderate to severe psoriasis.
- Milk thistle extract (standardized to 70 or 80 percent silymarin)— 420 milligrams of silymarin in three divided doses
  Action: Supports and promotes normal liver function[3]
- Psyllium husk powder—Mix one rounded teaspoonful in an 8-ounce glass of water or juice and down the hatch! Repeat this two to three times daily for 7 to 10 days.
  Actions: Helps cleanse the bowel and encourages normal elimination

DIETARY SUPPLEMENT RECOMMENDATIONS

- MaxEPA (fish oil)—8 to 10 grams daily with meals[4]
- Zinc (citrate or monomethionine)—30 milligrams daily[5]
- Selenium—200 micrograms daily[6]
- Vitamin E—400 IU daily
- Folic acid—500 micrograms daily[7]

DIETARY RECOMMENDATIONS

Reduce alcohol consumption, junk foods and animal fats. Follow a whole-foods diet, high in complex carbohydrates and fiber (lots of vegetables and fruits), combined with cold-water fish.

> ### For Psoriasis, Try Dr. Fish!
>
> As medical professionals, we've been trained in this country to impress our colleagues and the public with our grasp of the research literature. This includes filling up books with more references than actual text! Well, how about a study to make you laugh?
>
> In a medical report that sounds more suitable for the *Twilight Zone* or even *Geek Love*, researchers in Kangal, Turkey, report on a new breakthrough in treating psoriasis. Psoriasis patients are instructed to bathe in hot springs. As opposed to the uninhabited pools we're used to, these hot springs are inhabited by fish of the Cyprinidae family. As the patient bathes, the friendly fish actually nibble on their psoriatic scales and soften them so they can be removed without trauma to the underlying skin. Business is great in Kangal thanks to Dr. Fish.[8]

VITILIGO

Vitiligo is a skin disease that causes patches of skin to lose their normal pigment. It usually appears around the mouth, eyes, and nose as well as the bony prominences of the elbows, knees, and hands.

Vitiligo is caused by an absence of pigment-producing cells called *melanocytes*. Although the exact reason is still unknown, it is widely believed that these cells are destroyed by the body's immune system.

Note: None of the following treatments works rapidly. Allow 6 to 9 months of initial use before making a final evaluation.

HERBAL PRESCRIPTIONS

- St. John's wort extract (standardized for hypericin content)—1.0 milligram of hypericin daily
  Action: Hypericin makes the skin more sensitive to ultraviolet light from the sun and other sources. This may serve to activate surviving

melanocytes. Be careful, however; vitiligo lesions can burn easily with overexposure to the sun

- Khella extract (*Ammi visnaga*)—Daily dose of the extract should provide approximately 100 milligrams of the active constituent khellin[1]
  Action: Like psoralen drugs, khellin stimulates the repigmentation of the skin in some individuals with vitiligo. Higher doses of 120 to 160 milligrams of khellin can cause nausea, insomnia, and an increase in liver enzymes. Your doctor should monitor you closely if you take khella for vitiligo.

NUTRITIONAL SUPPLEMENT CONSIDERATIONS[2]
- Folic acid—2 milligrams twice daily
- Vitamin C—500 milligrams twice daily
- Vitamin B_{12}—1,000 micrograms by intramuscular injection every 2 weeks. This should be performed only by a trained health care professional.

DIETARY CONSIDERATIONS
Some people with vitiligo have been found to produce less than normal amounts of stomach acid.[3] This leads to poor digestion of many nutrients, including vitamin B_{12}. Try adding herbal digestive bitters before each meal (see the discussion in Part 4).

OTHER SKIN CONDITIONS

ATHLETE'S FOOT (TINEA PEDIS)
- Tea tree oil cream (10 to 15 percent concentration)—Apply topically to the affected area two to three times daily[1]

FUNGAL INFECTION OF THE NAILS (ONYCHOMYCOSIS)
- Tea tree oil—Apply full strength to the affected nail twice daily. Trimming the nail back as much as possible will help with optimal delivery of the tea tree oil.[1]

SHINGLES (*HERPES ZOSTER*)

Topical Preparations: Apply to Affected Area Four Times Daily

- Glycyrrhizic acid ointment (from licorice root)—Helps speed the healing of lesions[1]
- Capsaicin ointment (0.025 percent concentration)—Be sure to avoid contact with eyes or mouth, as this stuff is hot! Capsaicin reduces the nerve pain (neuralgia) that often follows an outbreak of shingles.[2,3]

Urinary Tract

Related Chapter in Part 5

- Cranberry
- Echinacea
- *Ginkgo biloba*

Recurrent Urinary Tract Infections

Attempting to decide what constitutes "recurrent" with regard to urinary tract infections (UTIs) is not easy.[1] The textbook *General Urology* gets right to the point by stating, "Chronic cystitis (urinary tract infection) is confusing because it means different things to different people: some physicians use the term exclusively to mean unresolved or persistent bladder infections, whereas others use it to mean three or more bouts of bladder infection occurring in the course of one year."[2]

While the definition for recurrent UTIs is somewhat elusive, the hard facts of women suffering from the condition are not. Women suffering from UTIs account for approximately 5.2 million visits to physicians' offices each year. One of five women in the United States will suffer a UTI at some time in her life and of these, 3 percent will experience recurrent disease. Finally, 20 percent of women treated for a simple UTI will suffer a repeat bout.

Two common symptoms of UTI are burning, painful urination and frequent urination. However, recurrent UTIs pose more serious health risks, including scarring of the bladder wall. Pregnant women suffering from UTI run an increased risk of kidney infection due to anatomical pressure on the bladder.[3]

As was noted under "Cranberry" in Part 5, the guilty party in the majority of bacterial-induced UTIs is *Escherichia coli* (called *E. coli* for short), a common inhabitant of the gastrointestinal tract. Most recurrent UTIs can be linked to this organism.

HERBAL PRESCRIPTIONS

- Cranberry juice extract—300 to 400 milligrams of an encapsulated, concentrated extract in the morning and evening. Ample intake of water throughout the day is also recommended

  Actions: Inhibits the adherence of *E. coli* to the lining of the bladder and helps clear the bacteria from the urine

- *Echinacea purpurea* (expressed juice of the herb or encapsulated dried juice)—40 drops of the juice three times daily or one capsule of the dried juice three or four times daily for 6 to 8 weeks

  Action: Helps restore healthy immune function in individuals with recurrent infections, especially those who have taken antibiotics for long periods of time

OTHER HERBAL CONSIDERATIONS

- Goldenseal root—500 milligrams two to three times daily for 14 to 21 days

  Action: Weak antimicrobial activity without the side effects of antibiotics. Actions may complement the inhibitory action of cranberry against *E. coli.*[4]

- Marshmallow root—900 milligrams two to three times daily

  Action: Soothing effect (demulcent) on irritated tissue

NUTRITIONAL SUPPLEMENT CONSIDERATIONS

- Vitamin C—1 to 2 grams daily
- Acidophilus/bifidus capsules or powder—Recommended for both oral and vaginal applications[5]

DIETARY RECOMMENDATIONS

Drink four to five 8-ounce servings of water daily. Decrease simple carbohydrates (refined sugar) and artificial sweeteners. Get on an anti-diet soda crusade!

Support for Kidney Function while Taking Immune-Suppressive Drugs

People who have had kidney transplants are often in a Catch-22 situation. To prevent the body's immune system from rejecting the transplanted kidney, they are given a drug that suppresses the immune system. The most common choice is cyclosporin. Cyclosporin does its job effectively on the immune system, but it has a negative trade-off—it impairs kidney function over time. Two natural medicines may counter this side effect.

- *Ginkgo biloba* extract—120 to 160 milligrams daily in two to three divided doses[1]
- MaxEPA (fish oil)—6 grams daily with meals (each capsule contains 750 milligrams of fish oil)[2]

Herbal Medicine Resources

WITH the vast array of herbal products currently available, health care consumers are clamoring to find credible information to further their education in this area. Since many of these herbal medicines are used for conditions requiring careful medical monitoring, finding a physician with training or experience in the use of herbs is also important.

ORGANIZATIONS OFFERING HERBAL MEDICINE INFORMATION

American Botanical Council

P.O. Box 201660
Austin, Texas 78720
(512) 331-8868; fax (512) 331-1924

Headed by Mark Blumenthal, the hardest working man in the herb world, the American Botanical Council produces educational materials for both the public and professionals. They copublish *HerbalGram* with the Herb Research Foundation. The American Botanical Council also has an excellent list of books on herbal medicine.

American Herbalists Guild

P.O. Box 1683
Soquel, California 95073
phone/fax (408) 464-2441

A professional organization that represents the goals and voices of herbalists. Offers referral services for the herbal community and the public.

Herb Research Foundation
1007 Pearl Street, Suite 200
Boulder, Colorado 80302
(303) 449-2265; fax (303) 449-7849

This nonprofit organization is dedicated to the dissemination of reliable information on herbs. The Herb Research Foundation offers published summaries on specific herbs and also herbal approaches to certain health conditions.

HEALTH CARE PROFESSIONAL REFERRAL

American Association of Naturopathic Physicians
2366 Eastlake Avenue East, Suite 322
Seattle, Washington 98102
(206) 323-7610; fax (206) 323-7612

Want to know if there's a naturopathic physician in your area? The American Association of Naturopathic Physicians is the place to call. Their referral line will give you a local listing of naturopaths.

American Holistic Medical Association
4101 Lake Boone Trail #201
Raleigh, North Carolina 26707
(919) 787-5146

An eclectic collection of medical doctors, osteopathic physicians, naturopathic physicians, and nurses, the American Holistic Medical Association promotes the use of alternative and complementary therapies in medical practice. Its current president is that well-known Prima author Alan Gaby.

PROFESSIONAL SCHOOLS TEACHING HERBAL MEDICINE

Bastyr University
144 NE 54th Street
Seattle, Washington 98105
(206) 523-9585

National College of Naturopathic Medicine
11231 SE Market Street
Portland, Oregon 97216
(503) 255-4860

**Southwest College of Naturopathic
Medicine and Health Sciences**
6535 East Osborn
Scottsdale, Arizona 85251
(602) 990-7424

The Canadian College of Naturopathic Medicine
60 Berl Avenue
Estobicoke, Ontario, Canada M8Y 3C7
(416) 251-5261

MY FAVORITE BOOKS ON HERBAL MEDICINE

Weiss RF: *Herbal Medicine.* Ab Arcanum, Gothenberg, Sweden, 1988.
Tyler VE: *Herbs of Choice: The Therapeutic Use of Phytomedicinals.* Pharmaceutical Products Press, New York, 1994.
Werbach MR and Murray MT: *Botanical Influences on Illness: A Sourcebook of Clinical Research.* Third Line Press, Tarzana, California, 1994.

Note: The first three books listed are available from the American Botanical Council.

Foster S and Chongxi Y: *Herbal Emissaries: Bringing Chinese Herbs to the West.* Healing Arts Press, Rochester, Vermont, 1993.
Hoffman D: *The Herbal Handbook: A User's Guide to Medical Herbalism.* Healing Arts Press, Rochester, Vermont, 1988.
Mills SY: *Out of the Earth: The Essential Book of Herbal Medicine.* Viking Arkana, London, 1991.

FAVORITE NONHERB BOOKS

One Hundred Years of Solitude, Gabriel Garcia Marquez
The English Patient, Michael Ondaatje

Herbal Medicine Resources

Mama Day, Gloria Naylor
Geek Love, Katherine Dunn
Beloved, Toni Morrison
To the Wedding, John Berger
The Crossing, Cormac McCarthy
Very Old Bones, William Kennedy
Paris Trout, Pete Dexter
The Book of Laughter and Forgetting, Milan Kundera
Middle Passage, Charles Johnson
Postcards, E. Annie Proulx

References

PART 1: THE CHANGING FACE OF HERBAL MEDICINE

1. Eisenberg DM, Kessler RC, et al.: Unconventional medicine in the United States: Prevalence, costs and patterns of use. *New Engl J Med* 328:246–252, 1993.
2. Akerele O: WHO guidelines for the assessment of herbal medicines. *Fitoterapia* 63:99–110, 1992.
3. Israelson L: Summary of the Dietary Supplement Health and Education Act of 1994. *Quart Rev Nat Med* Spring:73–80, 1995.

PART 2: EUROPEAN PHYTOTHERAPY: A RATIONAL MODEL FOR THE FUTURE

1. Grünwald J: The European phytomedicines market: Figures, trends, analyses. *HerbalGram* 34:60–65, 1995.

PART 4: CATEGORIES OF HERBAL MEDICINES

1. Brekhman II and Dardymov IV: New substances of plant origin which increase nonspecific resistance. *Annu Rev Pharmacol* 9:419–430, 1969.
2. Wagner H, Nörr H, and Winterhoff H: Plant adaptogens. *Phytomedicine* 1:63–76, 1994.
3. Harman D: Free radicals in aging. *Molecular Cell Biochem* 84:155–161, 1988.
4. Diplock AT: Antioxidant nutrients and disease prevention: An overview. *Am J Clin Nutr* 53(Suppl.):373–379, 1991.
5. Bindoli A, Cavallini L, and Sliprandi N: Inhibitory action of silymarin on lipid peroxide formation in rat liver mitochondria and microsomes. *Biochem Pharmacol* 26:2405–2409, 1977.
6. Frankel EN, Kramer J, et al.: Inhibition of oxidation of human low-density lipoprotein by phenolic substances in red wine. *Lancet* 341:454–457, 1993.
7. Hertog MG, Feskens EJ, et al.: Dietary antioxidant flavonoids and risk of coronary heart disease: The Zutphen elderly study. *Lancet* 342:1007–1011, 1993.
8. Tyler VE: *Herbs of Choice: The Therapeutic Use of Phytomedicinals.* Pharmaceutical Products Press, New York, 1994, pp. 54–60.
9. Weiss RF: *Herbal Medicine.* Ab Arcanum, Gothenburg, Sweden, 1988, pp. 75–78.

10. Hoffman D: *The Herbal Handbook: A User's Guide to Medical Herbalism.* Healing Arts Press, Rochester, Vermont, 1988, pp. 54–57.

11. Ridker PM and McDermott WV: Comfrey herb tea and hepatic veno-occlusive disease. *Lancet* ii:657–658, 1989

12. Tyler VE: *Herbs of Choice: The Therapeutic Use of Phytomedicinals.* Pharmaceutical Products Press, New York, 1994, pp. 90–91.

13. Lien EJ and Gao H: Higher plant polysaccharides and their pharmacological activities. *International Journal of Oriental Medicine* 15:123–140, 1990.

14. Pastors JG, Blaidsell PW, et al.: Psyllium fiber reduces rise in postprandial glucose and insulin concentrations in patients with non-insulin-dependent diabetes. *Am J Clin Nutr* 53:1431–1435, 1991.

15. Passmore AP, Wilson-Davies K, et al.: Chronic constipation in long stay elderly patients: A comparison of lactulose and a senna-fiber combination. *Br Med J* 307:769–771, 1993.

PART 5:   COMMONLY PRESCRIBED HERBAL MEDICINES

BILBERRY

1. Nakayama T, Yamada M, et al.: Suppression of oxygen-induced cytotoxicity by flavonoids. *Biochem Pharmacol* 45:265–267, 1993.

2. Husain SR, Cillard J, and Cillard P: Hydroxyl radical scavenging activity of flavonoids. *Phytochemistry* 26:2489–2491, 1987.

3. Cunio L: *Vaccinium myrtillus. Aust J Med Herbalism* 5:81–85, 1993.

4. Tyler VE: *Herbs of Choice: The Therapeutic Use of Phytomedicinals.* Pharmaceutical Products Press, New York, 1994.

5. Baj A, Bombardelli E, et al.: Qualitative and quantitative evaluation of *Vaccinium myrtillus* anthocyanins by high-resolution gas chromotography and high-performance liquid chromotography. *J Chromatography* 279:365–372, 1983.

6. Pizzorno JE and Murray MT: *A Textbook of Natural Medicine.* John Bastyr College Publications, Seattle, Washington, 1985, V: VacMyr-1.

7. Bonati A: How and why should we standardize phytopharmaceutical drugs for clinical validation? *J Ethnopharmacol* 32:195–197, 1991.

8. Alfieri R and Sole P: Influence des anthocyanosides administres par voie parenterale sur l'adaptoelectroretinogramme du lapin. *CR Soc Biol* 158:2338, 1964.

9. Vaughan D and Asbury T: *General Ophthalmology.* Lange Medical Publications, Los Altos, California, pp. 163–164.

10. Salvayre R, Braquet P, et al.: Comparison of the scavenger effect of bilberry anthocyanosides with various flavonoids. *Proceed Int Bioflavonoid Symposium,* Munich, 1981, pp. 437–442.

11. Lietti A and Forni G: Studies on *Vaccinium myrtillus* anthocyanosides. I. Vasoprotective and anti-inflammatory activity. *Arzneim-Forsch Drug Res* 26:829–832, 1976.

12. Mian E, Curri SB, et al.: Anthocyanosides and the walls of microvessels: Further aspects of the mechanism of action of their protective effect in syndromes due to abnormal capillary fragility. *Minerva Med* 68:3565–3581, 1977.

13. Colantuoni A, Bertuglia S, et al.: Effects of *Vaccinium myrtillus* anthocyanosides on arterial vasomotion. *Arzneim-Forsch Drug Res* 41:905–909, 1991.

14. Pulliero G, Montin S, et al.: *Ex vivo* study of the inhibitory effects of *Vaccinium myrtillus* anthocyanosides on human platelet aggregation. *Fitoterapia* 60:69–75, 1989.

15. Monbiosse JC, Braquest P, et al.: Non-enzymatic degradation of acid-soluble calf skin collagen by superoxide ion: Protective effect of flavonoids. *Biochem Pharmacol* 32:53–58, 1983.

16. Rao CN, Rao VH, and Steinman B: Influence of bioflavonoids on the collagen metabolism in rats with adjuvant induced arthritis. *Ital J Biochem* 30:54–62, 1981.

17. Terrase J and Moinade S: Premiers resultats obtenus avec un nouveau facteur vitamonique P, les anthocyanosides, extaits du *Vaccinium myrtillus*. *Presse Med* 72:397–400, 1964.

18. Sala D, Rolando M, et al.: Effect of anthocyanosides on visual performance at low illumination. *Minerva Oftalmol* 21:283–285, 1979.

19. Gandolfo E: Perimetric follow-up of myopic patients treated with anthocyanosides and beta-carotene. *Boll Ocul* 69:57–71, 1990.

20. Scharrer A and Ober M: Anthocyanosides in the treatment of retinopathies. *Klin Monatsbl Augenheilkd Beih* 178:386–389, 1981.

21. Werbach MR and Murray MT: *Botanical Influences on Illness*. Third Line Press, Tarzana, California, pp. 271–272, 1994.

22. Grismond GL: Treatment of pregnancy-induced phlebopathies. *Minerva Gynecol* 33:221–230, 1981.

CHAMOMILE

1. Mann C and Staba EJ: The chemistry, pharmacology, and commercial formulations of chamomile. In: *Herbs, Spices, and Medicinal Plants: Recent Advances in Botany, Horticulture, and Pharmacology*, Vol. 1 (Craker LE and Simon JE, eds.). Oryx Press, Phoenix, Arizona, 1986, pp. 235–280.

2. Tyler VE: *Herbs of Choice: The Therapeutic Use of Phytomedicinals*. Pharmaceutical Products Press, New York, 1994, pp. 57–59.

3. Foster S: *Herbal Renaissance*. Gibbs-Smith Publisher, Salt Lake City, Utah, 1994, pp. 64–67.

4. Grieve M: *A Modern Herbal*. Dover Publications, New York, 1971, pp. 185–188.

5. Tyler VE: *The Honest Herbal*. Pharmaceutical Products Press, New York, 1993, pp. 83–86.

6. Wichtl M: *Herbal Drugs and Phytopharmaceuticals*. CRC Press, Boca Raton, Florida, 1994, pp. 322–325.

7. Jakolev V, Isaac O, et al.: Pharmacological investigations with compounds of chamomile. II. New investigations on the antiphlogistic effects of (–)-α-bisabolol and bisabolol oxides. *Planta Med* 35:125–140, 1979.

8. Jakolev V, Isaac O, and Flaskamp E: Pharmacological investigations with compounds of chamomile. VI. Investigations on the antiphlogistic effects of chamazulene and matricine. *Planta Med* 49:67–73, 1983.

9. Della Loggia R, Tubaro A, et al.: The role of flavonoids in the antiinflammatory activity of *Chamomilla recutita*. In: *Plant Flavonoids in Biology and Medicine: Biochemical, Pharmacological, and Structure–Activity Relationships* (Cody V, Middleton E, and Harborne JB, eds.). Alan R. Liss, New York, pp. 481–4, 1986.

10. Achterrath-Tuckerman U, Kunde R, et al.: Pharmacological investigations with compounds of chamomile. V. Investigations on the spasmolytic effect of compounds of chamomile and Kamillosan® on the isolated guinea pig ileum. *Planta Med* 39:38–50, 1980.

11. Weiss RF: *Herbal Medicine*. Ab Arcanum, Gothenberg, Sweden, 1988, pp. 1–11.

12. Tyler VE: Phytomedicines in Western Europe: Their potential impact on herbal medicine in the United States. *HerbalGram* 30:24–30, 67–68, 1994.

13. *Matricaria flos*. European Scientific Cooperative on Phytotherapy (ESCOP) Monograph, October 1990.

14. Mills SY: *Out of the Earth: The Essential Book of Herbal Medicine.* Viking Press, London, 1991, pp. 448–451.
15. Nasemann T: Kamillosan® therapy in dermatology. *Z Allg Med* 25:1105–1106, 1975.
16. Aggag ME and Yousef RT: Study of the antimicrobial activity of chamomile oil. *Planta Med* 22:140–144, 1972.
17. Bradley PR, ed.: Matricaria flower. In: *British Herbal Compendium,* Vol. 1. British Herbal Medicine Association, Bournemouth, Dorset, England 1992, pp. 154–157.
18. Glowania HJ, Raulin C, and Swoboda M: The effect of chamomile on wound healing—a controlled clinical experimental double-blind trail. *Z Hautkrankh* 62: 1262–71, 1987.
19. Nasemann T: op cit. 1975.
21. Monograph, *Matricariae flos. Bundesanzeiger*, March 3, 1990.
22. Mann C and Staba EJ: The chemistry, pharmacology, and commercial formulations of chamomile. In: *Herbs, Spices, and Medicinal Plants: Recent Advances in Botany, Horticulture, and Pharmacology,* Vol. 1 (Craker LE and Simon JE, eds.). Oryx Press, Phoenix, Arizona, 1986, pp. 235–280.

CRANBERRY

1. Blatherwick NR and Long ML: Studies on urinary acidity. II. The increased acidity produced by eating prunes and cranberries. *J Biol Chem* 57:815, 1923.
2. Bodel PT, Cotran R, and Kass EH: Cranberry juice and the antibacterial action of hippuric acid. *J Lab Clin Med* 54:881–888, 1959.
3. Moen DV: Observations on the effectiveness of cranberry juice in urinary tract infections. *Wis Med J* 61:282–283, 1962.
4. Papas PN, Brusch CA, and Ceresia GC: Cranberry juice in the treatment of urinary tract infections. *Southwest Med* 47:17–20, 1966.
5. Schaefer AJ: Recurrent urinary tract infection in the female patient. *Urology* 32 (Suppl.):12–15, 1988.
6. Bettman LR: Pathogenesis of urinary tract infections: Host susceptibility and bacterial virulence factors. *Urology* 32 (Suppl.):9–11, 1988.
7. Sobota AE: Inhibition of bacterial adherence by cranberry juice: Potential use for the treatment of urinary tract infections. *J Urol* 131:1013–1016, 1984.
8. Schmidt DR and Sobota AE: An examination of the anti-adherence activity of cranberry juice on urinary and nonurinary bacterial isolates. *Microbios* 55:173–181, 1988.
9. Zafiri D, Ofek I, et al.: Inhibitory activity of cranberry juice on adherence of type 1 and type P fimbriated *Escherichia coli* to eucaryotic cells. *Antimicrob Agents Chemother* 33:92–98, 1989.
10. Ofek I, Goldhar J, et al.: Anti-*Escherichia coli* adhesion activity of cranberry and blueberry juices. *New Engl J Med* 324:1599, 1991.
11. Avorn J, Monane M, et al.: Reduction of bacteriuria and pyuria after ingestion of cranberry juice. *JAMA* 271:751–754, 1994.
12. Gibson L, Pike L, and Kilbourn JP: Effectiveness of cranberry juice in preventing urinary tract infections in long-term care facility patients. *J Naturopath Med* 2:45–47, 1991.

ECHINACEA

1. Melchart D, Linde K, et al.: Immunomodulation with echinacea—a systemic review of controlled clinical trials. *Phytomedicine* 1:245–254, 1994.
2. Hobbs C: Echinacea: A literature review. *HerbalGram* 30:33–48, 1994.

3. Foster S: Echinacea Education Monograph. *Quart Rev Nat Med* Winter:19–28, 1993.

4. Foster S: *Echinacea, Nature's Immune Enhancer*. Healing Arts Press, Rochester, Vermont, 1991.

5. Stimpel M, Proksch A, et al.: Macrophage activation and induction of macrophage cytotoxicity by purified polysaccharide fractions from the plant *Echinacea purpurea*. *Infect Immunity* 46:845–849, 1984.

6. Leuttig B, Steinmüller C, et al.: Macrophage activation by the polysaccharide arabinogalactan isolated from plant cell cultures of *Echinacea purpurea*. *J Natl Cancer Inst* 81:669–675, 1989.

7. Kuhn O: Echinacin® and phagocyte reaction. *Arzneim-Forsch Drug Res* 3:194–200, 1953.

8. Wagner H and Proksch A: Immunomodulatory drugs of fungi and higher plants. In: *Economic and Medicinal Plant Research*, Vol. 1 (Farnsworth N, Hikino H, and Wagner H, eds.). Academic Press, Orlando, Florida, 1985, pp. 113–155.

9. Gaisbauer M, Schleich T, et al.: Phagocytic activity of granulocytes using chemiluminescence measurement. *Arzneim-Forsch Drug Res* 40:594–598, 1990.

10. Schoenberger D: The influence of immune-stimulating effects of pressed juice from *Echinacea purpurea* on the course and severity of colds. *Forum Immunol* 8:2–12, 1992.

11. Braunig B, Dorn M, et al.: *Echinacea purpurea* root for strengthening the immune response in flu-like infections. *Zeitschrift Phytother* 13:7–13, 1992.

12. Coeugniet E and Kühnast R: Recurrent candidiasis: Adjuvant immunotherapy with different formulations of Echinacin®. *Therapiewoche* 36:3352–3358, 1986.

13. Monograph, *Echinacea purpurea* herba. *Bundesanzeiger*, March 2, 1989.

ELEUTHERO (SIBERIAN GINSENG)

1. Baranov AI: Medicinal uses of ginseng and related plant in the Soviet Union: Recent trends in the Soviet literature. *J Ethnopharmacol* 6:339–353, 1982.

2. Foster S and Chingxi Y: *Herbal Emissaries*. Healing Arts Press, Rochester, Vermont, 1992, pp. 73–79.

3. Brekhman II and Dardymov IV: New substances of plant origin which increase non-specific resistance. *Annu Rev Pharmacol* 4:419–430, 1969.

4. Brekhman II: *Man and Biologically Active Substances*. Pergamon Press, Oxford, 1980.

5. Collisson RJ: Siberian ginseng (*Eleutherococcus senticosus*). *Br J Phytother* 2:61–71, 1991.

6. Farnsworth NR, Kinghorn AD, Soejarto DD, and Waller DP: Siberian ginseng (*Eleutherococcus senticosus*): Current status as an adaptogen. In: *Economic and Medicinal Plant Research*, Vol. 1 (Wagner H, Hikino HZ, and Farnsworth NR, eds.). Academic Press, London, 1985, pp. 155–215.

7. Hikino H, Takahashi M, et al.: Isolation and hypoglycemic activity of eleutherans A, B, C, D, E, F and G: Glycans of *Eleutherococcus senticosus* roots. *J Nat Prod* 49:293–297, 1986.

8. Tintera JW: The hypoadrenocortical state and its management. *NY State J Med* 55:1869–1876, 1955.

9. Wagner H, Nörr H, and Winterhoff H: Plant adaptogens. *Phytomedicine* 1:63–76, 1994.

10. Farnsworth NR, Kinghorn AD, Soejarto DD, and Waller DP: Siberian ginseng (*Eleutherococcus senticosus*): Current status as an adaptogen. In: *Economic and Medicinal Plant Research*, Vol. 1 (Wagner H, Hikino HZ, and Farnsworth NR, eds.). Academic Press, London, 1985, pp. 155–215.

11. Fulder S: The drug that builds Russians. *New Sci* 21:576–579, 1980.

12. Asano K, Takahashi T, et al.: Effect of *Eleutherococcus senticosus* extract on human working capacity. *Planta Med* 37:175–177, 1986.

13. McNaughton L: A comparison of Chinese and Russian ginseng as ergogenic aids to improve various facets of physical fitness. *Int Clin Nutr Rev* 9: 32–5, 1989.
14. Gubchenko PP and Fruentov NK: Comparative study of the effectiveness of *Eleutherococcus* and other plant adaptogens as remedies for increasing the work capacity of flight personnel. In: *New Data on Eleutherococcus: Proceedings of the Second International Symposium on Eleutherococcus*, Moscow, 1984, pp. 240–251.
15. Collisson RJ: Siberian ginseng (*Eleutherococcus senticosus*). *Br J Phytother* 2:61–71, 1991.
16. Ben-Hur E and Fulder S: Effect of P. ginseng saponins and Eleutherococcus S. on survival of cultured mammalian cells after ionizing radiation. *Am J Chin Med* 9:48–56, 1981.
17. Bohn B, Nebe CT, and Birr C: Flow-cytometric studies with *Eleutherococcus senticosus* extract as an immunomodulating agent. *Arzneim-Forsch Drug Res* 37:1193–1196, 1987.
18. Brekhman II: Eleutherococcus: 20 Years of Research and Clinical Applications. Presentation at the 1st International Symposium on Eleutherococcus, Hamburg, Germany, May 29, 1980.
19. Zykov MP and Protasova SF: Prospects of immunostimulating vaccination against influenza including the use of *Eleutherococcus* and other preparations of plants. In: *New Data on Eleutherococcus: Proceedings of the Second International Symposium on Eleutherococcus*, Moscow, 1984, pp. 164–169.
20. Yarameko KV: The main aspects of the use of *Eleutherococcus* extract in oncology. In: *New Data on Eleutherococcus and Other Adaptogens*. The Far Eastern Scientific Center, USSR Academy of Sciences. Vladivostok, USSR, 1981, pp. 75–78.
21. Institute of Oncology, Ministry of Health, Georgia, USSR. Reported in: Brekhman II: *Eleutherococcus: Clinical Data*. USSR Foreign Trade Publication, Medexport, USSR, 1970.
22. Kupin VI, Polevaya EB and Sorokin AM: Increased immunologic reactivity of lymphocytes in oncologic patients treated with *Eleutherococcus* extract. In: *New Data on Eleutherococcus: Proceedings of the Second International Symposium on Eleutherococcus*, Moscow, 1984, pp. 294–300.
23. Sutton F: Personal communication, 1984.

EVENING PRIMROSE

1. Kesteloot H, Lesaffre E, and Joossens JV: Dairy fat, saturated animal fat, and cancer risk. *Prevent Med* 20:226–236, 1991.
2. Erasmus E: *Fats and Oils*. Alive Books, Vancouver, British Columbia, Canada, 1986, pp. 34–44.
3. Horrobin DF and Manku MS: Clinical biochemistry of essential fatty acids. In: *Omega-6 Essential Fatty Acids: Pathophysiology and Roles in Clinical Medicine*. Alan R. Liss, New York, 1990, pp. 21–54.
4. Horrobin DF: Gamma linolenic acid: An intermediate in essential fatty acid metabolism with potential as an ethical pharmaceutical and as a food. *Rev Contemp Pharmacother* 1:1–45, 1990.
5. Tilvis RS and Miettinen TA: Fatty acid composition of serum lipids, erythrocytes and platelets in insulin-dependent women. *J Clin Endocrinol Metab* 61:741–745, 1985.
6. Gibson RA and Rassias G: Infant nutrition and human milk. In: *Omega-6 Essential Fatty Acids: Pathophysiology and Roles in Clinical Medicine*. Alan R. Liss, New York, 1990, pp. 283–293.
7. Oil of evening primrose. *Lawrence Review of Natural Products,* November 1993.
8. Jenkins DK, Mitchell JC, et al.: Effects of different sources of gamma-linolenic acid on the formation of essential fatty acid and prostanoid metabolism. *Med Sci Res* 16:525–526, 1988.
9. Barre DE, Holub BJ, and Chapkin RS: The effect of borage oil supplementation on human platelet aggregation, thromboxane B2, prostaglandin E1, and E2 formation. *Nutr Res* 13:739–751, 1993.

10. Horrobin DF: Nutritional and medical importance of gamma-linolenic acid. *Prog Lipid Res* 31:163–194, 1992.

11. Manku MS, Horrobin DF, et al.: Essential fatty acids in the plasma phospholipids of patients with atopic eczema. *Br J Dermatol* 110:643–648, 1984.

12. Grulee CG and Sanford HH: The influence of breast and artificial feeding on infantile eczema. *J Pediatr* 9:223–225, 1936.

13. Businco L, Ioppi M, et al.: Breast milk from mothers of children with newly developed eczema has low levels of long chain polyunsaturated fatty acids. *J Allergy Clin Immunol* 91:1134–1139, 1993.

14. Cant A, Shay J, and Horrobin DF: The effect of maternal supplementation with linoleic and gamma-linolenic acids on the fat composition and content of human milk: A placebo-controlled trial. *J Nutr Sci Vitaminol* 37:573–579, 1991.

15. Morse PF, Horrobin DF, et al.: Meta-analysis of placebo-controlled studies of the efficacy of Epogam in the treatment of atopic eczema. Relationship between plasma essential fatty acid changes and clinical response. *Br J Dermatol* 121:75–90, 1989.

16. Bordoni A, Biagi PL, et al.: Evening primrose oil (Efamol) in the treatment of children with atopic eczema. *Drugs Exp Clin Res* 14:291–297, 1987.

17. Berth-Jones J and Graham-Brown RAC: Placebo-controlled trial of essential fatty acid supplementation in atopic dermatitis. *Lancet* 341:1557–1560, 1993.

18. Horrobin DF and Morse PF: Evening primrose oil and atopic eczema (letter to the Editor). *Lancet* 345:260–261, 1995.

19. Horrobin DF: Gamma linolenic acid: An intermediate in essential fatty acid metabolism with potential as an ethical pharmaceutical and as a food. *Rev Contemp Pharmacother* 1:1–45, 1990.

20. Reichert RG: Evening primrose oil and diabetic neuropathy. *Quart Rev Nat Med* Summer:141–145, 1995.

21. Jamal GA and Charmichael H: The effect of gamma-linolenic acid on human diabetic peripheral neuropathy: A double-blind placebo-controlled trial. *Diabetic Med* 7:319–323, 1990.

22. Keen H, Payan J, et al.: Treatment of diabetic neuropathy with gamma-linolenic acid. *Diabetes Care* 16:8–15, 1993.

23. Brush MG, Watson SJ, et al.: Abnormal essential fatty acid levels in plasma of women with premenstrual syndrome. *Am J Obstet Gynecol* 150:363–366, 1984.

24. Horrobin DF, Manku MS, et al.: Abnormalities in plasma essential fatty acid levels in women with premenstrual syndrome and with nonmalignant breast disease. *J Nutr Med* 2:259–264, 1991.

25. McFayden IJ, Forest AP, et al.: Cyclical breast pain—some observations and the difficulties in treatment. *Brit J Clinical Practice* 46:161–164, 1992.

26. Gateley CA, Niers M, et al.: Drug treatments for mastalgia: 17-year experience in the Cardiff mastalgia clinic. *J R Soc Med* 85:12–15, 1992.

27. Pye JK, Mansel RE, and Hughes LE: Clinical experience of drug treatment for mastalgia. *Lancet* ii:373–377, 1985.

28. Cyclical breast pain—what works and what doesn't. *Drug Therapeut Bull* 30:1–3, 1992.

29. Collins A, Cerin A, et al.: Essential fatty acids in the treatment of premenstrual syndrome. *Obstet Gynecol* 81:93–98, 1993.

30. O'Brien PM and Massil H: Premenstrual syndrome: Clinical studies on essential fatty acids. In: *Omega-6 Essential Fatty Acids: Pathophysiology and Roles in Clinical Medicine.* Alan R. Liss, New York, 1990, pp. 523–545.

31. Brenner RR: Nutritional and hormonal factors influencing desaturation of essential fatty acids. *Prog Lipid Res* 20:41–48, 1982.

References

FEVERFEW

1. Feverfew. *Lawrence Review of Natural Products*, September, 1994.
2. Hobbs C: Feverfew (*Tanacetum parthenium*). *HerbalGram* 20:26–35, 1989.
3. Awang DVC: Herbal medicine, feverfew. *Canadian Pharm J* 122:266–270, 1989.
4. Hepinstall S, Awang DVC, et al.: Parthenolide content and bioactivity of feverfew (*Tanacetum parthenium*). Estimation of commercial and authenticated feverfew products. *J Pharm Pharmacol* 44:391–395, 1992.
5. Hannington E: Migraine: The platelet hypothesis after 10 years. *Biomed Pharmacother* 43:719–726, 1989.
6. Hepinstall S, White A, et al.: Extracts of feverfew inhibit granule secretion in blood platelets and polymorphonuclear leukocytes. *Lancet* i:1071–1074, 1985.
7. Makheja AN and Bailery JM: A platelet phospholipase inhibitor from the medicinal herb feverfew (*Tanacetum parthenium*). *Prostaglandins, Leukotrienes Med* 8:653–660, 1982.
8. Pugh WJ and Sambo K: Prostaglandin synthetase inhibitors in feverfew. *J Pharm Pharmacol* 40:743–745, 1988.
9. Sumner H, Salan U, et al.: Inhibition of 5-lipoxygenase and cyclo-oxygenase in leukocytes by feverfew. *Biochem Pharmacol* 43:2313–2320, 1992.
10. Pattrick M, Hepinstall S, and Doherty M: Feverfew in rheumatoid arthritis: A double blind, placebo controlled study. *Ann Rheum Dis* 48:547–549, 1989.
11. Johnson ES, Kadam NP, et al.: Efficacy of feverfew as prophylactic treatment of migraine. *Br Med J* 291:569–573, 1985.
12. Murphy JJ, Hepinstall S, and Mitchell JR: Randomized double-blind placebo-controlled trial of feverfew in migraine prevention. *Lancet* ii:189–192, 1988.

GARLIC

1. Deveny K: Garlic pills are potent drugstore sellers. *Wall Street Journal,* October 1, 1992.
2. Foster S and Chongxi Y: *Herbal Emissaries: Bringing Chinese Herbs to the West.* Healing Arts Press, Rochester, Vermont, 1992, pp. 86–92.
3. Fulder S and Blackwood J: *Garlic: Nature's Original Remedy.* Healing Arts Press, Rochester, Vermont, 1991, pp. 15–25.
4. Leung AY: *Encyclopedia of Common Natural Ingredients Used in Food, Drugs and Cosmetics.* John Wiley & Sons, New York, 1980, pp. 176–179.
5. Lawson LD, Wang ZJ, and Hughes BG: Identification and HPLC quantitation of the sulfides and dialk(en)yl thiosulfinates in commercial garlic products. *Planta Med* 57:363–370, 1991.
6. Hughes BG and Lawson LD: Antimicrobial effects of *Allium sativum* L. (garlic), *Allium ampeloprasum* L. (elephant garlic), and *Allium cepa* L. (onion), garlic compounds and commercial garlic supplement products. *Phytother Res* 5:154–158, 1991.
7. Lawson LD and Hughes BG: Characterization of the formation of allicin and other thiosulfinates from garlic. *Planta Med* 58:345–350, 1992.
8. Tyler VE: *Herbs of Choice: The Therapeutic Use of Phytomedicinals.* Pharmaceutical Products Press, New York, 1994, pp. 104–108.
9. Josling P, Walerpa A, and Grunwald J, eds.: The action of garlic in the pathogenesis of atherosclerosis: Selected abstracts from the 4th and International Congress on Phytotherapy. *Eur J Clin Res* 3A:1–12, 1992.
10. Kleijnen J, Knipschild P, and Ter Riet G: Garlic, onion and cardiovascular risk factors. A review of the evidence from human experiments with emphasis on commercially available preparations. *Br J Clin Pharmacol* 28:535–544, 1989.

11. Gebhardt R: Multiple inhibitory effects of garlic extracts on cholesterol biosynthesis in hepatocytes. *Lipids* 28:613–619, 1993.

12. Gebhardt R, Beck H, and Wagner KG: Inhibition of cholesterol biosynthesis by allicin and ajoene in rat hepatocytes and HepG2 cells. *Biochim Biophys Acta* 1213:57–62, 1994.

13. Reuter HD: Garlic (*Allium sativum* L.) in the prevention and treatment of atherosclerosis. *Br J Phytother* 3:3–9, 1993/1994.

14. Legnani C, Frascaro M, et al.: Effects of a dried garlic preparation on fibrinolysis and platelet aggregation in healthy subjects. *Arzneim-Forsch Drug Res* 43:119–122, 1993.

15. Apitz-Castro R, Badimon JJ, and Badimon L: Effect of ajoene, the major antiplatelet compound from garlic, on platelet thrombus formation. *Thromb Res* 68:145–155, 1992.

16. Garlic. *Lawrence Review Natural Products,* April 1994.

17. Pareddy SR and Rosenberg JM: Does garlic have useful medicinal purposes? *Hosp Pharm Rep* 8:27, 1993.

18. Weber ND, Anderson DO, et al.: *In vitro* virucidal effects of *Allium sativum* (garlic) extract and compounds. *Planta Med* 58:417–423, 1992.

19. Nai-lan G, Dao-pei L, et al.: Demonstrations of the anti-viral activity of garlic extract against human cytomegalovirus in vitro. *Chin Med J* 106:93–96, 1993.

20. Shoji S, Furuishi K, et al.: Allyl compounds selectively killed human immunodeficiency virus (type-1)[r3]infected cells. *Biochem Biophys Res Commun* 194:610–621, 1993.

21. Ghannoum MA: Studies on the anticandidal mode of action of *Allium sativum* (garlic). *J Gen Microbiol* 134:2917–2924, 1988.

22. Hughes BG and Lawson LD: Antimicrobial effects of *Allium sativum* L. (garlic), *Allium ampeloprasum* L. (elephant garlic), and *Allium cepa* L. (onion), garlic compounds and commercial garlic supplement products. *Phytother Res* 5:154–158, 1991.

23. Lin XY, Liu JZ, and Milner JA: Dietary garlic suppresses DNA adducts caused by N-nitroso compounds. *Carcinogenesis* 15: 349–52, 1994.

24. Ip C, Lisk DJ, and Stoewsand GS: Mammary cancer prevention by regular garlic and selenium-enriched garlic. *Nutr Cancer* 17:279–286, 1992.

25. Dwivedi C, Rohlfs S, et al.: Chemoprevention of chemically induced skin tumor development by diallyl sulfide and diallyl disulfide. *Pharmaceutical Res* 9:1668–1670, 1992.

26. Mader FH: Treatment of hyperlipidemia with garlic-powder tablets. *Arzneim-Forsch Drug Res* 40:1111–1116, 1990.

27. Vorberg G and Schneider B: Therapy with garlic: Results of a placebo-controlled, double-blind study. *Br J Clin Pract* 44 (Suppl. 69):7–11, 1990.

28. Jain AK, Vargas R, et al.: Can garlic reduce serum lipids? A controlled clinical study. *Am J Med* 94:632–635, 1993.

29. Silagy C and Neil A: Garlic as a lipid lowering agent—a meta-analysis. *J R Coll Physicians London* 28:39–45, 1994.

30. Warshafsky S, Kramer RS, and Sivak SL: Effect of garlic on total serum cholesterol. *Ann Int Med* 119:599–605, 1993.

31. Holzgartner H, Schmidt U, and Kuhn U: Comparison of the efficacy and tolerance of a garlic preparation vs. bezafibrate. *Arzneim-Forsch Drug Res* 42:1473–1477, 1992.

32. Silagy C and Neil AW: A meta-analysis of the effect of garlic on blood pressure. *J Hypertens* 12:463–468, 1994.

33. Kieswatter H, Jung F, et al.: Effects of garlic coated tablets in peripheral arterial occlusive disease. *Clin Invest* 71:383–386, 1993.

34. Despande RG, Khan MB, et al.: Inhibition of *Mycobacterium avium* complex isolates from AIDS patients by garlic (*Allium sativum*). *J Antimicrob Chemother* 32:623–626, 1993.

References

35. Davis LE, Shen J, and Royer RE: *In vitro* synergism of concentrated *Allium sativum* extract and amphotericin B against *Cryptococcus neoformans*. *Planta Med* 60:546–549, 1994.
36. Steinmetz KA, Kushi LH, et al.: Vegetables, fruit, and colon cancer in the Iowa women's health study. *Am J Epidemiol* 139:1–5, 1994.
37. Dorant E, vander Brandt PA, et al.: Garlic and its significance for the prevention of cancer in humans: A critical view. *Br J Cancer* 67:424–429, 1993.
38. Mennella JA and Beauchamp GK: The effects of repeated exposure to garlic-flavored milk on the nursling's behavior. *Pediatr Res* 34:805–808, 1993.

GINGER

1. Awang DVC: Ginger. *Can Pharm J* 125:309–311, 1992.
2. Foster S and Chongxi Y: *Herbal Emissaries: Bringing Chinese Herbs to the West.* Healing Arts Press, Rochester, Vermont, 1992, pp. 92–102.
3. Foster S and Chongxi Y: *Herbal Emissaries: Bringing Chinese Herbs to the West.* Healing Arts Press, Rochester, Vermont, 1992, pp. 92–102.
4. Hikino H: Research on oriental medicinal plants. In: *Economic and Medicinal Plant Research,* Vol. 1 (Wagner H, Hikino H, and Farnsworth N, eds.). Academic Press, New York, 1985.
5. Tyler VE: *Herbs of Choice: The Therapeutic Use of Phytomedicinals.* Pharmaceutical Products Press, New York, 1994, pp. 39–42.
6. Bradley PR (ed.). *British Herbal Compendium,* Vol. 1. British Herbal Medicine Association, Bournemouth, Dorset, England, 1992, pp. 112–114.
7. Yamahara J, Huang Q, et al.: Gastrointestinal motility enhancing effect of ginger and its active constituents. *Chem Pharm Bull* 38:430–431, 1990.
8. Yamahara J, Miki K, et al.: Cholagogic effect of ginger and its active constituents. *J Ethnopharmacol* 13:217–225, 1985.
9. Al-Yahya MA, Rafatullah S, et al.: Gastroprotective activity of ginger in albino rats. *Am J Chin Med* 17:51–56, 1989.
10. Kawai T, Kinoshita K, et al.: Anti-emetic principles of *Magnolia obovata* bark and *Zingiber officinale* rhizome. *Planta Med* 60:17–20, 1994.
11. Suekawa M, Ishige A, et al.: Pharmacological studies on ginger. I. Pharmacological actions of pungent constituents, (6)-gingerol and (6)-shogaol. *J Pharmacobio Dyn* 7:836–848, 1984.
12. Holtmann S, Clarke AH, et al.: The anti-motion sickness mechanism of ginger. *Acta Oto-Laryngol* 108:168–174, 1989.
13. Backon J: Ginger: Inhibition of thromboxane synthetase and stimulation of prostacyclin. Relevance for medicine and psychiatry. *Med Hypotheses* 20: 271–278, 1986.
14. Verma Sk, Singh J, et al.: Effect of ginger on platelet aggregation in man. *Indian J Med Res* 98:240–242, 1994.
15. Kuchi F, Iwakami S, et al.: Inhibition of prostaglandin and leukotriene biosynthesis by gingerols and diarylheptanoids. *Chem Pharm Bull* 40:387–391, 1992.
16. Onogi T, Minami M, et al.: Capsaicin-like effect of (6)-shogaol on substance P-containing primary afferents of rats: A possible mechanism of its analgesic action. *Neuropharmacology* 31:1165–1169, 1992.
17. Mowrey DB and Clayson DE: Motion sickness, ginger, and psychophysics. *Lancet* i:655–657, 1982.
18. Grontved A, Brask T, et al.: Ginger root against seasickness. *Acta Oto-Laryngol* 105:45–49, 1988.

19. Stewart JJ, Wood MJ, et al.: Effects of ginger on motion sickness susceptibility and gastric function. *Pharmacology* 42:111–120, 1991.

20. Fischer-Rasmussen W, Kjaer SK, et al.: Ginger treatment of hyperemesis gravidarum. *Eur J Obstet Gynecol Reprod Biol* 38:19–24, 1990.

21. Phillips S, Ruggier R, and Hutchison SE: *Zingiber officinale* (ginger)—an antiemetic for day case surgery. *Anaesthesia* 48:715–717, 1993.

22. Bone ME and Wilkinson DJ: Ginger root—a new antiemetic. *Anaesthesia* 45:669–671, 1990.

23. Srivastava KC and Mustafa T: Ginger (*Zingiber officinale*) in rheumatism and musculoskeletal disorders. *Med Hypotheses* 39:342–348, 1992.

24. Mustafa T and Srivastava KC: Ginger (*Zingiber officinale*) in migraine headache. *J Ethnopharmacol* 29:267–273, 1990.

25. Monograph, *Zingiberis rhizoma* (ginger root). *Bundesanzeiger* May 5, 1988.

GINKGO BILOBA

1. Busse W: History and chemistry of *Ginkgo biloba*. *Rev Bras Neurol* 30 (Suppl. 1):3S–6S, 1994.

2. DeFeudis FV: *Ginkgo biloba Extract (EGb 761): Pharmacological Activities and Clinical Applications.* Elsevier, Paris, 1991, pp. 3–5.

3. Drieu K: Preparation and definition of *Ginkgo biloba* extract. In: *Rokan (Ginkgo biloba): Recent Results in Pharmacology and Clinic* (Fünfgeld EW, ed.). Springer-Verlag, Berlin, 1988, pp. 32–36.

4. *Ginkgolides: Chemistry, Biology, Pharmacology and Clinical Perspectives,* Vol. 1 (Braquet P, ed.). JR Prous Science Publishers, Barcelona, Spain, 1989.

5. *Ginkgolides: Chemistry, Biology, Pharmacology and Clinical Perspectives,* Vol. 2 (Braquet P, ed). JR Prous Science Publishers, Barcelona, 1989.

6. Krieglstein J: Neuroprotective properties of *Ginkgo biloba*—constituents. *Z Phytother* 15:92–96, 1994.

7. Bruno C, Cuppini R, et al.: Regeneration of motor nerves in bilobalide-treated rats. *Planta Med* 59:302–307, 1993.

8. Clostre F: From the body to the cellular membranes: The different levels of pharmacological action of *Ginkgo biloba* extract. In: *Rokan (Ginkgo biloba): Recent Results in Phamacology and Clinic* (Fünfgeld EW, ed.). Springer-Verlag, Berlin, 1988, pp. 180–198.

9. Jung F, Mrowietz C, et al.: Effect of *Ginkgo biloba* on fluidity of blood and peripheral microcirculation in volunteers. *Arzneim-Forsch Drug Res* 40:589–593, 1990.

10. Kleijnen J and Knipschild P: *Ginkgo biloba* for cerebral insufficiency. *Br J Clin Pharmacol* 34:352–358, 1992.

11. Harman D: Free radicals in aging. *Mol Cell Biochem* 84:155–161, 1988.

12. Ferrandini C, Droy-Lefaix MT, and Christen Y (eds.). *Ginkgo biloba Extract (EGb 761) as a Free Radical Scavenger.* Elsevier, Paris, 1993.

13. Harman D: Free radical theory of aging: A hypothesis on pathogenesis of senile dementia of the Alzheimer's type. *Age* 16:23–30, 1993.

14. Lamant V, Mauco G, et al.: Inhibition of the metabolism of platelet activating factor (PAF-acether) by three specific antagonists from *Ginkgo biloba*. *Biochem Pharmacol* 36:2749–2752, 1987.

15. Kroegel C: The potential pathophysiological role of platelet-activating factor in human disease. *Klin Wochenschr* 66:373–378, 1988.

16. Kroegel C, Kortsik C, et al.: The pathophysiological role and therapeutic implications of platelet activating factor in diseases of aging. *Drugs Aging* 2:345–55, 1992.

17. Krieglstein J: Neuroprotective properties of *Ginkgo biloba*—constituents. *Z Phytother* 15:92–96, 1994.

18. Stein DG and Hoffman SW: Chronic administration of *Ginkgo biloba* extract (EGb 761) can enhance recovery from traumatic brain injury. In: *Effects of Ginkgo biloba Extract (EGb 761) on the Central Nervous System* (Christen Y, Costentin J, and Lacour M, eds.). Elsevier, Paris, 1992, pp. 95–104.

19. Kleijnen J and Knipschild P: *Ginkgo biloba. Lancet* 340:1136–1139, 1992.

20. Voberg G: *Ginkgo biloba* extract (GBE): A long-term study of chronic cerebral insufficiency in geriatric patients. *Clin Trials J* 22:149–157, 1985.

21. Rai GS, Shovlin C, and Wesnes K: A double-blind, placebo controlled study of *Ginkgo biloba* extract (Tanakan®) in elderly outpatients with mild to moderate memory impairment. *Curr Med Res Opin* 12:350–355, 1991.

22. Mancini M, Agozzino B, and Bompani R: Clinical and therapeutic effects of *Ginkgo biloba* extract (GBE) versus placebo in the treatment of psychoorganic senile dementia of arteriosclerotic origin. *Gaz Med Ital* 152:69–80, 1993.

23. Lesser IM, Mena I, et al.: Reduction in cerebral blood flow in older depressed patients. *Arch Gen Psychiatr* 51:677–686, 1994.

24. Schubert H and Halama P: Depressive episode primarily unresponsive to therapy in elderly patients: Efficacy of *Ginkgo biloba* extract (EGb 761) in combination with antidepressants. *Geriatr Forsch* 3:45–53, 1993.

25. Hofferberth B: The efficacy of EGb 761 in patients with senile dementia of the Alzheimer type: A double-blind, placebo-controlled study on different levels of investigation. *Hum Psychopharmacol* 9:215–222, 1994.

26. Kanowski S, Herrman WM, et al.: Efficacy and tolerability of the *Ginkgo biloba* extract EGb 761 in outpatients with presenile and senile Alzheimer-type dementia and multi-infarct dementia. Abstract from the Sixth Congress of the International Psychogeriatric Association, Berlin, September 5–10, 1993.

27. Bauer U: Six-month double-blind randomized clinical trial of *Ginkgo biloba* extract versus placebo in two parallel groups of patients suffering from peripheral arterial insufficiency. *Arzneim-Forsch Drug Res* 34:716–720, 1984.

28. Schneider B: *Ginkgo biloba* extract in peripheral arterial disease: Meta-analysis of controlled clinical trials. *Arzneim-Forsch Drug Res* 42:428–436, 1992.

29. DeFeudis FV: *Ginkgo biloba Extract (EGb 761): Pharmacological Activities and Clinical Applications.* Elsevier, Paris, 1991, pp. 143–146.

30. Monograph, *Ginkgo biloba* leaves (dry extract). *Bundesanzieger,* June 21, 1994.

ASIAN GINSENG

1. Foster S: Three ginsengs: Asian, American, and Siberian. *The Herb Companion,* June/July 1995, pp. 75–77.

2. Duke JA: *Ginseng: A Concise Handbook.* Reference Publications, Algonac, Michigan, 1989.

3. Foster S and Chongxi Y: *Herbal Emissaries: Bringing Chinese Herbs to the West.* Healing Arts Press, Rochester, Vermont, 1992, pp. 102–112.

4. Hu SY: Knowledge of ginseng from Chinese records. *J Chin Univ Hong Kong* 4:283–305, 1977.

5. Hu SY: The genus *Panax* (ginseng) in Chinese medicine. *Econ Bot* 30:11–28, 1976.

6. Foster S and Chongxi Y: op cit., 1992.

7. Hikino H: Traditional remedies and modern assessment: The case of ginseng. In: *The Medicinal Plant Industry* (Wijeskera R, ed.), CRC Press, Boca Raton, Florida, 1991, pp. 149–66.

8. Shibata S, Tanaka O, et al.: Chemistry and pharmacology of *Panax*. In: *Economic and Medicinal Plant Research,* Vol. 1 (Wagner H, Hikino H, and Farnsworth NR, eds.), Academic Press, London, 1985, pp. 217–284.

9. Mowrey DB: Understanding standardized ginseng extracts. *Townsend Lett Doctors* October: 505–509, 1989.

10. Tomoda M, Hirabayashi K, et al.: Characterization of two novel polysaccharides having immunological activities from the root of *Panax ginseng. Biol Pharm Bull* 16:1087–1090, 1993.

11. Brekhman II and Dardymov IV: New substances of plant origin which increase non-specific resistance. *Annu Rev Pharmacol* 4:419–430, 1969.

12. Wagner H, Nörr H, and Winterhoff H: Plant adaptogens. *Phytomedicine* 1:63–76, 1994.

13. Hiai S, Yokoyama H, et al.: Stimulation of pituitary–adrenocortical system by ginseng saponin. *Endocrinol Jpn* 26:661–665, 1979.

14. Fulder SJ: Ginseng and the hypothalamic–pituitary control of stress. *Am J Chin Med* 9:112–118, 1981.

15. Petkov VD and Mosharrof AH: Age- and individual-related specificities in the effects of standardized ginseng extract on learning and memory (experiments in rats). *Phytother Res* 1:80–84, 1987.

16. D' Angelo L, Grimaldi R, et al.: A double-blind, placebo-controlled clinical study of a standardized ginseng extract on psychomotor performance in healthy volunteers. *J Ethnopharmacol* 16:15–22, 1986.

17. Medvedev MA: The effect of ginseng on the working performance of radio operators. In: *Papers on the Study of Ginseng and Other Medicinal Plants of the Far East,* Vol. 5. Primorskoe Knizhone Izdatelsvo, Vladivostok, USSR, 1963.

18. Owen RT: Ginseng—a pharmacological profile. *Drugs Today* 17:343–351, 1981.

19. Forgo I: The duration of effect of the standardized ginseng extract G115 in healthy competitive athletes. *Notabene Medici* 15:636–640, 1985.

20. McNaughton L: A comparison of Chinese and Russian ginseng as ergogenic aids to improve various facets of physical fitness. *Int Clin Nutr Rev* 9:32–35, 1989.

21. Pieralisi G, Rapari P, and Vecchiet L: Effects of a standardized ginseng extract combined with dimethylaminoethanol bitartrate, vitamins, minerals, and trace elements on physical performance during exercise. *Clin Ther* 13:372–382, 1991.

22. Avakia EV and Evonuk E: Effects of *Panax ginseng* extract on tissue glycogen and adrenal cholesterol depletion during prolonged exercise. *Planta Med* 36:43–48, 1979.

23. Zhang T, Hoshino M, et al.: Ginseng root: Evidence for numerous regulatory peptides and insulinotropic activity. *Biomed Res* 11:49–54, 1990.

24. Suzuki Y and Hikino H: Mechanisms of hypoglycemic activity of panaxans A and B, glycans of *Panax ginseng* roots: Effects on plasma levels, secretion, sensitivity and binding of insulin in mice. *Phytother Res* 3:20–24, 1989.

25. Waki I, Kyo H, et al.: Effects of a hypoglycemic component of ginseng radix on insulin biosynthesis in normal and diabetic animals. *J Pharmacobio Dyn* 5:547–554, 1982.

26. Ben-Hur E and Fulder S: Effect of *Panax ginseng* saponins and *Eleutherococcus senticosus* on survival of cultured mammalian cells after ionizing radiation. *Am J Chin Med* 9:48–56, 1981.

27. Kim HS, Jang CG, and Lee MK: Antinarcotic effects of the standardized ginseng extract G115 on morphine. *Planta Med* 56:158–163, 1990.

28. Voskresensky ON, Devayathina TA, et al.: Effect of *Eleutherococcus* and ginseng on the development of free radical pathology. In: *New Data on Eleutherococcus, Proceedings of the 2nd International Symposium on Eleutherococcus.* Moscow, 1984, pp. 141–145.

References

317

29. Kim H, Chen X, and Gillis CN: Ginsenosides protect pulmonary vascular endothelium against free radical-induced jnjury. *Biochem Biophys Res Commun* 189:670–676, 1992.
30. Yamamoto M, Uemura T, et al.: Serum HDL-cholesterol-increasing and fatty liver-improving actions of *Panax ginseng* in high cholesterol diet-fed rats with clinical effect on hyperlipidemia in man. *Am J Chin Med* 11:1–4, 1983.
31. Yun TK and Choi SY: A case-control study of ginseng intake and cancer. *Int J Epidemiol* 19:871–876, 1990.
32. Tode T, Kikuchi Y, et al.: Inhibitory effects by oral administration of ginsenoside Rh2 on the growth of human ovarian cancer cells in nude mice. *J Cancer Res Clin Oncol* 120:24–26, 1993.
33. Hau DM and You ZS: Therapeutic effects of ginseng and mitomycin C on experimental liver tumors. *Int J Oriental Med* 15:10–14, 1990.
34. Yun YS, Lee YS, et al.: Inhibition of autochthonous tumor by ethanol insoluble fraction from *Panax ginseng* as an immunomodulator. *Planta Med* 59:521–524, 1993.
35. Scaglione F, Ferrara F, et al.: Immunomodulatory effects of two extracts of *Panax ginseng* C.A. Meyer. *Drugs Exp Clin Res* 16:537–542, 1990.
36. Siegel RK: Ginseng abuse syndrome. *JAMA* 241:1614–1615, 1979.
37. Tyler VE: *Herbs of Choice: The Therapeutic Use of Phytomedicinals.* Pharmaceutical Products Press, New York, 1994, pp. 171–174.

HAWTHORN

1. Hamon NW: Hawthorns: The genus *Crataegus. Can Pharm J* 121:708–709, 724, 1988.
2. Wichtl M: *Herbal Drugs and Phytopharmaceuticals.* CRC Press, Boca Raton, Florida, pp. 161–166.
3. Grieve M: *A Modern Herbal.* Dover Publications, New York, 1971, pp. 385–386.
4. Loew D: Pharmacological and clinical results with *Crataegus* special extracts in cardiac insufficiency. *European Scientific Cooperative on Phytotherapy Phytotelegram* 6:20–26, 1994.
5. Rewerski VW, Piechocki T, et al.: Some pharmacological properties of oligomeric procyanidin isolated from hawthorn (*Crataegus oxyacantha*). *Arzneim-Forsch Drug Res* 17:490–491, 1967.
6. Weiss RF: *Herbal Medicine.* Ab Arcanum, Gothenberg, Sweden, 1988, pp. 162–169.
7. Maevers VW and Hensel H: Changes in local myocardial blood flow following oral administration of a *Crataegus* extract to non-anesthetized dogs. *Arzneim-Forsch Drug Res* 24:783–785, 1974.
8. Ammon HP and Handel M: *Crataegus*: Toxicology and pharmacology. *Planta Med* 43:101–120, 1981.
9. Wagner H and Grevel J: Cardiotonic drugs. IV. Cardiotonic amines from *Crataegus oxyacantha*. *Planta Med* 45:98–101, 1982.
10. Nasa Y, Hashizume H, et al.: Protective effect of *Crataegus* extract on the cardiac mechanical dysfunction in isolated perfused working rat heart. *Arzneim-Forsch Drug Res* 43:945–949, 1993.
11. Weikl A and Noh HS: The influence of *Crataegus* on global cardiac insufficiency. *Herz Gefäße* 11:516–524, 1993.
12. Schlegelmilch R and Heywood R: Toxicity of *Crataegus* (hawthorn) extract (WS 1442). *J Am Coll Toxicol* 13:103–111, 1994.
13. Blesken VR: Use of *Crataegus* in cardiology. *Fortschr Med* 15:290–292, 1992.
14. Leuchtgens H: *Crataegus* special extract (WS 1442) in cardiac insufficiency. *Fortschr Med* 111:352–354, 1993.
15. Reuter H: *Crataegus* as a herbal cardiac. *Z Phytother* 15:73–81, 1994.

16. Schmidt U, Kuhn U, et al.: Efficacy of the hawthorn (*Crataegus*) preparation LI 132 in 78 patients with chronic congestive heart failure defined as NYHA functional class II. *Phytomedicine* 1:17–24, 1994.

17. Zapfe G, Aßmus KD, and Noh HS: Placebo–controlled multicenter study with *Crataegus* special extract WS 1442: Clinical results in the treatment of NYHA II cardiac insufficiency. Presented at the 5th Congress on Phytotherapy, Bonn, Germany, June 11, 1993 (in press).

18. Tauchert M, Ploch M, and Hubner WD: Effectiveness of hawthorn extract LI 132 compared with the ACE inhibitor Captopril: Multicenter double-blind study with 132 NYHA stage II. *Muench Med Wochenschr* 136 (Suppl.):S27–S33, 1994.

19. Hanack T and Bruckel MH: The treatment of mild stable forms of angina pectoris using Crategutt® novo. *Therapiewoche* 33:4331–4333, 1983.

20. Nasa Y, Hashizume H, et al.: Protective effect of *Crataegus* extract on the cardiac mechanical dysfunction in isolated perfused working rat heart. *Arzneim-Forsch Drug Res* 43:945–949, 1993.

21. Bahorun T, Trotin F, et al.: Antioxidant activities of *Crataegus monogyna* extracts. *Planta Med* 60:323–328, 1994.

KAVA-KAVA

1. Singh YN: Kava: An overview. *J Ethnopharmacol* 37:13–45, 1992.

2. Newell WH: The kava ceremony in Tonga. *J Polynesian Soc* 56:364–417, 1947.

3. Singh YN: *Kava: A Bibliography.* Pacific Information Center, University of the South Pacific, Suva, Fiji, 1986.

4. Lebot V, Merlin M, and Lindstrom L: *Kava: The Pacific Drug.* Yale University Press, New Haven, Connecticut, 1992.

5. Murray MT: Natural anxiolytics—kava and L.72 anti-anxiety formula. *Am J Nat Med* 1:10–14, 1994.

6. Weiss RF: *Herbal Medicine.* Ab Arcanum, Gothenberg, Sweden, 1988, p. 298.

7. Lewin L: *Uber Piper methysticum (Kawa).* A. Hirschwald, Berlin, 1886.

8. Meyer HJ: Pharmacology of kava. In: *Ethnopharmacoligcal Search for Psychoactive Drugs* (Efron DH, Holmstedt B, and Kline NS, eds.). Raven Press, New York, 1979, pp. 133–140.

9. Bone K: Kava—a safe herbal treatment for anxiety. *Br J Phytother* 3:145–153, 1994.

10. Buckley JP, Furgiulel AR, and O'Hara MJ: Pharmacology of kava. In: *Ethnopharmacological Search for Psychoactive Drugs* (Efron DH, Holmstedt B, and Kline NS, eds.). Raven Press, New York, 1979, pp. 141–151.

11. Davies LP, Drew CA, et al.: Kava pyrones and resin: Studies on GABAA, GABAB and benzodiazepine binding sites in rodent brain. *Pharmacol Toxicol* 71:120–126, 1992.

12. Holm E, Staedt U, et al.: Studies on the profile of the neurophysiological effects of D,L–kavain: Cerebral sites of action and sleep-wakefulness-rhythm in animals. *Arzneim-Forsch Drug Res* 41:673–683, 1991.

13. Jamieson DD and Duffield PH: The antinociceptive actions of kava components in mice. *Clin Exp Pharmacol Physiol* 17:495–508, 1990.

14. Kretzschmar R and Meyer HJ: Vergleichende unterschungen über die antikonvulsive wirksamkeit der pyronverbindungen aus *Piper methysticum* Forst. *Arch Int Pharmacodyn Ther* 177:261–77, 1969.

15. Backhauß and Krieglstein J: Extract of kava (*Piper methysticum*) and its methysticin constituents protect brain tissue against ischemic damage to rodents. *Eur J Pharmacol* 215:265–269, 1992.

References.

16. Johnson D, Frauendorf A, et al.: Neurophysiological active profile and tolerance of kava extract WS 1490. *Therapiewoche Neurologie Psychiatr* 5:349–354, 1991.

17. Saletu B, Grünberger J, et al.: EEG-brain mapping, psychometric and psychophysiological studies on the central effects of kavain—a kava plant derivative. *Hum Psychopharmacol* 4:169–190, 1989.

18. Munte TF, Heinze HJ, et al.: Effects of oxazepam and an extract of kava roots (*Piper methysticum*) on event-related potentials in a word-recognition task. *Pharmacoelectro-encephalography* 27:46–53, 1993.

19. Kinzler E, Krömer J, and Lehmann E: Efficacy of kava special extract in patients with conditions of anxiety, tension and excitation of non-psychotic origin. *Arzneim–Forsch Drug Res* 41:584-588, 1991.

20. Warnecke G: Psychosomatic disorders in the female climacterium: Clinical efficacy and tolerance of kava extract WS 1490. *Fortsch Med* 109:119–122, 1991.

21. Scholing WE and Clausen HD: On the effect of D,L-kavain: Experience with neuronika. *Med Klin* 72:1301–1306, 1977.

22. Kindenberg VD and Pitule-Schödel H: D,L-Kavain in comparison with oxazepam in anxiety states. *Fortschr Med* 108:49–54, 1990.

23. Monograph, Kava–Kava rhizome (*Piperis methystici Rhizoma*). *Bundesanzeiger*, June 1, 1990.

24. Herberg KW: Effect of special extract WS 1490 combined with ethyl alcohol on safety-relevant performance parameters. *Blutalkohol* 30:96–105, 1993.

MILK THISTLE

1. Culpepper N: *The English Physician Enlarged*. H. Colbert, London, 1787.

2. Felter HW and Lloyd JU: *King's American Dispensary*. Original printing 1898; reprint by Eclectic Medical Publications, Portland, Oregon, 1983.

3. Wagner H, Horhammer L, and Munster R: The chemistry of silymarin (silybin), the active principle of the fruits of *Silybum marianum* (L.) Gaertn. *Arzneim-Forsch Drug Res* 18:688–696, 1968.

4. Pelter A and Hansel R: The structure of silibinin (*Silybum* substance E6)—the first flavonolignan. *Tetrahedron Lett* 25:2911–2916, 1968.

5. Hikino H, Kiso Y, et al.: Antihepatotoxic actions of flavonolignans from *Silybum marianum* fruits. *Planta Med* 50:248–250, 1984.

6. Faulstich H, Jahn W, and Wieland T: Silibinin inhibition of amatoxin uptake in the perfused rat liver. *Arzneim-Forsch Drug Res* 30:452–454, 1980.

7. Tuchweber B, Sieck R, and Trost W: Prevention by silibinin of phalloidin induced hepatotoxicity. *Toxicol Appl Pharmacol* 51:265–275, 1979.

8. Campos R, Garrido A, et al.: Silibinin dihemisuccinate protects against glutathione depletion and lipid peroxidation induced by acetaminophen on rat liver. *Planta Med* 55:417–419, 1989.

9. Feher J, Lang I, et al.: Free radicals in tissue damage in liver diseases and therapeutic approach. *Tokai J Exp Clin Med* 11:121–134, 1986.

10. Valenzuela A, Aspillaga M, et al.: Selectivity of silymarin on the increase of the glutathione content in different tissues of the rat. *Planta Med* 55:42–42, 1989.

11. Muzes G, Deak G, et al.: Effect of the bioflavonoid silymarin on the in vitro activity and expression of superoxide dismutase (SOD) enzyme. *Acta Physiol Hung* 78:3–9, 1991.

12. Maguilo E, Scevola D, and Carosi GP: Studies on the regenerative capacity of the liver in rats subjected to partial hepatectomy and treated with silymarin. *Arzneim-Forsch Drug Res* 23:161–167, 1973.

References

13. Sonnenbichler J and Zetl I: Stimulating influence of a flavonolignan derivative on proliferation, RNA synthesis and protein synthesis in liver cells. In: *Assessment and Management of Hepatobiliary Disease* (Okolicsanyi L, Csomos G, and Crepaldi G, eds.). Springer-Verlag, Berlin, 1987, pp. 265–272.

14. Sonnenbichler J, Goldberg M, et al.: Stimulating effects of silibinin on the DNA-synthesis in partially hepatectomized rat livers: Non-response in hepatoma and other malignant cell lines. *Biochem Pharmacol* 35:538–541, 1986.

15. Albrecht M, Frerick H, et al.: Therapy of toxic liver pathologies with Legalon®. *Z Klin Med* 47:87–92, 1992.

16. Salmi HA and Sama S: Effect of silymarin on chemical, functional and morphological alterations of the liver. *Scand J Gastroenterol* 17:517–521, 1982.

17. DiMario FR, Farini L, et al.: The effects of silymarin on the liver function parameters of patients with alcohol-induced liver disease: A double-blind study. In: *Der Toxisch-metabolische Leberschaden* (De Ritis F, Csomos G, and Braatz R, eds.). Hans. Verl-Kontor, Lubeck, Germany, 1981, pp. 54–58.

18. Leng-Peschlow E: Alcohol-related liver diseases—use of Legalon® for therapy. *Pharmedicum* 2:22–27, 1994.

19. Ferenci R, Dragosics B, et al.: Randomized controlled trial of silymarin treatment in patients with cirrhosis of the liver. *J Hepatol* 9:105–113, 1989.

20. Berenguer J and Carrasco D: Double-blind trial of silymarin versus placebo in the treatment of chronic hepatitis. *Muench Med Wochenschr* 119:240–260, 1977.

21. Poser G: Experience in the treatment of chronic hepatopathies with silymarin. *Arzneim-Forsch Drug Res* 21:1209–1212, 1971.

22. Leng-Peschlow E and Strenge-Hesse (Madaus AG): Personal communication, 1995.

23. Palasciano G, Portincasa P, et al.: The effect of silymarin on plasma levels of malondialdehyde in patients receiving long-term treatment with psychotropic drugs. *Curr Ther Res* 55:537–545, 1994.

St. John's Wort

1. Wichtl M: *Herbal Drugs and Phytopharmaceuticals*. CRC Press, Boca Raton, Florida, 1994, pp. 273–275.

2. Hobbs C: St. John's wort, *Hypericum perforatum* L. *HerbalGram* 18/19:24–33, 1989.

3. Weiss RF: *Herbal Medicine*. Ab Arcanum, Gothenberg, Sweden, 1988, pp. 295–297.

4. Brown DJ: *Hypericum perforatum*. In: *A Textbook of Natural Medicine* (Pizzorno JP and Murray MT, eds.). John Bastyr College Publications, Seattle, Washington, 1991.

5. Reichert RG: St. John's wort for depression. *Q Rev Nat Med* Spring:17–18, 1994.

6. Suzuki O, et al.: Inhibition of monoamine oxidase by hypericin. *Planta Med* 50:272–274, 1984.

7. Holzl J, Demisch L, and Gollnik B: Investigations about antidepressive and mood changing effects of *Hypericum perforatum*. *Planta Med* 55:643, 1989.

8. Lavie D: Antiviral pharmaceutical compositions containing hypericin or pseudohypericin. European Patent Application No. 87111467.4, filed August 8, 1987, European Patent Office, Publ. No. 0 256 A2. 175–7, 1987.

9. Someya H: Effect of a constituent of *Hypericum erectum* on infection and multiplication of Epstein-Barr virus. *J Tokyo Med Coll* 43:815–826, 1985.

10. Moraleda G, Wu TT, et al.: Inhibition of duck hepatitis B virus replication by hypericin. *Antiviral Res* 20:235–247, 1993.

11. Meruelo D, Lavie G, and Lavie D: Therapeutic agents with dramatic antiretroviral activity and little toxicity at effective doses: Aromatic polycyclic diones hypericin and pseudohypericin. *Proc Natl Acad Sci USA* 85:5230–5234, 1988.

12. Lavie G, Valentine F, et al.: Studies of the mechanism of action of the antiretroviral agents hypericin and pseudohypericin. *Proc Natl Acad Sci USA* 86:5963–5967, 1989.

13. Hudson JB, Harris L, and Towers GHN: The importance of light in the anti-HIV effect of hypericin. *Antiviral Res* 20:173–178, 1993.

14. Gurummadhva R, Udupa AL, et al.: Calendula and hypericum: Two homeopathic drugs promoting wound healing in rats. *Fitoterapia* 62:508–510, 1991.

15. Sakar MK and Tamer AU: Antimicrobial activity of different extracts from some *Hypericum* species. *Fitoterapia* 61:464–466, 1990.

16. Muldner VH and Zöller M: Antidepressive effect of hypericum extract standardized to the active hypericin complex: Biochemistry and clinical studies. *Arzneim-Forsch Drug Res* 34:918–920, 1984.

17. Reh C and Laux P: Hypericum Extrakt bei Depressionen—eine wirksame Alternative. *Therapiewoche* 42:1576–1581, 1992.

18. Harrer G and Sommer H: Treatment of mild/moderate depressions with *Hypericum*. *Phytomedicine* 1:3–8, 1994.

19. James J: Hypericum: Common herb shows antiretroviral activity. *AIDS Treatment News* 63:1–5, 1988.

20. James J: Hypericin/St. John's wort: Experience so far. *AIDS Treatment News* 74:1–6, 1989.

21. Payne DL: Unpublished observations. Fall, 1989.

22. James J: Hypericin results: Community Research Alliance Study. *AIDS Treatment News* 96:2–4, 1990.

23. Araya OS and Ford EJ: An investigation of the type of photosensitization caused by the ingestion of St. John's wort (*Hypericum perforatum*) by calves. *J Comp Pathol Ther* 91:135–41, 1981.

24. Monograph, *Hyperici herba* (St. John's wort). *Bundesanzeiger*, December 5, 1984.

SAW PALMETTO

1. Saw palmetto. *Lawrence Review of Natural Products,* March 1994.

2. Tyler VE: *The Honest Herbal*. Pharmaceutical Products Press, New York, pp. 285–287, 1993.

3. Duke JA: *Handbook of Medicinal Herbs*. CRC Press, Boca Raton, Florida, 1985.

4. Geller J: Overview of benign prostatic hypertrophy. *Urology* 34 (Suppl.):57–68, 1989.

5. Bartsch W, Klein H, et al.: Enzymes of androgen formation and degradation in the human prostate. *Ann NY Acad Sci* 595:53–66, 1990.

6. Tenover JS: Prostates, pates, and pimples. The potential medical uses of steroid 5-α-reductase inhibitors. *Endocrinol Metab Clin North Am* 20:893–903, 1991.

7. Duker EM, Kopansi L, and Schweikert HU: Inhibition of 5-α-reductase activity by extracts from *Sabal serrulata*. *Planta Med* 55:587, 1989.

8. Koch E and Biber A: Pharmacological effects of *Sabal* and *Urtica* extracts as a basis for a rational medication of benign prostatic hyperplasia. *Urologe B* 34:3–8, 1994.

9. Niederprüm HJ, Schweikert HU, and Zanker KS: Testosterone 5-α-reductase inhibition by free fatty acids from *Sabal serrulata* fruits. *Phytomedicine* 1:127–133, 1994.

10. Strauch G, Perles P, et al.: Comparison of finasteride and *Serenoa repens* in the inhibition of 5-α-reductase in healthy male volunteers. *Eur Urol* 26:247–252, 1994.

11. DiSilverio F, D'Eramo G, et al.: Evidence that *Serenoa repens* extract displays an antiestrogenic activity in prostatic tissue of benign prostatic hypertrophy patients. *Eur Urol* 21:309–314, 1992.

12. Breau W, Hagenlocher M, et al.: Antiphlogistic activity of an extract from *Sabal serrulata* fruits prepared by supercritical carbon dioxide: In vitro inhibition of the cyclooxygenase and 5-lipoxygenase metabolism. *Arzneim-Forsch Drug Res* 42:547–551, 1992.

13. Champault G, Bonnard AM, et al.: The medical treatment of prostatic adenoma—a controlled study: PA-109 versus placebo in 110 patients. *Ann Urol* 6:407–410, 1984.

14. Tasca A, Barulli M, et al.: Treatment of obstructive symptomology caused by prostatic adenoma with an extract of *Serenoa repens*: Double-blind clinical study vs. placebo. *Minerva Urologica e Nefrologica* 37:87–91, 1985.

15. Semino MA, Lozano JL, et al.: Symptomatic treatment of benign prostatic hypertrophy. Comparative study of prazosin and *Serenoa repens*. *Arch Esp Urol* 45:211–213, 1992.

16. Braeckman J: The extract of *Serenoa repens* in the treatment of benign prostatic hyperplasia: A multicenter open study. *Curr Ther Res* 55:776–785, 1994.

17. Romics I, Wschmitz H, and Frang D: Experience in treating benign prostatic hypertrophy with *Sabal serrulata* for one year. *Int Urol Nephrol* 25:565–569, 1993.

18. Dathe G and Schmid H: Phytotherapy of benign prostatic hyperplasia (BPH) with extractum *Serenoa repens*. *Urologe B* 31:220–223, 1991.

19. Schneider HJ, Honold E, and Mashur T: Treatment of benign prostatic hyperplasia. Results of a surveillance study in the practices of urological specialists using a combined plant-based preparation. *Fortschr Med* 113:37–40, 1995.

20. Anonymous: Two studies supporting phytotherapy in cases of BPH. *Ärzte Zeitung* 15:27–28, 1995.

VALERIAN

1. Hobbs C: Valerian—a literature review. *HerbalGram* 21:19–34, 1989.

2. Bradley PR (ed.). *British Herbal Compendium*. British Herbal Medicine Association, London, 1992, pp. 214–217.

3. Monograph, *Valeriana* radix (valerian root). *European Scientific Cooperative for Phytotherapy*, 1992.

4. Holzl J and Godau P: Receptor binding studies with *Valeriana officinalis* on the benzodiazepine receptor. *Planta Med* 55:642, 1989.

5. Mennini T, Bernasconi P, et al.: In vitro study on the interaction of extracts and pure compounds from *Valeriana officinalis* roots with GABA, benzodiazepine and barbiturate receptors. *Fitoterapia* 64:291–300, 1993.

6. Bixler EO, Kales A, et al.: Prevalence of sleep disorders in the Los Angeles metropolitan area. *Am J Psychiatr* 136:1257–1262, 1979.

7. Leathwood PD and Chauffard F: Aqueous extract of valerian reduces latency to fall asleep in man. *Planta Med* 51:144–148, 1985.

8. Leathwood PD, Chauffard F, et al.: Aqueous extract of valerian root (*Valeriana officinalis* L.) improves sleep quality in man. *Pharmacol Biochem Behav* 17:65–71, 1982.

9. Lindahl O and Lindwall L: Double blind study of a valerian preparation. *Pharmacol Biochem Behav* 32:1065–1066, 1989.

10. Dressing H, Riemann D, et al.: Insomnia: Are valerian/balm combinations of equal value to benzodiazepine? *Therapiewoche* 42:726–736, 1992.

11. Brown D: Valerian: A possible substitute for benzodiazepines. *Q Rev Nat Med* Winter:17–18, 1993.

12. Monograph, *Valeriana* radix. Commission E, May 15, 1985 (amended March 13, 1990).

13. Albrecht M, Berger W, et al.: Psychopharmaceuticals and safety in traffic. *Z Allg Med* 71:1215–1221, 1995.

VITEX AGNUS-CASTUS

1. Böhnert KJ and Hahn G: Phytotherapy in gynecology and obstetrics—*Vitex agnus-castus*. *Erfahrungsheilkunde* 39:494–502, 1990.
2. Monographs, *Agni casti fructus* (chaste tree fruits). *Bundesanzeiger* No. 90, May 15, 1985 and No. 226, December 2, 1992.
3. Propping D, Katzorke T, and Belkien L: Diagnosis and therapy of corpus luteum insufficiency in general practice. *Therapiewoche* 38:2992–3001, 1988.
4. Muhlenstedt D, Bohnet JP, et al.: Short luteal phase and prolactin. *Int J Fertil* 23:213–217, 1978.
5. Weiss RF: *Herbal Medicine*. Ab Arcanum, Gothenburg, Sweden, 1988, pp. 317–318.
6. Amann W: Removing an obstipation using Agnolyt®. *Ther Gegenw* 104:1263–1265, 1965.
7. Sliutz G, Speiser P, et al.: Agnus castus extracts inhibit prolactin secretion of rat pituitary cells. *Horm Metab Res* 25:253–255, 1993.
8. Dittmar FW, Böhnert KJ, et al.: Premenstrual syndrome: Treatment with a phytopharmaceutical. *Therapiewoche Gynäkol* 5:60–68, 1992.
9. Peteres-Welte C and Albrecht M: Menstrual abnormalities and PMS: *Vitex agnus-castus*. *Therapiewoche Gynäkol* 7:49–52, 1994.
10. Coeugniet E, Elek E, and Kühnast R: Premenstrual syndrome (PMS) and its treatment. *Ärztezeitschr Naturheilverf* 27:619–622, 1986.
11. Probst V and Roth OA: On a plant extract with a hormone-like effect. *Dtsch Med Wochenschr* 79:1271–1274, 1954.
12. Loch EG and Kayser E: Diagnosis and treatment of dyshormonal menstrual periods in the general practice. *Gynäkol Praxis* 14:489–495, 1990.
13. Propping D and Katzorke T: Treatment of corpus luteum insufficiency. *Z Allg Med* 63:932–933, 1987.
14. Propping D, Katzorke T, Belkien L: Diagnosis and therapy of corpus luteum insufficiency in general practice. *Therapiewoche* 38:2992–3001, 1988.
15. Milewicz A, Gejdel E, et al.: *Vitex agnus-castus* in the treatment of luteal phase defects due to hyperprolactinemia: Results of a randomized placebo-controlled double-blind study. *Arzneim-Forsch Drug Res* 43:752–756, 1993.

PART 6:   HERBAL PRESCRIPTIONS FOR COMMON HEALTH CONDITIONS

CARDIOVASCULAR SYSTEM

Angina

1. Kamikawa T, Kobayashi A, et al.: Effects of coenzyme Q-10 on exercise tolerance in stable angina pectoris. *Am J Cardiol* 56:247, 1985.
2. Kamikawa T, Suzuki Y, et al.: Effects of L-carnitine on exercise tolerance in patients with stable angina pectoris. *Jpn Heart J* 25:587–597, 1984.
3. Cohen L and Kitzes R: Magnesium sulfate in the treatment of variant angina. *Magnesium* 3:46–49, 1984.

Cerebrovascular Insufficiency

1. Lesser IM, Mena I, et al.: Reduction of cerebral blood flow in older depressed patients. *Arch Gen Psychiatr* 51:677–686, 1994.
2. Kleijnen J and Knipschild P: *Ginkgo biloba* for cerebral insufficiency. *Br J Clin Pharmacol* 34:352–358, 1992.
3. Selhub J, Jaques PF, et al.: Association between plasma homocysteine concentrations and extracranial carotid-artery stenosis. *New Engl J Med* 332:286–291, 1985.

Congestive Heart Failure

1. Morisco C, Trimarco C, and Condorelli M: Effect of coenzyme Q-10 therapy in patients with congestive heart failure: A long-term multicenter randomized study. *Clin Invest* 71:S134–S136, 1993.
2. Mancini M, Rengo F, et al.: Controlled study on the therapeutic efficacy of propionyl-L-carnitine in patients with congestive heart failure. *Arzneim-Forsch Drug Res* 42:1101–1104, 1992.
3. Azuma J, Suwamura A, et al.: Therapeutic effect of taurine in congestive heart failure: A double blind crossover trail. *Clin Cardiol* 8:278–282, 1985.

Hypercholesterolemia (High Cholesterol)

1. Verma SK and Bordia A: Effect of *Commiphora mukul* (gum guggul) in patients with hyperlipidemia with special reference to HDL–cholesterol. *Indian J Med Res* 87:356–360, 1988.
2. Sharma RD, Raghuram TC, and Rao VD: Hypolipidemic effect of fenugreek seeds. A clinical study. *Phytother Res* 5:145–147, 1991.
3. McKenney JM, Proctor JD, et al.: A comparison of the efficacy and toxic effects of sustained- vs. immediate-release niacin in hypercholesterolemic patients. *JAMA* 271:672–677, 1994.

Intermittent Claudication

1. Drabaek H, Mehlsen J, et al.: A botanical compound, Padma 28, increases walking distance in stable intermittent claudication. *Angiology* 44:863–867, 1993.
2. Haeger K: Long-term study of α-tocopherol in intermittent claudication. *Ann NY Acad Sci* 393:369–375, 1982.
3. O'Hara J, Jolly PN, and Nicol CG: The therapeutic efficacy of inositol nicotinate (Hexopal) in intermittent claudication: A controlled trial. *Br J Clin Pract* 42:377–383, 1988.
4. Brevetti G, Chiariello M, et al.: Increases in walking distance in patients with peripheral vascular disease treated with L-carnitine: A double-blind, cross-over study. *Circulation* 77:767–773, 1988.

Raynaud's Disease

1. Nguyen F, d'Arbigny P, et al.: In vitro hemorheological effect of standardized *Ginkgo biloba* extract (EGb 761). In: *Advances in Ginkgo biloba Extract Research*, Vol. 3: *Cardiovascular Effect of Ginkgo biloba Extract (EGb 761)* (Clostre F and DeFeudis FV, eds.). Elsevier, Paris, 1994, pp. 39–47.
2. Belch JJF, et al.: Evening primrose oil (Efamol) as a treatment for cold-induced vasospasm (Raynaud's phenomenon). *Prog Lipid Res* 25:335–340, 1986.
3. Sunderland GT, Belch JJF, et al.: A double-blind randomized placebo-controlled trial of Hexopal in primary Raynaud's disease. *Clin Rheum* 7:46–49, 1988.

Varicose Veins

1. Hitzenberger G: The therapeutic effectiveness of chestnut extract. *Wien Med Wochenschr* 139:385–389, 1989.
2. Cappelli R, Nicora M, and Di Perri T: Use of extract of *Ruscus aculeatus* in venous disease of the lower limbs. *Drugs Exp Clin Res* 14:277–283, 1988.

DIGESTIVE SYSTEM

Alcohol–Related Liver Disease

1. Bulanov AE, Polozhentseva MI, and Yatskov LP: Anti-alcoholic effect of *eleutherococcus*. In: *New Data on Eleutherococcus, Proceedings of the 2nd International Symposium on Eleutherococcus*. Moscow, 1984, pp. 175–183.
2. Kubo S, Ohkura Y, et al.: Effect of Gomisin A (TJN-101) on liver regeneration. *Planta Med* 58:489–492, 1992.

Constipation

1. Kinnunen O and Salokannel J: Constipation in elderly long-term stay patients: Its treatment by magnesium hydroxide and bulk-laxative. *Ann Clin Res* 19:321–323, 1987.

Diarrhea

1. Loeb H, Vandenplas Y, et al.: Tannin-rich pod for treatment of acute–onset diarrhea. *J Pediatr Gastroenterol Nutr* 8:480–485, 1989.
2. Tyler VE: *Herbs of Choice: The Therapeutic Use of Phytomedicinals*. Pharmaceutical Products Press, New York. 1994, pp. 51–54.
3. Isolauri E, Juntunen M, et al.: A human *Lactobacillus* strain (*Lactobacillus casei* sp. strain GG) promotes recovery from acute diarrhea in children. *Pediatrics* 88:90–97, 1991.
4. Oksanen PJ, Salminen S, et al.: Prevention of travelers' diarrhea by *Lactobacillus* GG. *Ann Med* 23:53–56, 1990.

Heartburn

1. Segal I, Hale M, et al.: Pathological effects of pellagra on the esophagus. *Nutr Cancer* 14:233–238, 1990.

Irritable Bowel Syndrome

1. Somerville K, Richmond C, and Bell G: Delayed response peppermint oil capsules (Colpermin) for the spastic colon syndrome: A pharmacokinetic study. *Br J Pharm* 18:638–640, 1984.
2. Dew MJ, Evnas BK, and Rhodes J: Peppermint oil for the irritable bowel syndrome: A multicenter trial. *Br J Clin Pract* 38:394–398, 1984.
3. Whorwell PJ, Prior A, and Feregher EB: Controlled trial of hypnotherapy in the treatment of severe refractory irritable bowel syndrome. *Lancet* ii:1232–1234, 1984.
4. Blanchard EB, Grenne B, et al.: Relaxation training as a treatment for irritable bowel syndrome. *Biofeedback and Self-Regul* 18:125–132, 1993.
5. Shaw G, Srivastava ED, et al.: Stress management for irritable bowel syndrome: A controlled trial. *Digestion* 50:36–42, 1991.

Peptic Ulcer Disease

1. Wilson JAC: A comparison of carbenoxolone sodium and deglycyrrhizinated licorice in the treatment of gastric ulcer in the ambulant patient. *Br J Clin Pract* 25:563–566, 1972.
2. Brogden RN, Speight TM, and Avery GS: Deglycyrrhizinated licorice: A report of its pharmacological properties and therapeutic efficacy in peptic ulcer. *Drugs* 8:330–339, 1974.
3. Wendt P, Reiman H, et al.: The use of flavonoids as inhibitors of histidine decarboxylase in gastric diseases: Experimental and clinical studies. *Naunyn–Schmeidebergs Arch Pharmakol* 313 (Suppl.):238, 1980.
4. Frommer DJ: The healing of gastric ulcers by zinc sulphate. *Med J Aust* 2:793, 1975.
5. Jimenez E, Bosch F, et al.: Meta-analysis of efficacy of zinc acexamate in peptic ulcer. *Digestion* 51:18–26, 1992.
6. Sobala GM, Schorah CJ, et al.: Ascorbic acid in the human stomach. *Gastroenterology* 97:357–363, 1989.
7. Al-Somal N, Coley KE, et al.: Susceptibility of *Helicobacter pylori* to the antibacterial activity of manuka honey. *J R Soc Med* 87:9–12, 1994.

EARS, NOSE, AND THROAT

Ear Infections (Recurrent)

1. Diamant M and Diamant B: Abuse and timing of use of antibiotics in acute otitis media. *Arch Otolaryngol* 100:226–232, 1974.
2. Strachan DP, Jarvis MJ, and Feyerabend C: Passive smoking, salivary cotinine concentrations, and middle ear effusion in 7 year old children. *Br Med J* 298:1549–1552, 1989.
3. Balli R: Controlled trial on the use of oral acetylcysteine in the treatment of glue-ear following drainage. *Eur J Respir Dis* 61 (Suppl. 111):158, 1980.
4. Backon J: Prolonged breastfeeding for at least 4 months protects against otitis media. *Pediatrics* 91:867–872, 1993.
5. Saarinen UM: Prolonged breast feeding as prophylaxis for recurrent otitis media. *Acta Pediatr Scand* 71:567–571, 1982.
6. Hurst DS: Allergy management of refractory serous otitis media. *Otolaryngol Head Neck Surg* 102:664–669, 1990.

Tinnitus and Hearing Loss

1. Moller AR: Pathophysiology of tinnitus. *Ann Otol Rhinol Laryngol* 93:39–44, 1984.
2. Coles R: Trial of an extract of *Ginkgo biloba* for tinnitus and hearing loss. *Clin Otolaryngol* 13:501–502, 1988.
3. Shemesh Z, Attias J, et al.: Vitamin B_{12} deficiency in patients with chronic tinnitus and noise-induced hearing loss. *Am J Otolaryngol* 14:94–99, 1993.
4. Shambaugh GE: Zinc for tinnitus, imbalance, and hearing loss in the elderly. *Am J Otolaryngol* 7:467–467, 1986.
5. Brown DJ: Alternative approaches to tinnitus, Meniere's disease and hearing loss. *Let's Live*, October 1993, p. 80.
6. Marion MS and Cevette MJ: Tinnitus. *Mayo Clin Proc* 66:614–620, 1991.

Hay Fever

1. Mittman P: Randomized double–blind study of freeze-dried *Urtica diocia* in the treatment of allergic rhinitis. *Planta Med* 56:44–47, 1990.

2. Middleton E and Drzewicki G: Effect of ascorbic acid and flavonoids on human basophil release. *J Allerg Clin Immunol* Jan. 1992, p. 278.
3. Clemetson CA: Histamine and ascorbic acid in human blood. *J Nutr* 110: 662–668, 1980.

Sinus Infections (Recurrent)

1. Panosetti E, Pidoux JM, and Lehmann W: Clinical trial with oral acetylcysteine in chronic sinusitis. *Eur J Respir Dis* 61 (Suppl. 111):159, 1980.

ENDOCRINE SYSTEM

Diabetes

1. Madar Z, Abel R, et al.: Glucose–lowering effect of fenugreek in non-insulin dependent diabetics. *Eur J Clin Nutr* 42:51–54, 1988.
2. Sharma RD, Raghuram TC, and Rao NS: Effect of fenugreek seed on blood glucose and serum lipids in type I diabetes. *Eur J Clin Nutr* 44:301–306, 1990.
3. Shanmugasundaram ERB, Rajeswari G, et al.: Use of *Gymnema sylvestre* leaf extract in the control of blood glucose in insulin–dependent diabetes mellitus. *J Ethnopharmacol* 30:281–294, 1990.
4. Baskaran K, Ahamath BK, et al.: Antidiabetic effect of a leaf extract from *Gymnema sylvestre* in non-insulin dependent diabetes mellitus patients. *J Ethnopharmacol* 30:295–305, 1990.
5. Varma SD: Diabetic cataracts and flavonoids. *Science* 1985:205, 1977.
6. Lysy J and Zimmerman J: Ascorbic acid status in diabetes mellitus. *Nutr Res* 12:713–20, 1992.
7. Anderson RA, Polansky MM, et al.: Supplemental chromium effects glucose, insulin, glucagon, and urinary chromium losses in subjects consuming controlled low–chromium diets. *Am J Clin Nutr* 54:909–916, 1991.
8. Rude RK: Magnesium deficiency and diabetes mellitus. *Postgrad Med* 92:217–224, 1992.
9. Mocchegiani E, Boemi M, et al.: Zinc-dependent low thymic hormone level in type I diabetes. *Diabetes* 12:932–937, 1989.
10. Ceriello A, Giugliano D, et al.: Vitamin E reduction of protein glycosylation in diabetes. *Diabetes Care* 14:68–72, 1991.
11. Poicot F, Reimers JI, and Andersen HU: Nicotinamide—biological actions and therapeutic potential in diabetes prevention. *Diabetologica* 36:574–576, 1993.

Stress and Fatigue (Adrenal Exhaustion)

1. Selye H: The general adaptation syndrome and the diseases of adaptation. *J Clin Endocrinol* 6:117, 1946.
2. Tintera JW: The hypoadrenocortical state and its management. *NY State Med J* 55:1869–1876, 1955.

EYES

Cataracts

1. Leske MC and Sperduto RD: The epidemiology of senile cataracts: A review. *Am J Epidemiol* 118:152–165, 1983.
2. U.S. Department of Health and Human Services: Report of the Cataract Panel, Vol. 2, part 3. *Vision Research, a National Plan.* NIH Publication No. 83-2473. Washington, D.C.: U.S. Department of Health and Human Services, 1983.

3. Bravetti G: Preventive medical treatment of senile cataract with vitamin E and anthocyanosides: Clinical evaluation. *Ann Ottamol Clin Ocul* 115:109, 1989.
4. Robertson JM, Donner AP, and Trevithick JR: A possible role for vitamins C and E in cataract prevention. *Am J Clin Nutr* 53 (Suppl.):346–351, 1991.
5. Various nutrients studied for cataract prevention. *Geriatrics* 46:24, 1991.

Diabetic Retinopathy
1. Droy-Lefaix MT and Doly M: EGb 761, a retina free-radical scavenger. In: *Effects of Ginkgo biloba Extract (EGb 761) on the Central Nervous System* (Christen Y, Costentin M, and Lacour M, eds.). Elsevier, Paris, 1992, pp. 7–17.

Macular Degeneration
1. Farber ME and Farber AS: Macular degeneration: A devastating but treatable disease. *Postgrad Med* 88:181–183, 1990.
2. Lebuisson DA, Leroy L , and Reigal G: Treatment of senile macular degeneration with *Ginkgo biloba* extract: A preliminary double-blind study versus placebo. In: *Rökan (Ginkgo biloba): Recent Results in Pharmacology and Clinic* (Fünfgeld EW, ed.). Springer-Verlag, Berlin, 1988, pp. 231–236.
3. Seddon JM, Ajani UA, et al.: Dietary carotenoids, vitamins A, C, E, and advanced age-related macular degeneration. *JAMA* 272:143–20, 1994.
4. Newsome DA, Swartz M, et al.: Oral zinc in macular degeneration. *Arch Ophthamol* 106:192–198, 1988.
5. Micossi, Beecher GR, et al.: Carotenoid analyses of selected raw and cooked foods associated with a lower risk of cancer. *J Natl Cancer Inst* 82:282–285, 1990.

Other Eye Conditions
Dry Eyes Associated with Sjögren's Syndrome
1. Campbell A and MacEwen CG: Systemic treatment of Sjögren's syndrome and the sicca syndrome with Efamol (evening primrose oil), vitamin C and pyridoxine. In: *Clinical Uses of Essential Fatty Acids* (Horrobin DF, ed.). Eden Press, 1982, pp. 129–137.

Uveitis
1. Lavine JB: Suppression of chronic uveitis with the platelet-activating factor antagonist *Ginkgo biloba*. *Quart Rev Nat Med* Summer:5–6, 1993.

FEMALE HEALTH CONDITIONS

Fibrocystic Breast Disease
1. London RS, Sundarram GS, et al.: Mammary dysplasia: Endocrine parameters and tocopherol therapy. *Nutr Res* 2:243–247, 1982.
2. Minton JP, Foecking MK, et al.: Caffeine, cyclic nucleotides, and breast disease. *Surgery* 86:105–109, 1979.
3. Minton JP and Abou–Issa H: Clinical and biochemical studies on methylxanthine-related fibrocystic breast disease. *Surgery* 90:299–304, 1981.

Hot Flashes

1. Duker EM: Effects of extracts from *Cimicifuga racemosa* on gonadotropin release in menopausal women and ovariectomized rats. *Planta Med* 57:420–424, 1991.
2. Reitz R: *Menopause: A Positive Approach.* Penguin Books, New York, 1979.
3. Messina M and Barnes S: The roles of soy products in reducing risk of cancer. *J Natl Cancer Inst* 83:541–546, 1991.
4. Reichert R: Phytoestrogens. *Q Rev Nat Med* Spring:27–33, 1994.

Infertility

1. Judd AM, MacLeod RM, and Login IS: Zinc acutely, selectively and reversibly inhibits prolactin secretion. *Brain Res* 294:190–192, 1984.
2. MacIntosh EN: Treatment of women with galactorrhea–amenorrhea syndrome with pyridoxine. *J Clin Endocrinol Metab* 42:1192–1195, 1976.

Morning Sickness during Pregnancy

1. Gaby A: B_6 *the Natural Healer.* Keats Publishing, New Canaan, Connecticut, 1984, pp. 37–55.

Premenstrual Syndrome

1. Qi-bing M, Jing-yi T, and Bo C: Advance in the pharmacological studies of radix *Angelica sinensis* (oliv) diels (Chinese danggui). *Chin Med J* 104:776–781, 1991.
2. London RS, Bradley L, and Chiamori NY: Effect of nutritional supplement on premenstrual symptomology in women with premenstrual syndrome: A double–blind longitudinal study. *J Am Coll Nutr* 10:494–499, 1991.
3. Abraham GE and Hargrove JT: Effect of vitamin B_6 on premenstrual symptomology in women with premenstrual tension syndrome: A double–blind crossover study. *Infertility* 3:155–165, 1980.
4. Facchinetti F, Borella P, et al.: Oral magnesium successfully relieves premenstrual mood changes. *Obstet Gynecol* 78:177–181, 1991.
5. London RS, Murphy L, et al.: Efficacy of α-tocopherol in the treatment of the premenstrual syndrome. *J Reprod Med* 32:400–404, 1987.

Vaginal Yeast Infections (Recurrent)

1. Belaiche P: Treatment of vaginal yeast infections of *Candida albicans* with the essential oil of *Malaleuca alternifolia. Phytotherapie* 15:15–16, 1985.
2. Blackwell AL: Tea tree oil and anaerobic (bacterial) vaginosis. *Lancet* 337:300, 1991.
3. Hilton E, Isenberg HD, et al.: Ingestion of yogurt containing *Lactobacillus acidophilus* as prophylaxis for candidal vaginitis. *Ann Intern Med* 116:353–357, 1992.

IMMUNE SYSTEM

Chronic Fatigue Syndrome

1. Demitrack MA, Dale JK, et al.: Evidence for impaired activation of the hypothalamic–pituitary–adrenal axis in patients with chronic fatigue syndrome. *J Clin Endocrinol Metab* 73:1224–1234, 1991.
2. Jeffries WM: Mild adrenocortical deficiency, chronic allergies, autoimmune disorders and the chronic fatigue syndrome: A continuation of the cortisone story. *Med Hypotheses* 42:183–189, 1994.

3. Homes GP, Kaplan JE, et al.: Chronic fatigue syndrome: A working case definition. *Ann Intern Med* 108:387–389, 1988.

4. Tintera JW: The hypoadrenocortical state and its management. *NY State J Med* 55:1869–1876, 1955.

5. Lloyd A, Hickie I, et al.: Cell-mediated immunity in patients with chronic fatigue syndrome, healthy control subjects and patients with major depression. *Clin Exp Immunol* 87:76–79, 1992.

6. Klimas NG, Slavato FR, et al.: Immunologic abnormalities in chronic fatigue syndrome. *J Clin Microbiol* 28:1403–1410, 1990.

7. Behan PO, Behan WM, and Horrobin DF: Effect of high doses of essential fatty acids on the postviral fatigue syndrome. *Acta Neurol Scand* 82:209–216, 1990.

8. Cox IM, Campbell MJ, and Dowson D: Red blood cell magnesium and chronic fatigue syndrome. *Lancet* 337:757–760, 1991.

9. Diet may be the key to beating chronic fatigue syndrome. *Seattle, Post–Intelligencer,* September 9, 1992, p. C6.

10. Lathan SR: Chronic fatigue? Consider hypothyroidism. *Phys Sports Med* 19:67–70, 1991.

Colds and Flu

1. Werbach MR: *Nutritional Influences on Illness*. Third Line Press, Tarzana, California, 1993, pp. 367–375.

HIV Infection/AIDS

1. Lee-Huang S, Huang PL, et al.: MAP 30: A new inhibitor of HIV–infection and replication. *FEBS Lett* 272:12–18, 1990.

2. Li CJ, Zhang LJ, et al.: Three inhibitors of type 1 human immunodeficiency virus long terminal repeat-directed gene expression and virus replication. *Proc Natl Acad Sci USA* 90:1839–1842, 1993.

3. Mori K, Sakai H, et al.: Effects of glycyrrhizin (SNMC: Stronger Neo-Minohagen) in hemophilia patients with HIV infection. *Tohoku J Exp Med* 158:25–35, 1989.

4. Bohn B, Nebe CT, and Birr C: Flow-cytometric studies with *Eleutherococcus senticosus* as an immunomodulatory agent. *Arzneim–Forsch Drug Res* 37:1193–1196, 1987.

5. Lau BHS, Ong PY, et al.: Chinese medicinal herbs for immunodeficiency. *Int Clin Nutr Rev* 10:430–434, 1990.

6. Ikehara S, Kawamura H, et al.: Effects of medicinal plants on hemopoietic cells. In: *Microbial Infections* (Friedman H, ed.). Plenum Press, New York, 1992, pp. 319–330.

7. Nai-lan G, Dao-pei L, et al.: Demonstrations of the anti-viral activity of garlic extract against human cytomegalovirus in vitro. *Chin Med J* 106:93–96, 1993.

8. Ghannoum MA: Studies on the anticandidal mode of action of *Allium sativum* (garlic). *J Gen Microbiol* 134:2917–2924, 1988.

9. Despande RG, Kahn MG, et al.: Inhibition of *Mycobacterium avium complex* isolates from AIDS patients by garlic (*Allium sativum*). *J Antimicrob Chemother* 32:623–626, 1993.

10. Dworkin BM: Selenium deficiency in HIV infection and the acquired immunodeficiency syndrome. *Chemico Biol Interact* 91:199–205, 1994.

11. Wang Y and Watson RR: Is vitamin E supplementation a useful agent in AIDS therapy? *Prog Food Nutr Sci* 17:351–375, 1993.

12. Harakeh S, Niedzwiecki A, and Jariwalla RJ: Mechanistic aspects of ascorbate inhibition of human immunodeficiency virus. *Chemico Biol Interact* 91:207–215, 1994.

13. Remacha AF, Riera A, et al.: Vitamin B_{12} abnormalities in HIV–infected patients. *Eur J Hematol* 47:60–64, 1991.
14. Boudes P, Zittoun J, and Sobel A: Folate, vitamin B_{12}, and HIV infection. *Lancet* 335:1401–1402, 1990.

MALE HEALTH CONDITIONS

Benign Prostate Enlargement

1. Geller J: Overview of benign prostatic hypertrophy. *Urology* 34 (Suppl.):57–68, 1989.
2. Koch E and Biber A: Pharmacological effects of sabal and urtica extracts as a basis for a rational medication of benign prostatic hyperplasia. *Urologe B* 334:90–95, 1994.
3. Brown DJ: The male dilemma: Relief for prostate problems. *Total Health* June 1990, pp. 40, 58.
4. Ross JK, Pusateri DJ, and Schultz TD: Dietary and hormonal evaluation of men at different risks for prostate cancer: Fiber intake, excretion, and composition, with in-vitro evidence for an association between steroid hormones and specific fiber components. *Am J Clin Nutr* 51:365–370, 1990.
5. Pusateri DJ, Roth WT, et al.: Dietary and hormonal evaluation of men at different risks for prostate cancer: Plasma and fecal hormone–nutrient interrelationships. *Am J Clin Nutr* 51:371–377, 1990.
6. Aldercreutz H, Markkanen H, and Watanabe S: Plasma concentrations of phyto-estrogens in Japanese men. *Lancet* 342:1209–1210, 1993.

Impotence

1. Sohn M and Sikora R: *Ginkgo biloba* extract in the therapy of erectile dysfunction. *J Sex Educ Ther* 17:53–61, 1991.
2. Sikora R, Sohn M, et al.: *Ginkgo biloba* extract in the therapy of erectile dysfunction. *J Urol* 141:188A, 1989.
3. Riley AJ, Goodman RE, et al.: Double-blind trial of yohimbine hydrochloride in the treatment of erection inadequacy. *Sex Marital Ther* 4:17–26, 1989.
4. Waynberg J: Aphrodisiacs: Contribution to the clinical validation of the traditional use of *Ptychopetalum guyanna*. Presented at the First International Congress on Ethnopharmacology, Strasbourg, France, June 5–9, 1990.

MOUTH AND GUMS

Canker Sores

1. Das SK, Gulati AK, and Singh VP: Deglycyrrhizinated licorice in aphthous ulcers. *J Assoc Physicians India* 37:647, 1989.
2. Wray DW, Ferguson MM, et al.: Nutritional deficiencies in recurrent aphthae. *J Oral Pathol* 7:418–423, 1978.
3. Nolan A, McIntosh WB, et al.: Recurrent aphthous ulceration: Vitamin B_1, B_2, and B_6 status and response to replacement therapy. *J Oral Pathol Med* 20:389–391, 1991.
4. Wray D: A double-blind trial of systemic zinc sulfate in recurrent aphthous stomatitis. *Oral Surg* 53:469, 1982.
5. Wray D: Gluten-sensitive recurrent aphthous stomatitis. *Digest Dis Sci* 26:737, 1981.
6. Andrews VH and Hall HR: The effects of relaxation/imagery training on recurrent aphthous stomatitis: A preliminary study. *Psychosom Med* 52:526–535, 1990.

References

Cold Sores

1. Wöbling RH and Leonhardt K: Local therapy of herpes simplex with dried extract from *Melissa officinalis*. *Phytomedicine* 1:25–31, 1994.
2. Griffith RS, et al.: Success of L-lysine therapy in frequently recurrent herpes simplex infection. *Dermatologica* 175:183–190, 1987.
3. Terezhealmy G, Bottomley W, and Pellu G: The use of water-soluble bioflavonoid–ascorbic acid complex in the treatment of recurrent herpes labialis. *Oral Surg* 45:56–62, 1978.

Periodontal Disease

1. Godowski KC: Antimicrobial action of sanguinarine. *J Clin Dent* 1:96–101, 1989.
2. Werbach MR and Murray MT: *Botanical Influences on Illness*. Third Line Press, Tarzana, California, 1994, pp. 268–270.
3. Serfaty R and Itic J: Comparative trial with natural herbal mouthwash versus chlorhexidine in gingivitis. *J Clin Dent* 1:A34, 1988.
4. Yamnkell S and Emling RC: Two–month evaluation of Parodontax dentifrice. *J Clin Dent* 1:A41, 1988.
5. Leggott PJ, Robertson PB, et al.: Effects of ascorbic acid depletion and supplementation on periodontal health and subgingival microflora in humans. *J Dent Res* 70:1531–1536, 1991.
6. Harrap GJ, Saxton C, and Best J: Inhibition of plaque growth by zinc salts. *J Periodont Res* 55:634–642, 1983.
7. Wilkinson EG: Adjunctive treatment of periodontal disease with coenzyme Q10. *Res Commun Chem Pathol Pharmacol* 14:715, 1978.

MUSCULOSKELETAL SYSTEM

Rheumatoid Arthritis

1. Belch JJF, Ansell D, et al.: Effects of altering dietary essential fatty acids on requirements for non-steroidal anti-inflammatory drugs in patients with rheumatoid arthritis: A double-blind, placebo-controlled study. *Ann Rheum Dis* 47:96–104, 1988.
2. Taussig SJ and Batkin S: Bromelain, the enzyme complex of pineapple (*Ananas comosus*) and its clinical application. An update. *J Ethnopharmacol* 22:191–203, 1988.
3. Deal CL, Schnitzer TJ, et al.: Treatment of arthritis with topical capsaicin: A double-blind trial. *Clin Ther* 13:383–395, 1991.
4. Heliövaara M, Knekt P, et al.: Serum antioxidants and risk of rheumatoid arthritis. *Ann Rheum Dis* 53:51–53, 1994.
5. Werbach MR: *Nutritional Influences on Illness*. Third Line Press, Tarzana, California, 1993, pp. 570–584.
6. Kjeldsen-Kragh J, Haugen M, et al.: Controlled trial of fasting and one-year vegetarian diet in rheumatoid arthritis. *Lancet* ii:899–902, 1991.
7. Peltonen R, Kjeldsen-Kragh J, et al.: Changes of fecal flora in rheumatoid arthritis during fasting and one-year vegetarian diet. *Br J Rheum* 33:638–643, 1994.

Sprains and Strains

1. Rothhaar J and Thiel W: Percutaneous gel therapy for blunt sports injuries. *Med Welt* 33:1006–1010, 1982.
2. Calabrese C and Preston P: Report of the results of a double–blind, randomized, single-dose trial of topical 2% escin gel versus placebo in the acute treatment of experimentally induced hematoma in volunteers. *Planta Med* 59:394–397, 1993.

References

3. Cirelli MG: Five years of experience with bromelains in therapy of edema and inflammation in postoperative tissue reaction, skin infections and trauma. *Clin Med* 74:55–59, 1967.
4. Srimal R and Dhawan B: Pharmacology of diferuloyl methane (curcumin), a non-steroidal anti-inflammatory agent. *J Pharm Pharmacol* 25:447–452, 1973.

NERVOUS SYSTEM

Alzheimer's Disease

1. Petkov VD, Belcheva S, et al.: Participation of the serotonergic system in the memory effects of *Ginkgo biloba* L. and *Panax ginseng* C.A. Mey. *Phytother Res* 8:470–477, 1994.
2. Bottiglieri T, Hyland K, et al.: Enhancement of recovery from psychiatric illness by methylfolate. *Lancet* 336:1579–1580, 1990.
3. Lowinger P: Cobalamin and organic mood syndrome. *J Neuropsychiatr* 2:467, 1991.
4. Joosten E, van den Berg A, et al.: Metabolic evidence that deficiencies of vitamin B_{12}, folate, and vitamin B_6 occur commonly in elderly people. *Am J Clin Nutr* 58:468–476, 1993.
5. Bell IR, Edman JS, et al.: Plasma homocysteine in vascular disease and in nonvascular dementia of depressed elderly people. *Acta Psychiatr Scand* 86:386–390, 1992.
6. Behl C, Davis J, et al.: Vitamin E protects nerve cells from amyloid beta–protein toxicity. *Biochem Biophys Res Commun* 186:944–950, 1992.
7. Berr C, Nicole A, et al.: Selenium and oxygen-metabolizing enzymes in elderly community residents: A pilot epidemiological study. *J Am Geriatr Soc* 41:143–148, 1993.
8. Spagnoli A, Lucca U, et al.: Long-term acetyl–L–carnitine treatment in Alzheimer's disease. *Neurology* 41:1726–1732, 1991.

Attention-Deficit Hyperactivity Disorder

1. Pihl RO, and Peterson, JB: Attention Deficit Hyperactivity Disorder, Childhood Conduct Disorder, and Alcoholism. *Alcohol Health Research World* 15:25–31, 1991.
2. Colquhoun I and Bunday S: A lack of essential fatty acids as a possible cause of hyperactivity in children. *Med Hypotheses* 7:673–679, 1981.
3. Bhagavan HH, Coleman M, and Coursin DB: The effect of pyridoxine hydrochloride on blood serotonin and pyridoxil phosphate contents in hyperactive children. *Pediatrics* 55:437–441, 1975.
4. Ward NI, Soulsbury KA, et al.: The influence of the chemical additive tartrazine on the zinc status of hyperactive children—a double-blind placebo-controlled study. *J Nutr Med* 1:51–57, 1990.
5. Mertz W: Chromium occurrence and function in biological systems. *Physiol Rev* 49:163–239, 1969.
6. Zametkin AJ, Nordahl TE, et al.: Cerebral glucose metabolism in adults with hyperactivity of childhood onset. *New Engl J Med* 323:1361–1366, 1990.
7. Swain A, Soutter V, et al.: Salicylates, oligoantigenic diets and behavior. *Lancet iii,* July 6, 1985, pp. 41–2, 1985.
8. Egger J, Stolla A, and McEwen LM: Controlled trial of hyposensitisation in children with food-induced hyperkinetic syndrome. *Lancet* 339:1150–1153, 1992.

Depression

1. Bell IR, Edman JS, et al.: Brief communication: vitamin B_1, B_2, and B_6 augmentation of tricyclic antidepressant treatment in geriatric depression with cognitive dysfunction. *J Am Coll Nutr* 11:159–163, 1992.

References

2. Bottiglieri T, Hyland K, et al.: Enhancement of recovery from psychiatric illness by methylfolate. *Lancet* 336:1579–1580, 1990.

3. Lowinger P: Cobalamin and organic mood syndrome. *J Neuropsychiatr* 2:467, 1991.

4. Joosten E, van den Berg A, et al.: Metabolic evidence that deficiencies of vitamin B_{12}, folate, and vitamin B_6 occur commonly in elderly people. *Am J Clin Nutr* 58:468–476, 1993.

5. Bell IR, Edman JS, et al.: Plasma homocysteine in vascular disease and in nonvascular dementia of depressed elderly people. *Acta Psychiatr Scand* 86:386–90, 1992.

Insomnia

1. Wichtl M: *Herbal Drugs and Phytopharmaceuticals*. CRC Press, Boca Raton, Florida, pp. 363–365.

Migraine Headache

1. DeFeudis FV: *Ginkgo biloba Extract (EGb 761): Pharmacological Activities and Clinical Applications*. Elsevier, Paris, 1991, p. 142.

2. Gallai V, Sarchielli P, et al.: Red blood cell magnesium levels in migraine patients. *Cephalagia* 13:94–98, 1993.

3. McCarren T, Hitzemann R, et al.: Amelioration of severe migraine by fish oil (omega-3) fatty acids. *Am J Clin Nutr* 41:874a, 1985.

4. Egger J, Carter CM, et al.: Is migraine food allergy? A double-blind controlled trial of oligoantigenic diet treatment. *Lancet* October 15, 1983, pp. 865–869.

RESPIRATORY TRACT

Asthma

1. Spitzer WO, Suissa S, et al.: The use of beta–agonists and the risk of death and near death from asthma. *New Engl J Med* 326:501–506, 1992.

2. Pearce N, Crane J, et al.: Beta agonists and asthma mortality: Déjà vu. *Clin Exp Allergy* 21:401–410, 1991.

3. Crane J, Pearce N, et al.: Worldwide worsening of wheezing—is the cure the cause? *Lancet* 339:814, 1992.

4. Wilkens JH, Wilkens H, et al.: Effect of PAF–antagonist (BN 52063) on bronchoconstriction and platelet activation during exercise–induced asthma. *Br J Clin Pharm* 29:85–101, 1990.

5. Guinot P, Brambilla C, et al.: Effect of BN 52063, a specific PAF-acether antagonist, on bronchial provocation test to allergens in asthmatic patients: A preliminary test. *Prostaglandins* 34:723–731, 1987.

6. Middleton E and Drzewiecki G: Naturally occurring flavonoids and human basophil histamine release. *Int Arch Allergy Appl Immunol* 77:155–157, 1985.

7. Tyler VE: *Herbs of Choice: The Therapeutic Use of Phytomedicinals*. Pharmaceutical Products Press, New York, 1994, pp. 88–89.

8. Werbach MR and Murray MT: *Botanical Influences on Illness*. Third Line Press, Tarzana, California, 1994, p. 86.

9. Collipp PJ, Goldzier S, et al.: Pyridoxine treatment of childhood bronchial asthma. *Ann Allergy* 35:93–97, 1975.

10. Anah CO, Jarike LN, and Baig HA: High dose ascorbic acid in Nigerian asthmatics. *Trop Geogr Med* 32:132–137, 1980.

References

11. Hasselmark L, Malmgren R, et al.: Selenium supplementation in intrinsic asthma. *Allergy* 48:30–36, 1993.

12. Dorsh W, Wagner H, et al.: Antiasthmatic effects of onions: Alk(en)ylsulfinothic acid alk(en)ylesters inhibit histamine release, leukotriene and thromboxane biosynthesis in vitro and counteract PAF- and allergen-induced bronchial obstruction in vivo. *Biochem Pharmacol* 37:4479–4485, 1988.

13. Wright AL, Holberg CJ, et al.: Breast feeding and lower respiratory tract illness in the first year of life. *Br Med J* 299:946–949, 1989.

14. Singh V, Wisniewski A, et al.: Effect of yoga breathing exercises (pranayama) on airway reactivity in subjects with asthma. *Lancet* 335:1381–133, 1990.

15. Chilmonczyx BA, Salmun LM, et al.: Association between exposure to environmental tobacco smoke and exacerbations of asthma in children. *New Engl J Med* 328:1665–1669, 1993.

16. Lindahl O, Lindwall L, et al.: Vegan regimen with reduced medication in the treatment of bronchial asthma. *J Asthma* 22:45–55, 1985.

Coughs

1. Tyler VE: *Herbs of Choice: The Therapeutic Use of Phytomedicinals.* Pharmaceutical Products Press, New York, 1994, pp. 90–93.

2. Schilcher H and Elzer M: *Drosera* (Sundew): A proven antitussive. *Z Phyother* 14:50–54, 1993.

3. Czygan FC and Hansel R: Thyme species as cough medicines. *Z Phytother* 14:104–110, 1993.

SKIN CONDITIONS

Acne

1. Bassett IB, Pannowitz DL, and Barnetson RSC: A comparative study of tea-tree oil versus benzoyl peroxide in the treatment of acne. *Med J Aust* 153:455–458, 1990.

2. Kligman AM, Mills OH, et al.: Oral vitamin A in acne vulgaris. *Int J Dermatol* 20:278–285, 1981.

3. Michaelsson G, Juhlin L, and Vahlquist A: Effects of oral zinc and vitamin A in acne. *Arch Dermatol* 113:31–36, 1977.

4. Michaelsson G, Juhlin L, and Ljunghall K: A double-blind study of the effect of zinc and oxytetracycline in acne vulgaris. *Br J Dermatol* 97:561–565, 1977.

5. Michaelsson G and Edqvist LE: Erythrocyte glutathione peroxidase activity in acne vulgaris and the effect of selenium and vitamin E treatment. *Acta Derm Venereol* 64:9–14, 1984.

6. Snider BL and Dieteman DF: Pyridoxine therapy for premenstrual acne flare. *Arch Dermatol* 110:130–131, 1974.

Eczema

1. Sheehan MP and Atherton DJ: One-year follow up of children treated with Chinese medical herbs for atopic eczema. *Br J Dermatol* 130:488–493, 1994.

2. Sheehan MP, Rustin MHA, et al.: Efficacy of traditional Chinese herbal therapy in adult atopic dermatitis. *Lancet* 340:13–17, 1992.

3. Laux P and Oschmann R: Witch hazel—*Hamamelis virgincia* L. *Z Phytother* 14:155–166, 1993.

4. Evans FQ: The rational use of glycyrrhetinic acid in dermatology. *Br J Clin Pract* 12:269–279, 1958.

5. Teelucksingh S, Mackie ADR, et al.: Potentiation of hydrocortisone activity in the skin by glycyrrhetinic acid. *Lancet* 335:1060–1063, 1990.

6. Hörmann HP and Korting HC: Evidence for the efficacy and safety of topical herbal drugs in dermatology. I. Anti-inflammatory agents. *Phytomedicine* 1:161–171, 1994.
7. Sloper KS, Wadsworth J, and Brostoff J: Children with atopic eczema. I. Clinical response to food elimination and subsequent double-blind food challenge. *Q Rev Med* 292:677–693, 1991.

Psoriasis

1. Ellis CN, Berberian B, et al.: A double-blind evaluation of topical capsaicin in pruritic psoriasis. *J Am Acad Dermatol* 29:438–442, 1993.
2. Bernstein JE, Parish LC, et al.: Effects of topically applied capsaicin on moderate and severe psoriasis vulgaris. *J Am Acad Dermatol* 15:504–507, 1986.
3. Werbach MR and Murray MT: *Botanical Influences on Illness*. Third Line Press, Tarzana, California, 1994, pp. 289–290.
4. Kragballe K and Fogh K: A low-fat diet supplemented with dietary fish oil (Max-EPA) results in improvement of psoriasis and in formation of leukotriene B5. *Acta Derm Venereol* 69:23–28, 1989.
5. Donadini A, et al.: Plasma levels of zinc, copper, and nickel in healthy controls and in psoriatic patients. *Acta Vitaminol Enzymol* 2:9–16, 1980.
6. Michaelsson G, Berne B, et al.: Selenium in whole blood and plasma is decreased in patients with moderate and severe psoriasis. *Acta Derm Venereol* 69:29–34, 1989.
7. Fry L, McDonald A, et al.: The mechanism of folate deficiency in psoriasis. *Br J Dermatol* 84:539–544, 1971.
8. Under L, Sli Akpinar M, and Yanikoglu A: "Doctor fish" and psoriasis. *Lancet* 335:470–471, 1990.

Vitiligo

1. Abdel-Fattah A, Aboul-Enein MN, et al.: An approach to the treatment of vitiligo by khellin. *Dermatologica* 165:136–140, 1982.
2. Montes LF, Diaz ML, et al.: Folic acid and vitamin B12 in vitiligo: A nutritional approach. *Cutis* 50:39–42, 1992.
3. Howitz J and Schwartz M: Vitiligo, acholrhydria, and pernicious anemia. *Lancet* 1:1331–1335, 1971.

Athlete's Foot (Tinea Pedis)

1. Tong MM, Altman PM, and Barnetson RSC: Tea tree oil in the treatment of tinea pedis. *Austr J Dermatol* 33:145–149, 1992.

Fungal Infections of the Nails (Onychomycosis)

1. Buck DS, Nidorf DM, and Addino JG: Comparison of two topical preparations for the treatment of onychomycosis: *Malaleuca alternifolia* (tea tree) oil and clotrimazole. *J Family Pract* 38:601–605, 1994.

Shingles

1. Baba M and Shigeta S: Antiviral activity of glycyrrhizin against varicella-zoster virus in vitro. *Antiviral Res* 7:99–107, 1987.
2. Peikert A, et al.: Topical 0.025% capsaicin in chronic post-herpetic neuralgia: Efficacy, predictors of response and long-term course. *J Neurol* 238:452–456, 1991.
3. Watson CP, et al.: Post-herpetic neuralgia and topical capsaicin. *Pain* 33:333–340, 1988.

References

URINARY TRACT

Urinary Tract Infections (Recurrent)

1. Stamm WE and Turck M: Urinary tract infection, pyelonephritis, and related conditions. In: *Harrison's Principles of Internal Medicine* (Braunwald E, Isselbacher KJ, et al., eds.). McGraw-Hill, New York, 1987, pp. 1189–1194.
2. Meares EM: Nonspecific infections of the genitourinary tract. In: *General Urology* (Smith DR, ed.), Lange Medical Publications, Los Altos, California, 1981, pp. 177–227.
3. Krieger JN: Complications and treatment of urinary tract infections during pregnancy. *Urol Clin North Am* 13:685–693, 1986.
4. Sun D, Abraham SN, and Beachey EH: Influence of berberine sulfate on synthesis and expression of pap fimbrial adhesion in uropathogenic *Escherichia coli. Antimicrob Agents Chemother* 32:1274–1277, 1988.
5. Bruce AW and Reid G: Intravaginal instillation of lactobacilli for prevention of recurrent urinary tract infections. *Can J Microbiol* 34:339–343, 1988.

Support for Kidney Function while Taking Immune-Suppressive Drugs

1. Pirotzky E, Colliez P, et al.: Cyclosporin–induced nephrotoxicity: Preventive effect of a PAF-acether antagonist, BN 52063. *Transplant Proceed* 20 (Suppl. 3):665–669, 1988.
2. van der Heide JJ, Bilo HJ, et al.: Effect of dietary fish oil on renal function and rejection in cyclosporine–treated recipients of renal transplants. *New Engl J Med* 329:769–773, 1993.

Index

Ginkgo biloba, continued
    health care applications, 124–128
    medically active constituents, 119,
        121–122
    physiological effects, 122–123
    treatments, 126–127
Ginkgo flavone glycosides, 119, 121–122
Ginseng, *see* Asian ginseng; Eleuthero
Ginseng abuse syndrome, 137
Glasgow study, 86–87
Godau, P., 175
Gum disease, chamomile for, 53

H

Hawthorn, 139–144
    for angina pectoris, 143–144
    for congestive heart failure, 142–143
    contraindications, 140
    health care applications, 142–143
    history, 141
    physiological effects, 139, 141–142
    plant facts, 140–141
    treatments, 144
Hay fever, treatments for, 216
Headaches, *see* Migraine headaches
Head trauma, case study, 127
Health care
    Europe, herbal medicine in, 8–10
    role of herbal medicine, 15
    United States, herbal medicine
        in, 1–5
Hearing loss, *see* Tinnitus
Heart ailments, *see also specific ailments*
    hawthorn for, 142–144
Heartburn
    about, 207
    dietary recommendations, 208
    herbal prescriptions, 207–208
    nutritional supplements, 208
Helms, Jesse, 247
Hepatitis, *see* Liver disease
Herbal Emissaries: Bringing Chinese
    Herbs to the West, 131

The Herbal Handbook: A User's Guide to
    Medical Herbalsim, 27
Herbal Medicine, 8
Herbal medicines
    addictive properties, 19
    combinations, effectiveness of,
        22–23
    effectiveness, 13–14
    forms, effectiveness of, 20–23
    forms, equivalents, 22
    guidelines, 16–17, 39–40
    in health care system, 1–5
    hormonal properties, 19–20
    labelling, 14–15
    literature, resources, 25
    over-the-counter drugs taken with,
        15–16
    physician's attitudes, 14
    prescription drugs taken with, 15–16
    quality, determining, 23–24
    regulation, in Europe, 9–10
    regulation, in United States, 3–5
    role in health care, 1–15, 8–10, 15
    side effects, 17
    use by children, 18–19
    use in pregnancy, 17–18
Herbal powders, 20
Herpes zoster, treatments for, 296
High blood pressure, garlic for, 106
Hippocrates, 57, 160, 180
HIV, *see* Acquired immunodeficiency
    syndrome
Hoffman, Abbie, 29
Hoffman, David, 27
Holzl, J., 175
Hormones, in herbal medicines, 19–20
Hot flashes, *see also* Menopause
    about, 234
    dietary recommendations, 235
    herbal prescription, 235
    nutritional supplements, 235
    Vitex agnus-castus for, 184
Hu, S. Y., 131

Human immunodeficiency virus, *see*
    Acquired immunodeficiency
    syndrome
Hypercholesterolemia
    about, 194–195
    Asian ginseng for, 136
    dietary recommendations, 196
    garlic for, 105–106
    herbal prescriptions, 195
    nutritional supplements, 195–196
Hyperemesis gravidarum, ginger for,
    116–117
Hypericin, 161
    for AIDS, 162–163
Hyperplasia, *see* Benign prostatic
    hyperplasia
Hypertension, *see* High blood pressure
Hypoglycemia, Asian ginseng
    for, 135

I
Immune-suppressive drugs, herbal
    treatments with, 299
Immune system
    Asian ginseng for, 136–137
    echinacea for, 65
    eleuthero for, 74
Immunomodulators, 35–36, *see also*
    specific immunomodulators
Impotence
    about, 255–256
    herbal prescriptions, 256–257
    nutritional supplements, 257
Infections
    echinacea for, 66–67
    garlic for, 107
Infertility
    about, 236
    herbal prescription, 236
    nutritional supplements, 236
    Vitex agnus-castus for, 183
Inflammation, ginger for, 115
Infusions, 20

Inositol nicotinate, 195
Insomnia
    about, 279
    herbal prescriptions, 279
    valerian for, 176–177
Intermittent claudication
    about, 196
    dietary recommendations, 197
    garlic for, 106–107
    herbal prescriptions, 196
    lifestyle considerations, 197
    nutritional supplements, 196–197
International Psychogeriatic Association,
    125–126
Irritable bowel syndrome
    about, 208
    dietary recommendations, 209
    herbal prescriptions, 209
    lifestyle considerations, 210
    medical considerations, 210
    nutritional supplements, 209

J
James, John, 248
Jartous, Petrus, 132
*Journal of the American Medical
    Association*, 137

K
Kava α-pyrones, 145
Kava-kava, 145–150
    for anxiety, 149
    and brain, 148–149
    contraindications, 145–146, 150
    health care applications, 149–150
    history, 146–147
    medically active constituents, 148
    for menopause, 149–150
    for nervous tension, 149
    physiological effects, 148–149
    plant facts, 146
    treatments, 150
Kava lactones, 145

Index